Pediatric Critical Care Medicine

Editors

KATHLEEN L. MEERT
DANIEL A. NOTTERMAN

PEDIATRIC CLINICS OF NORTH AMERICA

www.pediatric.theclinics.com

Consulting Editor
BONITA F. STANTON

October 2017 • Volume 64 • Number 5

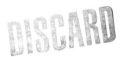

ELSEVIER

1600 John F. Kennedy Boulevard • Suite 1800 • Philadelphia, Pennsylvania, 19103-2899

http://www.theclinics.com

THE PEDIATRIC CLINICS OF NORTH AMERICA Volume 64, Number 5
October 2017 ISSN 0031-3955, ISBN-13: 978-0-323-54678-2

Editor: Kerry Holland
Developmental Editor: Casey Potter

The Pediatric Clinics of North America (ISSN 0031-3955) is published bimonthly by Elsevier Inc., 360 Park Avenue South, New York, NY 10010-1710. Months of issue are February, April, June, August, October, and December. Periodicals postage paid at New York, NY and additional mailing offices. Subscription prices are $208.00 per year (US individuals), $589.00 per year (US institutions), $281.00 per year (Canadian individuals), $784.00 per year (Canadian institutions), $338.00 per year (international individuals), $784.00 per year (international institutions), $100.00 per year (US students and residents), and $165.00 per year (international and Canadian residents and students). To receive students/resident rare, orders must be accompanied by name of affiliated institution, date of term, and the signature of program/residency coordinator on institution letterhead. Orders will be billed at individual rate until proof of status is received. Foreign air speed delivery is included in all Clinics subscription prices. All prices are subject to change without notice. **POSTMASTER:** Send address changes to The Pediatric Clinics of North America, Elsevier Health Sciences Division, Subscription Customer Service, 3251 Riverport Lane, Maryland Heights, MO 63043. **Customer Service: 1-800-654-2452 (US and Canada). From outside of the US and Canada: 1-314-447-8871. Fax: 1-314-447-8029. For print support, E-mail: JournalsCustomerService-usa@elsevier.com. For online support, E-mail: JournalsOnlineSupport-usa@elsevier.com.**

Reprints. For copies of 100 or more, of articles in this publication, please contact the Commercial Reprints Department, Elsevier Inc., 360 Park Avenue South, New York, NY 10010-1710. Tel.: 212-633-3874; Fax: 212-633-3820; E-mail: reprints@elsevier.com.

The Pediatric Clinics of North America is also published in Spanish by McGraw-Hill Inter-americana Editores S.A., Mexico City, Mexico; in Portuguese by Riechmann and Affonso Editores, Rua Comandante Coelho 1085, CEP 21250, Rio de Janeiro, Brazil; and in Greek by Althayia SA, Athens, Greece.

The Pediatric Clinics of North America is covered in MEDLINE/PubMed (Index Medicus), Excerpta Medica, Current Contents, Current Contents/Clinical Medicine, Science Citation Index, ASCA, ISI/BIOMED, and BIOSIS.

Printed in the United States of America.

PROGRAM OBJECTIVE
The goal of the *Pediatric Clinics of North America* is to keep practicing physicians and residents up to date with current clinical practice in pediatrics by providing timely articles reviewing the state-of-the-art in patient care.

TARGET AUDIENCE
All practicing pediatricians, physicians and healthcare professionals who provide patient care to pediatric patients.

LEARNING OBJECTIVES
Upon completion of this activity, participants will be able to:
1. Review topics in cardiopulmonary management in the pediatric intensive care unit (PICU).
2. Discuss mechanical ventilation in the PICU.
3. Recognize developments in pain management and other therapies in the PICU.

ACCREDITATION
The Elsevier Office of Continuing Medical Education (EOCME) is accredited by the Accreditation Council for Continuing Medical Education (ACCME) to provide continuing medical education for physicians.

The EOCME designates this enduring material for a maximum of 15 *AMA PRA Category 1 Credit*(s)™. Physicians should claim only the credit commensurate with the extent of their participation in the activity.

All other healthcare professionals requesting continuing education credit for this enduring material will be issued a certificate of participation.

DISCLOSURE OF CONFLICTS OF INTEREST
The EOCME assesses conflict of interest with its instructors, faculty, planners, and other individuals who are in a position to control the content of CME activities. All relevant conflicts of interest that are identified are thoroughly vetted by EOCME for fair balance, scientific objectivity, and patient care recommendations. EOCME is committed to providing its learners with CME activities that promote improvements or quality in healthcare and not a specific proprietary business or a commercial interest.

The planning committee, staff, authors and editors listed below have identified no financial relationships or relationships to products or devices they or their spouse/life partner have with commercial interest related to the content of this CME activity:
Omar Z. Ahmed, MD; Rajesh Aneja, MD; Michael J. Bell, MD; Robert A. Berg, MD; Yonca Bulut, MD; Randall S. Burd, MD, PhD; Joseph A. Carcillo, MD; Martha A.Q. Curley, RN, PhD, FAAN; Allan Doctor, MD; Anjali Fortna; Kristin C. Greathouse, MS, CPNP-AC; Mark W. Hall, MD; Sabrina M. Heidemann, MD; Julia Heneghan, MD; Kerry Holland; Peter Hovmand, PhD; Tammara L. Jenkins, MSN, RN, PCNS-BC; Todd J. Kilbaugh, MD; Santiago Lopez, MD; Chris Markham, MD; Kathleen L. Meert, MD, FCCM; Ryan W. Morgan, MD; Peter M. Mourani, MD; Jennifer A. Muszynski, MD; Vinay M. Nadkarni, MD, MS; Alison Nair, MD; Daniel A. Notterman, MA, MD, FAAP; Andrew Nowalk, MD; Anita K. Patel, MD; Bradley S. Podd, MD, PhD; Anil Sapru, MD, MAS; Dennis W. Simon, MDMarci K. Sontag, PhD; Eric A. Sribnick, MD, PhD; Bonita F. Stanton, MD; Markita L. Suttle, MD; Robert M. Sutton, MD, MSCE; Katherine A. Sward, RN, PhD; Robert F. Tamburro, MD, MSc; Rajan K. Thakkar, MD; Chani Traube, MD; Vignesh Viswanathan; Amy Williams; Jerry J Zimmerman, PhD, MD; Athena F. Zuppa, MD, MSCE.

The planning committee, staff, authors and editors listed below have identified financial relationships or relationships to products or devices they or their spouse/life partner have with commercial interest related to the content of this CME activity:
Phillippe Jouvet, MD, PhD has research support from Air Liquide Santé France.
Robinder G. Khemani, MD, MsCI is a consultant/advisor for OrangeMed Inc.
Christopher John L. Newth, MD, FRACP, FRCPC is a consultant/advisor for Koninklijke Philips N.V.
Murray M. Pollack, MD has research support from the National Institutes of Health.

UNAPPROVED/OFF-LABEL USE DISCLOSURE
The EOCME requires CME faculty to disclose to the participants:
1. When products or procedures being discussed are off-label, unlabelled, experimental, and/or investigational (not US Food and Drug Administration [FDA] approved); and
2. Any limitations on the information presented, such as data that are preliminary or that represent ongoing research, interim analyses, and/or unsupported opinions. Faculty may discuss information about

pharmaceutical agents that is outside of FDA-approved labelling. This information is intended solely for CME and is not intended to promote off-label use of these medications. If you have any questions, contact the medical affairs department of the manufacturer for the most recent prescribing information.

TO ENROLL

To enroll in the *Pediatric Clinics of North America* Continuing Medical Education program, call customer service at 1-800-654-2452 or sign up online at http://www.theclinics.com/home/cme. The CME program is available to subscribers for an additional annual fee of USD 290.

METHOD OF PARTICIPATION

In order to claim credit, participants must complete the following:
1. Complete enrolment as indicated above.
2. Read the activity.
3. Complete the CME Test and Evaluation. Participants must achieve a score of 70% on the test. All CME Tests and Evaluations must be completed online.

CME INQUIRIES/SPECIAL NEEDS

For all CME inquiries or special needs, please contact elsevierCME@elsevier.com.

Contributors

CONSULTING EDITOR

BONITA F. STANTON, MD
Founding Dean, Professor of Pediatrics, School of Medicine, Seton Hall University,
South Orange, New Jersey, USA

EDITORS

KATHLEEN L. MEERT, MD, FCCM
Chief, Division of Pediatric Critical Care Medicine, Department of Pediatrics, Children's
Hospital of Michigan, Wayne State University School of Medicine, Detroit, Michigan, USA

DANIEL A. NOTTERMAN, MA, MD, FAAP
Professor, Department of Molecular Biology, Princeton University, Princeton, New Jersey;
Professor of Clinical Pediatrics, Rutgers Robert Wood Johnson Medical School,
New Brunswick, New Jersey, USA

AUTHORS

OMAR Z. AHMED, MD
Fellow, Division of Trauma and Burn Surgery, Children's National Health System,
Washington, DC, USA

RAJESH ANEJA, MD
Professor, Department of Critical Care Medicine, Children's Hospital of Pittsburgh of
UPMC, University of Pittsburgh School of Medicine, Pittsburgh, Pennsylvania, USA

MICHAEL J. BELL, MD
Professor, Critical Care Medicine, Neurological Surgery, Pediatrics, University of
Pittsburgh, Pittsburgh, Pennsylvania, USA

ROBERT A. BERG, MD
Professor of Anesthesia, Critical Care, and Pediatrics, Department of Anesthesia and
Critical Care Medicine, Children's Hospital of Philadelphia, University of Pennsylvania
School of Medicine, Philadelphia, Pennsylvania, USA

YONCA BULUT, MD
Professor, Department of Pediatrics, David Geffen School of Medicine at UCLA,
Los Angeles, California, USA

RANDALL S. BURD, MD, PhD
Professor of Surgery and Pediatrics, The School of Medicine & Health Science, The
George Washington University, Chief, Division of Trauma and Burn Surgery, Children's
National Health System, Washington, DC, USA

JOSEPH A. CARCILLO, MD
Professor, Department of Critical Care Medicine, Children's Hospital of Pittsburgh of UPMC, University of Pittsburgh School of Medicine, Pittsburgh, Pennsylvania, USA

MARTHA A.Q. CURLEY, RN, PhD, FAAN
Ellen and Robert Kapito Professor in Nursing Science, Family & Community Health, School of Nursing, Anesthesia and Critical Care Medicine, Perelman School of Medicine, University of Pennsylvania School of Nursing, Philadelphia, Pennsylvania, USA

ALLAN DOCTOR, MD
Division of Critical Care Medicine, Department of Pediatrics, Washington University School of Medicine in St. Louis, St Louis, Missouri, USA

KRISTIN C. GREATHOUSE, MS, CPNP-AC
The Heart Center, Nationwide Children's Hospital, Columbus, Ohio, USA

MARK W. HALL, MD
Associate Professor, Department of Pediatrics, Division of Critical Care Medicine, Nationwide Children's Hospital, Columbus, Ohio, USA

SABRINA M. HEIDEMANN, MD
Professor, Department of Pediatrics, Wayne State University, Detroit, Michigan, USA

JULIA A. HENEGHAN, MD
Fellow, Critical Care Medicine, Children's National Health System, Washington, DC, USA

PETER HOVMAND, PhD
Social Systems Design Laboratory, Brown School at Washington University, St Louis, Missouri, USA

TAMMARA L. JENKINS, MSN, RN, PCNS-BC
Pediatric Trauma and Critical Illness Branch, Eunice Kennedy Shriver National Institute of Child Health and Human Development, National Institutes of Health, Bethesda, Maryland, USA

PHILIPPE A. JOUVET, MD, PhD
Professor of Pediatrics, Research Centre of the Sainte-Justine University Hospital, University of Montréal; Director of Pediatric Critical Care, Centre Hospitalier Universitaire Sainte-Justine, Montréal, Québec, Canada

ROBINDER G. KHEMANI, MD, MsCI
Associate Professor of Pediatrics, Keck School of Medicine at University of Southern California, Associate Director of Research, Department of Anesthesiology and Critical Care Medicine, Children's Hospital Los Angeles, Los Angeles, California, USA

TODD J. KILBAUGH, MD
Associate Professor of Anesthesia, Critical Care, and Pediatrics, Department of Anesthesia and Critical Care Medicine, Children's Hospital of Philadelphia, University of Pennsylvania School of Medicine, Philadelphia, Pennsylvania, USA

SANTIAGO LOPEZ, MD
Fellow, Department of Pediatrics, Division of Infectious Diseases, Children's Hospital of Pittsburgh of UPMC, University of Pittsburgh School of Medicine, Pittsburgh, Pennsylvania, USA

CHRIS MARKHAM, MD
Division of Critical Care Medicine, Department of Pediatrics, Washington University School of Medicine in St. Louis, St Louis, Missouri, USA

RYAN W. MORGAN, MD
Assistant Professor of Anesthesia, Critical Care, and Pediatrics, Department of Anesthesia and Critical Care Medicine, Children's Hospital of Philadelphia, University of Pennsylvania School of Medicine, Philadelphia, Pennsylvania, USA

PETER M. MOURANI, MD
Professor of Pediatrics, Section of Critical Care, University of Colorado Denver School of Medicine, Children's Hospital Colorado, Aurora, Colorado, USA

JENNIFER A. MUSZYNSKI, MD
Assistant Professor, Department of Pediatrics, Division of Critical Care Medicine, Nationwide Children's Hospital, Columbus, Ohio, USA

VINAY M. NADKARNI, MD, MS
Professor of Anesthesia, Critical Care, and Pediatrics, Department of Anesthesia and Critical Care Medicine, Children's Hospital of Philadelphia, University of Pennsylvania School of Medicine, Philadelphia, Pennsylvania, USA

ALISON NAIR, MD
Clinical Instructor, Department of Pediatrics, University of California San Francisco, San Francisco, California, USA

CHRISTOPHER JOHN L. NEWTH, MD, FRACP, FRCPC
Professor of Pediatrics, Keck School of Medicine at University of Southern California, Director of Research, Department of Anesthesiology and Critical Care Medicine, Children's Hospital Los Angeles, Los Angeles, California, USA

ANDREW NOWALK, MD
Associate Professor, Department of Pediatrics, Division of Infectious Diseases, Children's Hospital of Pittsburgh of UPMC, University of Pittsburgh School of Medicine, Pittsburgh, Pennsylvania, USA

ANITA K. PATEL, MD
Assistant Professor, Pediatrics, Children's National Health System, Washington, DC, USA

BRADLEY S. PODD, MD, PhD
Fellow, Department of Critical Care Medicine, Children's Hospital of Pittsburgh of UPMC, University of Pittsburgh School of Medicine, Pittsburgh, Pennsylvania, USA

MURRAY M. POLLACK, MD
Professor, Department of Pediatrics, The School of Medicine & Health Sciences, The George Washington University, Critical Care Medicine, Children's National Health System, Washington, DC, USA

ANIL SAPRU, MD, MAS
Associate Professor, Department of Pediatrics, University of California San Francisco, San Francisco, California, USA; Professor, Department of Pediatrics, David Geffen School of Medicine at UCLA, Los Angeles, California, USA

DENNIS W. SIMON, MD
Assistant Professor, Department of Critical Care Medicine, Children's Hospital of Pittsburgh of UPMC, University of Pittsburgh School of Medicine, Pittsburgh, Pennsylvania, USA

MARCI K. SONTAG, PhD
Associate Professor of Epidemiology, Colorado School of Public Health, University of Colorado Denver School of Medicine, Anschutz Medical Campus, Aurora, Colorado, USA

ERIC A. SRIBNICK, MD, PhD
Assistant Professor, Department of Neurosurgery, Nationwide Children's Hospital, Columbus, Ohio, USA

MARKITA L. SUTTLE, MD
Department of Critical Care Medicine, Nationwide Children's Hospital, Columbus, Ohio, USA

ROBERT M. SUTTON, MD, MSCE
Associate Professor of Anesthesia, Critical Care, and Pediatrics, Department of Anesthesia and Critical Care Medicine, Children's Hospital of Philadelphia, University of Pennsylvania School of Medicine, Philadelphia, Pennsylvania, USA

KATHERINE A. SWARD, RN, PhD
Associate Professor of Nursing, College of Nursing and Adjunct Associate Professor of Biomedical Informatics, Department of Biomedical Informatics, School of Medicine, University of Utah, Salt Lake City, Utah, USA

ROBERT F. TAMBURRO, MD, MSc
Pediatric Trauma and Critical Illness Branch, Eunice Kennedy Shriver National Institute of Child Health and Human Development, National Institutes of Health, Bethesda, Maryland, USA

RAJAN K. THAKKAR, MD
Assistant Professor, Department of Pediatric Surgery, Nationwide Children's Hospital, Columbus, Ohio, USA

CHANI TRAUBE, MD
Associate Professor, Pediatrics, Weill Cornell Medicine, New York, New York, USA

JERRY J. ZIMMERMAN, PhD, MD
Faculty, Pediatric Critical Care Medicine, Professor of Pediatrics and Anesthesiology, Seattle Children's Hospital, Harborview Medical Center, University of Washington School of Medicine, Seattle, Washington, USA

ATHENA F. ZUPPA, MD, MSCE
Associate Professor, Department of Pediatric Anesthesia and Critical Care Medicine, Perelman School of Medicine at the University of Pennsylvania; Director, Center for Clinical Pharmacology, Children's Hospital of Philadelphia Colket Translation research building, University of Pennsylvania School of Medicine, Philadelphia, Pennsylvania, USA

Contents

> Approximately 5000 to 10,000 children suffer an in-hospital cardiac arrest
> requiring cardiopulmonary resuscitation (CPR) each year in the United
> States. Importantly, 2% to 6% of all children admitted to pediatric inten-
> sive care units (ICUs) receive CPR, as do 4% to 6% of children admitted
> to pediatric cardiac ICUs. Survival from pediatric ICU cardiac arrest has
> improved substantially during the past 20 years presumably due to
> improved training methods, CPR quality, and post–resuscitation care.
> Extracorporeal life support CPR remains an important treatment option
> for both cardiac and noncardiac ICU patients.

> The management of critically ill pediatric patients with trauma poses many
> challenges because of the infrequency and diversity of severe injuries and
> a paucity of high-level evidence to guide the care for these uncommon
> events. This article discusses recent recommendations for early resuscita-
> tion and blood component therapy for hypovolemic pediatric patients with
> trauma. It also highlights the specific types of injuries that lead to severe
> injury in children and presents challenges related to their management.

> Transfusion decision making (TDM) in the critically ill requires consider-
> ation of: (1) anemia tolerance, which is linked to active pathology and to
> physiologic reserve, (2) differences in donor RBC physiology from that of
> native RBCs, and (3) relative risk from anemia-attributable oxygen delivery
> failure vs hazards of transfusion, itself. Current approaches to TDM (e.g.
> hemoglobin thresholds) do not: (1) differentiate between patients with
> similar anemia, but dissimilar pathology/physiology, and (2) guide transfu-
> sion timing and amount to efficacy-based goals (other than resolution of
> hemoglobin thresholds). Here, we explore approaches to TDM that
> address the above gaps.

phenotypes. The article discusses the literature on adjunctive anti-inflammatory and immune modulation therapies that, in addition to traditional organ support and infection source control, might be part of a personalized precision medicine approach to the reversal of each of these inflammatory pathobiology phenotypes.

Although many forms of critical illness are initiated by a proinflammatory stimulus, a compensatory anti-inflammatory response can occur with systemic inflammation. Immunoparalysis, an important form of acquired immunodeficiency, affects the innate and adaptive arms of the immune system. Immunoparalysis has been associated with increased risks for nosocomial infection and death in a variety of pediatric critical illnesses. Evidence suggests that immunoparalysis is reversible with immunostimulants. Highly standardized, prospective immune monitoring regimens are needed to better understand the immunologic effects of critical care treatment regimens and to enrich clinical trials with subjects most likely to benefit from immunostimulatory therapies.

Sedation is a mainstay of therapy for critically ill children. Although necessary in the care of the critically ill child, sedative drugs are associated with adverse effects, such as disruption of circadian rhythm, altered sleep, delirium, potential neurotoxicity, and immunosuppression. Optimal approaches to the sedation of the critically ill child should include identification of sedation targets and sedation interruptions, allowing for a more individualized approach to sedation. Further research is needed to better understand the relationship between critical illness and sedation pharmacokinetics and pharmacodynamics, the impact of sedation on immune function, and the genetic implications on drug disposition and response.

Delirium occurs frequently in the critically ill child. It is a syndrome characterized by an acute onset and fluctuating course, with behaviors that reflect a disturbance in awareness and cognition. Delirium represents global cerebral dysfunction due to the direct physiologic effects of an underlying medical illness or its treatment. Pediatric delirium is strongly associated with poor outcomes, including increased mortality, prolonged intensive care unit length of stay, longer time on mechanical ventilation, and increased cost of care. With heightened awareness, the pediatric intensivist can detect, treat, and prevent delirium in at-risk children.

Septic shock remains the major cause of childhood morbidity and mortality worldwide. Although early sepsis recognition, fluid resuscitation, timely administration of antimicrobials, and vasoactive-inotropic drug infusions are all key to achieving good sepsis outcomes, therapy using various steroid drug classes remains an attractive adjunctive intervention to minimize the duration of septic shock and transition to multiple organ dysfunction syndrome. All steroid drug classes possess biological plausibility to affect a beneficial clinical effect among children with septic shock, but none has undergone rigorous, prospective assessment in a large, high-quality pediatric interventional trial.

The focus of critical care has evolved from saving lives to preservation of function. Morbidity rates in pediatric critical care are approximately double mortality rates. Morbidity includes complications of disease and medical care. In pediatric critical care, functional status morbidity is an intermediate outcome in the progression toward death and is the result of the same factors associated with mortality, including physiologic profiles and case-mix factors. The Functional Status Scale developed by Collaborative Pediatric Critical Care Research Network is a validated, granular, age-independent measure of functional status that has proved valuable and practical even in large outcome studies.

Most childhood deaths in the United States occur in hospitals. Pediatric intensive care clinicians must anticipate and effectively treat dying children's pain and suffering and support the psychosocial and spiritual needs of families. These actions may help family members adjust to their loss, particularly bereaved parents who often experience reduced mental and physical health. Candid and compassionate communication is paramount to successful end-of-life (EOL) care as is creating an environment that fosters meaningful family interaction. EOL care in the pediatric intensive care unit is associated with challenging ethical issues, of which clinicians must maintain a sound and working understanding.

PEDIATRIC CLINICS OF NORTH AMERICA

Foreword

Pediatric Critical Care Medicine

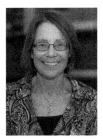

Bonita F. Stanton, MD
Consulting Editor

The arrival of a critically ill child in a hospital setting stimulates a cascade of well-coordinated actions crafted to first stabilize the child and second, almost simultaneously, initiate the steps needed to diagnose and treat the child. The staff of virtually all children's hospitals and the vast majority of general hospitals are well rehearsed in these steps so that regardless of when or where the child may be within that setting, he or she receives immediate and appropriate care. Once stabilized, the child is transferred to a setting devoted to children suffering from immediate life-threatening conditions, where they are treated by highly skilled and committed staff who specialize in the care of these sickest of children; this transfer process is now a routine component of modern children's hospitals. Attendings and residents throughout the hospital take great comfort from the knowledge that if, despite their best efforts on the general floors, a child's health deteriorates, critical care support is immediately accessible.

This finely orchestrated response is of recent origin, coinciding with the birth of the subspecialty of pediatric critical care. In earlier decades, reaction to a critically ill child was longer in coming, less likely to be scripted, and often did not best address the child's immediate life-threatening condition. Even when stabilized, the child was frequently not brought to a specialized setting as generally there were no settings devoted to critically ill children. Rather, beds or rooms within general wards may have been outfitted in some fashion to better address the needs of these children than in other rooms, but certainly not at the level we have come to associate with modern children's hospitals. While general hospitals with pediatric wards may not have pediatric critical care units, there is nonetheless great emphasis on immediate recognition, stabilization, and transfer of the child to a critical care setting.

Much of this highly precise and sophisticated script both leading up to and continuing with admission into the critical care unit has evolved over the last two decades, and so, many pediatricians practicing in the community have but limited notion as to what is occurring in modern critical care. In this issue of *Pediatric Clinics of North*

Pediatr Clin N Am 64 (2017) xv–xvi
http://dx.doi.org/10.1016/j.pcl.2017.07.002
0031-3955/17/© 2017 Published by Elsevier Inc.

pediatric.theclinics.com

America, we learn about the recent research pushing the frontiers of care for critically ill children and their families and their general pediatric care providers. Often families wish to better understand what is occurring in the critical care unit and turn to their pediatrician for explanation. Pediatricians practicing in the community for two or three decades may no longer be knowledgeable about critical care unit interventions. In this issue, we explain many of the new approaches to saving children with acute life-threatening conditions. Likewise, we talk about the innovations made in critical care settings that aid families in coping with the magnitude of the child's illness, thereby helping the families to be of greater comfort to their sick children. It is our expectation that general pediatricians who read this issue will be well prepared to address most of the questions of families of children in contemporary critical care units.

Bonita F. Stanton, MD
Steon Hall-Hackensack Meridian School of Medicine
Seton Hall University
400 South Orange Avenue
South Orange, NJ 07079, USA

E-mail address:
bonita.stanton@shu.edu

Preface

The Collaborative Pediatric Critical Care Research Network: Recent Progress and Future Directions

 CrossMark

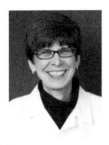
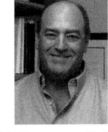

Kathleen L. Meert, MD, FCCM   Daniel A. Notterman, MA, MD, FAAP
Editors

The American Board of Pediatrics first recognized Pediatric Critical Care Medicine as a separate specialty in 1987. Since that time, the number of pediatric intensivists, pediatric intensive care units (PICUs), and PICU beds has continued to grow. Although mortality in PICUs has declined from more than 8% in 1987 to less than 3% today,[1,2] many survivors of pediatric critical illness suffer chronic illness or disability. Continued research will generate new paradigms of therapy and advance existing management in order to improve short- and long-term outcomes from pediatric critical illness.

Research in pediatric critical care has many barriers, including the wide range of critical illnesses and the small number of children with any one type of illness, insufficient knowledge regarding patient-centered and clinically relevant outcomes; limited research time and resources among intensivists, and lack of agreement within the critical care community regarding equipoise for some commonly used but unproven interventions.[3,4] Because of these and other research barriers, the practice of pediatric critical care has often relied on research findings from adult intensive care or other specialties without adequate investigation of benefit or harm to critically ill children.

http://dx.doi.org/10.1016/j.pcl.2017.07.001
0031-3955/17/© 2017 Published by Elsevier Inc.
pediatric.theclinics.com

In an effort to advance pediatric critical care research and thereby provide a scientific basis for pediatric critical care practice, the Eunice Kennedy Shriver National Institute of Child Health and Human Development (NICHD) established the Collaborative Pediatric Critical Care Research Network (CPCCRN) in 2004.[5] Clinical research sites and a data-coordinating center were identified through a competitive peer-review process. The CPCCRN was renewed in 2009 and 2014. As described in the initial request for applications, the purpose of the CPCCRN is to investigate the safety and efficacy of treatment and management strategies to care for critically ill children as well as the pathophysiologic basis of critical illness and injury in childhood.[5] The support provided by the NICHD has allowed the CPCCRN to conduct and participate in numerous multicenter studies, overcome many of the obstacles to critical care research, and foster a spirit of collaboration and mentoring among intensivists.

In this issue of *Pediatric Clinics of North America*, we have invited several investigators affiliated with the CPCCRN to provide an update on the current state of knowledge in their area of research. As might be expected from the wide range of illnesses and treatments encountered in PICUs, the range of research topics is also broad. Conditions reviewed in this issue include sepsis-induced multiple organ failure and associated inflammation pathobiology phenotypes, acute respiratory distress syndrome and its pathophysiology; trauma and the challenge of managing infrequent and diverse severe injuries in children; ventilator-associated pneumonia and the complex interaction between microbes, the environment, and the host immune response; immune paralysis due to critical illness and its detection and treatment; and delirium and its recognition, risk factors, and consequences. Treatment and supportive approaches reviewed include cardiopulmonary resuscitation and the utility of physiologic monitoring during resuscitation; transfusion decision making using a system dynamics model, mechanical ventilation and the use of computerized decision support, optimal sedation practices during critical illness, and corticosteroids and their role as adjunctive agents during pediatric sepsis. Outcomes reviewed include morbidity from critical illness and measurement tools, end-of-life and bereavement care in PICUs, and their potential long-term impact on parents and families.

As the specialty of Pediatric Critical Care Medicine continues to progress, so does its basic and applied research basis. Despite barriers, PICUs can be viewed as ideal settings for research, since they permit continuous physiologic monitoring of patients, routine use of invasive devices allowing biosample collection, and use of electronic medical records and are staffed by highly trained multidisciplinary personnel.[4] Some have proposed that PICUs become "learning health care systems" in which generation of new knowledge is integrated into usual clinical practice, and a culture of evidence-based learning and continual care improvement is fostered.[4] As investigators privileged to be affiliated with the CPCCRN, we hope the reviews presented in this issue inspire and energize the readers to continue to develop new hypotheses and novel approaches to address critical illness, conduct well-planned basic, translational, and clinical research, and disseminate and implement their research findings to advance our profession's mission of improving health outcomes for critically ill and injured children.

Kathleen L. Meert, MD, FCCM
Division of Pediatric Critical Care Medicine
Department of Pediatrics
Children's Hospital of Michigan/
Wayne State University
3901 Beaubien Boulevard
Detroit, MI 48201, USA

Daniel A. Notterman, MA, MD, FAAP
Department of Molecular Biology
Princeton University
219 Lewis Thomas Laboratory
Princeton, NJ 08544, USA

Department of Pediatrics
Rutgers Robert Wood Johnson Medical School
New Brunswick, NJ 08901, USA

E-mail addresses:
kmeert@med.wayne.edu (K.L. Meert)
dan1@princeton.edu (D.A. Notterman)

Cardiopulmonary Resuscitation in Pediatric and Cardiac Intensive Care Units

CrossMark

Robert M. Sutton, MD, MSCE*, Ryan W. Morgan, MD,
Todd J. Kilbaugh, MD, Vinay M. Nadkarni, MD, MS,
Robert A. Berg, MD

KEYWORDS

- Blood pressure • Carbon dioxide • Cardiac arrest • Intensive care • Pediatric
- Survival

KEY POINTS

- Survival outcomes after pediatric intensive care unit (ICU) cardiac arrest have been improving.
- Most in-hospital cardiopulmonary resuscitation (CPR) occurs in highly monitored patients in ICUs.
- The quality of CPR is associated with pediatric survival outcomes.
- Patient physiology can be used to monitor the resuscitation effort.
- Postarrest care is a key component of resuscitation care.

INTRODUCTION

In-hospital pediatric cardiac arrest (p-IHCA) affects approximately 5000 to 10,000 children per year in the United States.[1,2] Although survival outcomes have improved substantially over the past 20 years,[2,3] more work is needed. Nearly half of these children will not live to hospital discharge, and in those that do survive, new morbidity is common.[4] Cardiopulmonary resuscitation (CPR) delivered in compliance with recommended targets for chest compression rate and depth has been associated with improved event survival in children,[5] with the latest research highlighting physiologic-directed CPR as a promising CPR method to improve outcomes further.[6,7] In this article, the authors review the latest epidemiologic data regarding p-IHCA, highlight CPR quality and postarrest care as targets to improve survival outcomes, and discuss the use of

Disclosure Statement: The authors have nothing to disclose.
Department of Anesthesia and Critical Care Medicine, University of Pennsylvania School of Medicine, Children's Hospital of Philadelphia, 3401 Civic Center Boulevard, Philadelphia, PA 19104, USA
* Corresponding author. Children's Hospital of Philadelphia, 8th Floor Main Building: Suite 8566, Room 8570, 3401 Civic Center Boulevard, Philadelphia, PA 19104.
E-mail address: suttonr@email.chop.edu

patient physiology to guide resuscitation quality and potential areas of clinical care and research that may be targeted in the future to improve outcomes further.

DISCUSSION
Epidemiology of Pediatric Cardiac Arrest

p-IHCA is an important public health problem. Best estimates reveal that approximately 5000–10,000 children per year will be treated with CPR for a cardiac arrest at some point during their hospitalization.[1,2] More than half of these children will not live to hospital discharge, and in those who do survive, new morbidity is common.[4] Assuming a pediatric cardiac arrest survival rate of 40%, an average age at arrest of 6 years,[8] and a life expectancy of 78 years, p-IHCA accounts for *the loss of up to 400,000 quality-of-life years annually in the United States.*

Although the newest evidence still suggests that more than half of children will not live to hospital discharge after p-IHCA, this is a substantial improvement over the past 20 years. Of the pediatric patients who survive to hospital discharge, nearly three-quarters will have good neurologic outcome,[4] and more than 90% who survive to discharge are alive 1 year later.[9] Factors that influence outcome after p-IHCA include the following: (1) the preexisting condition of the child[8]; (2) the initial electrocardiographic (ECG) rhythm detected (ie, shockable rhythms have better outcomes[8,10]); (3) the quality of CPR provided during the resuscitation[5,11]; and (4) the quality-of-life supporting therapies during post–resuscitation care.[12,13]

Early warning scores and rapid response teams have successfully decreased the number p-IHCAs that occur on general medical wards outside of the intensive care unit (ICU).[14] In a large study using the American Heart Association's (AHA) Get with the Guidelines-Resuscitation (GWTG-R) registry, more than 95% of pediatric intensive care unit (PICU) and ward CPR events in the United States occurred in an ICU between 2005 and 2010.[15] Many of these ICU patients have invasive monitoring in place at the time of arrest to guide resuscitation quality. Nearly half of the children in the aforementioned GWTG-R study had arterial blood pressure monitoring in place at the time of the event. These data have substantial implications for CPR training that will be discussed in more detail later.

As this article intends to focus on ICU CPR, it is important to note that ICU CPR is common, affecting 1.4% to 1.8% of children in 2 large prospective studies.[2,4] This percentage has remained relatively constant over the past 20 to 30 years despite the growing proportion of p-IHCA occurring in ICUs, likely due to rapid increases in the size and number of PICUs.[16] Similar to p-IHCA that occurs outside of an ICU, hypotension and acute respiratory insufficiency are the most common immediate causes of arrest.[15] Fortunately, over time, outcomes have improved substantially in the ICU CPR population as well (**Table 1**). In the most recent study published in 2016 by the Collaborative Pediatric Critical Care Research Network (CPCCRN; a National Institute

Table 1
Intensive care unit cardiopulmonary resuscitation outcomes are improving

Author, Year	Setting	Patients	ROSC	Survival to Discharge, %
Berg et al,[4] 2016	All ICUs	139	78%	45
Berg et al,[15] 2013	All ICUs	5477	72%	38
Meaney et al,[63] 2006	All ICUs	464	50%	22
Slonim et al,[2] 1997	PICU	205	Not reported	14

of Child Health and Human Development–funded clinical network of 7 leading pediatric institutions[17]), nearly 80% of children who received ICU CPR attained return of circulation (ROC), 45% survived to hospital discharge, and 89% of survivors had favorable neurologic outcome defined by the Pediatric Cerebral Performance Category Scale. However, substantial new morbidity defined by the Functional Status Scale affected almost 30% of survivors, suggesting neurologic changes may be underestimated in the literature.[4] This study affirmed previous work that demonstrated a higher incidence of p-IHCA in cardiac patients compared with noncardiac patients.[18–21] However, in contrast to previous single-center and registry studies, this prospective trial demonstrated that survival outcomes were similar between these groups. Although shorter duration of CPR was associated with better outcome, 89% of children who survived after more than 30 minutes of CPR had a favorable neurologic outcome, indicating that long durations of CPR do not necessarily translate into a universally poor outcome for the child.

High-Quality Cardiopulmonary Resuscitation

One potential explanation of improved outcomes following p-IHCA may be related to a growing understanding of the effect of CPR quality on outcomes. High-quality CPR is best described by the AHA catch-phrase "PUSH HARD and PUSH FAST." Additional aspects of high-quality CPR include minimizing interruptions in chest compressions,[22] allowing full chest recoil between compressions,[23] and avoiding excessive ventilation.[24] There is a focus on delivery of chest compressions over ventilations, even in pediatrics where most events have a respiratory cause. This algorithm was best exemplified in the acronym change from Airway-Breathing-Circulation, or ABC, to Circulation-Airway-Breathing, or CAB in the 2010 iteration of the pediatric advanced life support (PALS) Guidelines. If compressions are delivered at an adequate rate, initiation of ventilation will theoretically be delayed by only about 18 seconds if a pediatric rescuer starts with chest compressions for children without an artificial airway. **Table 2** shows the most recent evidence-supported pediatric CPR targets.

Intra-Arrest Cardiopulmonary Resuscitation Quality Monitoring Technology

Innovative technology primarily using force transducers and accelerometers[25] has allowed resuscitation scientists to quantitatively measure the quality of CPR

Table 2	
2015 Cardiopulmonary resuscitation quality targets	
Metric	**Evidence-Based Target**
Depth: infant/children	PUSH HARD At least 1/3 the anterior-posterior diameter of the chest (~4 cm in infants and ~5 cm in children)
Depth: adolescents[a]	PUSH HARD At least 5 cm but no more than 6 cm
Rate	PUSH FAST 100–120/min
CPR fraction	Minimize interruptions Compressions provided for at least 80% of the arrest duration
Ventilation rate	Avoid excessive ventilation 10 breaths/min
Chest recoil	FULL chest recoil between all compressions

[a] Evidence of pubertal development.

performed during actual resuscitation attempts. This technology has provided important additions to the pediatric resuscitation knowledge base. First, providing high-quality CPR is difficult. Professional pediatric rescuers frequently fail to deliver the recommended chest compression depth and rate,[26] to avoid long pauses in CPR,[27] and to allow full chest recoil during compressions.[28] Second, when high-quality pediatric CPR is provided to patients, outcomes improve. Specifically, when rescuers achieve AHA guideline recommendations for CPR, patients are almost twice as likely to have excellent blood pressure during CPR[11] and 10 times as likely to survive for at least 24 hours after the event.[5] Finally, incorporation of CPR quality data into education and patient care is a vital component of any comprehensive resuscitation quality improvement program. In a single-center study, the combination of focused bedside training with audiovisual feedback before the resuscitation, automated defibrillator CPR feedback during the resuscitation, and post–cardiac arrest debriefing after the resuscitation improved guideline compliance and survival outcomes. In this study, favorable neurologic survival after PICU arrest improved from 29% to 50% with this approach.[29] Currently, a National Heart, Lung, and Blood Institute-funded clinical trial in the CPCCRN network is evaluating this resuscitation bundle of care to improve outcomes across 18 ICUs in the United States (ICU-RESUS: R01HL131544).

Point-of-Care Bedside Training

Traditional CPR training programs function under a high-intensity, low-frequency training paradigm. As such, trainees attend a lengthy CPR instruction class offered every 2 years to maintain their certification. Unfortunately, there is a substantial body of evidence showing decline of CPR skills as early as 3 months after conventional training.[30] In response, resuscitation scientists have evaluated an alternative CPR training approached termed "Rolling Refreshers": a point-of-care educational program that functions under a low-intensity, but high-frequency paradigm.[31] Rooted in adult educational theory, this new approach allows trainees to practice their CPR skills "on the job" in a brief (<2 minute) instruction. Studies have demonstrated this approach to improve initial skill acquisition and retention of both ICU and non-ICU providers alike during simulated resuscitation.[31,32] The AHA now offers Basic Life Support recertification through this transformational approach: http://cpr.heart.org/AHAECC/CPRAndECC/Training/RQI/UCM_476470_RQI.jsp.

Physiologic Monitoring During Cardiopulmonary Resuscitation

Traditionally, CPR training has focused on treatment of out-of-hospital cardiac arrests (OHCAs), mostly because the magnitude of OHCA was previously thought to be much greater than IHCA, and therefore, training was appropriately designed for a wide range of skill levels across both trained and untrained rescuers. As a result, the paradigm for optimal resuscitation was more "rescuer-centric" in that the rescuer was coached to provide a specific rate and depth of compression and to provide vasopressors at a fixed dosing interval across all patients, irrespective of the patient's underlying physiologic response to the resuscitation. However, newer data have suggested that in-hospital professional CPR is as common as out-of-hospital professional CPR,[33] and more importantly, that most IHCA occurs in ICUs where physiologic data are available to guide the resuscitation.[15] This statement is particularly true in pediatrics, where more than 95% of arrests now occur in ICUs compared with general wards. In response, both in a recent 2013 CPR Quality Consensus Statement[34] released by the AHA and in the 2015 PALS Guidelines,[35] physiologic monitoring during CPR was recommended with invasive hemodynamic targets favored over exhaled end tidal carbon dioxide ($ETCO_2$).

Arterial blood pressure

Achieving adequate coronary perfusion pressure (CPP), the mathematical difference between aortic and right atrial diastolic pressures, is an important determinant of successful resuscitation.[36] In preclinical models of p-IHCA, titration of vasopressor administration to CPP and adjustment of compression depth to systolic blood pressure resulted in improved survival.[6,7] Although CPP monitoring requires simultaneous measurement of diastolic blood pressure (DBP) and central venous pressure, DBP alone is a more clinically feasible surrogate marker of CPR quality. Therefore, in the most recent 2015 PALS Guidelines, use of the arterial waveform as a feedback device to evaluate chest compression quality was recommended in patients with an indwelling arterial catheter in place at the time of arrest. This recommendation acknowledges the substantial risk of interrupting CPR to place an arterial line for CPR quality monitoring. Specific target values in children have not been identified; however, a large multicenter trial in the CPCCRN network is ongoing to establish these targets (expected publication, 2017).

End tidal carbon dioxide

$ETCO_2$ reflects pulmonary blood flow and is thereby a marker of cardiac output (**Fig. 1**).[37] $ETCO_2$ values <10 mm Hg during cardiac arrest are associated with mortality, but higher $ETCO_2$ values do not always correspond to a successful resuscitation (ie, $ETCO_2$ is a good negative predictor).[38] $ETCO_2$ can also be used to detect return of spontaneous circulation (ROSC), because abrupt increases in $ETCO_2$ result from the increased pulmonary blood flow at ROSC. In adult studies, $ETCO_2$ values correlate with chest compression depth and ventilation rates.[39] Similar to arterial blood pressure–guided CPR described above, recent animal work has also demonstrated that $ETCO_2$-guided chest compressions are as effective as standard CPR optimized with other feedback modalities (eg, visual depth marker, video, verbal cues).[40] Although specific cutoff values are not known, monitoring of $ETCO_2$ may be considered to guide CPR quality (2015 PALS Guidelines).

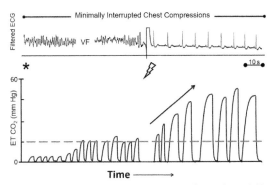

Fig. 1. CPR quality monitoring with $ETCO_2$. From onset of CPR (*asterisk*), note slow increase in $ETCO_2$ as minimally interrupted compressions are delivered. Dashed line represents 2010 PALS Guidelines recommendation to target at least 15 mm Hg. A defibrillation attempt is provided to this patient in VF (*lightning bolt*). Notice the brief interruption to delivery energy (<10 seconds), the conversion to a sinus rhythm with successful defibrillation, and the increase in $ETCO_2$ (>50 mm Hg) with ROSC (*arrow*). Note avoidance of excessive ventilation (goal 10 breaths/min). Filtered ECG provided to remove compression artifact from rhythm depiction. (*Data from* Aase SO, Eftestol T, Husoy JH, et al. CPR artifact removal from human ECG using optimal multichannel filtering. IEEE Trans Biomed Eng 2000;47(11):1440–9.)

Despite being recommended by the AHA, a recent large GWTG-R study demonstrated that providers rarely use physiology to guide the resuscitation effort.[41] Specifically, of 21,375 index events with an invasive airway in place at the time of the arrest, $ETCO_2$ was used to monitor quality in only 803 (4%). Similarly, of 7260 index events with an arterial catheter in place at the time of the arrest, DBP was used to monitor CPR quality in only 2145 (30%). In this propensity-matched cohort, use of physiologic monitoring was associated with a higher likelihood of ROSC, indicating that more widespread use may be one method to improve ICU CPR outcomes in the future.

Drugs During Cardiopulmonary Resuscitation

Epinephrine
Although recent adult evidence has suggested no benefit to epinephrine administration during OHCA resuscitation,[42] it is still recommended by the 2015 PALS Guidelines as a reasonable therapy. Epinephrine (recommended dose of 0.010 mg/kg) helps achieve ROSC by increasing systemic vascular resistance, which leads to a higher DBP and CPP.[43] Delayed administration of epinephrine has been associated with worse outcomes in a recent large pediatric registry study of patients with nonshockable rhythms, suggesting that when needed, early administration is better.[44] High-dose epinephrine (0.100 mg/kg) is not recommended because of its use being associated with higher mortality in a randomized pediatric cardiac arrest trial.[45]

Vasopressin
The 2015 Advance Cardiac Life Support Guidelines removed the use of vasopressin because of a lack of survival advantage over epinephrine alone.[46] Because of limited pediatric data and an association with lower rates of ROSC in a GWTG-R study,[47] routine vasopressin use is also not recommended during cardiac arrest in children. Experts will still consider administration in select resuscitation circumstances where adrenergic receptor stimulation may be detrimental (eg, pulmonary hypertension, arrhythmogenic states) or ineffective (eg, catecholamine-refractory shock).

Amiodarone versus lidocaine
The 2005 and 2010 PALS Guidelines recommended amiodarone over lidocaine for refractory ventricular fibrillation (VF) or pulseless ventricular tachycardia (pVT) based on pediatric case series/adult data. In contrast with this older data, a more recent GWTG-R study demonstrated improved ROSC with lidocaine compared with amiodarone.[48] As such, the 2015 PALS Guidelines state that either amiodarone or lidocaine is an appropriate pharmacologic choice for treatment of shock-refractory VF or pVT.

Airway Management

Tracheal intubation is emphasized as a basic tenet of CPR, especially for treatment of p-IHCA. However, tracheal intubation of critically ill children is increasingly recognized as high risk for precipitating cardiac arrest.[49] In addition, 2 large propensity-matched cohort studies demonstrate that tracheal intubation DURING cardiac arrest compared with no intubation is associated with decreased survival.[50,51] Further prospective studies are needed to determine the following: (1) why tracheal intubation during CPR can be dangerous (eg, prolonged pauses in chest compressions during intubation attempts or inadvertent esophageal intubations) in order to ameliorate adverse effects; and (2) whether the current emphasis on early invasive airway management for p-IHCA should be reevaluated.

Postarrest Care

The post–resuscitation phase should focus on limiting secondary injury. Management priorities should include attention to blood pressure goals; avoidance of extremes of oxygenation and ventilation; anticipation of and prevention of hyperthermia; and monitoring for and treatment of status epilepticus.

Blood pressure

Myocardial dysfunction and arterial hypotension occur commonly after successful resuscitation.[52] Hypotension after ROSC, defined as less than the fifth percentile for age, is associated with higher mortality.[13] In response, the most recent iteration of the PALS Guidelines recommended that when appropriate resources are available, providers should both continuously monitor invasive arterial pressure after ROSC and use parenteral fluids, inotropes, and vasopressors to avoid/treat hypotension (class I).

Temperature

Hyperthermia following cardiac arrest is common in children and is associated with poor neurologic outcome.[53] However, whether a patient should receive therapeutic hypothermia was a topic of recent study. Two large pediatric multicenter trials (https://www.thapca.org/) have now demonstrated no benefit to comatose patients post–cardiac arrest who were treated with therapeutic hypothermia (32°C–34°C) compared with those treated with therapeutic normothermia (36°C–37.5°C) for OHCA and IHCA, respectively.[54,55] As a result, the most recent PALS Guidelines recommended that for infants and children remaining comatose after cardiac arrest, that either maintenance of 5 days of continuous normothermia (36°C–37.5°C) or maintenance of 2 days of initial continuous hypothermia (32°C–34°C) followed by 3 days of continuous normothermia, were reasonable choices. Continuous measurement of temperature during the post–resuscitation period and aggressive treatment of fever (temperature of 38°C or more) were class I recommendations.

Oxygenation and ventilation

One large observational pediatric study found that the presence of normoxemia (Pao_2 $\geq$60 and <300 mm Hg) when compared with hyperoxemia (Pao_2 >300 mm Hg) after ROSC was associated with improved survival to PICU discharge.[56] In one observational study of p-IHCA, hypocapnia ($Paco_2$ <30 mm Hg) and hypercapnia ($Paco_2$ $\geq$50 mm Hg) were both associated with mortality.[12] As such, the most recent PALS Guidelines made recommendations to avoid extremes of oxygenation and ventilation, with the understanding that *hypoxemia* should be strictly avoided.

Glucose

Both hyperglycemia and hypoglycemia after adult cardiac arrest are associated with worse outcome.[57] Unfortunately, there is insufficient evidence to make a strong recommendation regarding glucose management in children after ROSC. If a decision is made to treat hyperglycemia after ROSC in pediatric patients, blood glucose concentrations should be monitored carefully, and hypoglycemia (<80 mg/dL) should be strictly avoided.

Seizures

Seizures are common after cardiac arrest, present in up to 30% of patients,[58] and certain electroencephalographic findings (abnormal background, burst suppression, and subclinical status epilepticus) are associated with worse neurologic outcome.[59] Therefore, most experts agree that close monitoring and treatment of status epilepticus in the post-ROSC phase are important, although there is a paucity of data showing that treatment of seizures improves outcomes. In making the decision to treat seizures in the postarrest period, side effects of antiepileptic drugs should be considered. Treating seizures only to induce severe systolic hypotension with benzodiazepines would likely be detrimental to the outcome of the child.

Extracorporeal Life Support Cardiopulmonary Resuscitation

No discussion of ICU CPR would be complete without mention of extracorporeal life support cardiopulmonary resuscitation (ECPR). In the aforementioned large CPCCRN study of ICU CPR, more than 15% of the 77% of patients who achieved ROC did so through use of extracorporeal life support instituted during CPR.[4] In children with medical or surgical cardiac diseases, ECPR has been shown to improve survival to hospital discharge[60] and can be effective even after prolonged episodes of CPR (>50 minutes).[61] In a recent GWTG-R study that looked at patients from all illness categories who received at least 10 minutes of CPR, ECPR had improved survival and favorable neurologic outcome at discharge compared with conventional CPR, even after propensity matching.[62] The most recent PALS Guidelines stated that ECPR may be considered for pediatric patients with cardiac diagnoses, but highlighted that existing ECMO protocols, expertise, and equipment should be in place. Most experts would agree that suitability for ECPR rescue should be individualized at the patient level, considering reversibility of the underlying process in the ultimate decision rather than focusing on a specific disease category such as cardiac versus noncardiac.

SUMMARY

ICU CPR is a significant problem. Fortunately, resuscitation science advances in both education and clinical care have improved ICU CPR outcomes substantially over the past 20 years. Critically ill children who receive CPR now have almost a 50% chance of leaving the hospital with favorable neurologic outcome.

REFERENCES

1. Knudson JD, Neish SR, Cabrera AG, et al. Prevalence and outcomes of pediatric in-hospital cardiopulmonary resuscitation in the United States: an analysis of the kids' inpatient database*. Crit Care Med 2012;40(11):2940–4.
2. Slonim AD, Patel KM, Ruttimann UE, et al. Cardiopulmonary resuscitation in pediatric intensive care units. Crit Care Med 1997;25(12):1951–5.
3. Girotra S, Spertus JA, Li Y, et al. Survival trends in pediatric in-hospital cardiac arrests: an analysis from get with the guidelines-resuscitation. Circ Cardiovasc Qual Outcomes 2013;6(1):42–9.
4. Berg RA, Nadkarni VM, Clark AE, et al. Incidence and outcomes of cardiopulmonary resuscitation in PICUs. Crit Care Med 2016;44(4):798–808.
5. Sutton RM, French B, Niles DE, et al. 2010 American Heart Association recommended compression depths during pediatric in-hospital resuscitations are associated with survival. Resuscitation 2014;85(9):1179–84.
6. Sutton RM, Friess SH, Naim MY, et al. Patient-centric blood pressure-targeted cardiopulmonary resuscitation improves survival from cardiac arrest. Am J Respir Crit Care Med 2014;190(11):1255–62.
7. Naim MY, Sutton RM, Friess SH, et al. Blood pressure- and coronary perfusion pressure-targeted cardiopulmonary resuscitation improves 24-hour survival from ventricular fibrillation cardiac arrest. Crit Care Med 2016;44(11):e1111–7.

8. Nadkarni VM, Larkin GL, Peberdy MA, et al. First documented rhythm and clinical outcome from in-hospital cardiac arrest among children and adults. JAMA 2006; 295(1):50–7.
9. Michiels EA, Dumas F, Quan L, et al. Long-term outcomes following pediatric out-of-hospital cardiac arrest*. Pediatr Crit Care Med 2013;14(8):755–60.
10. Samson RA, Nadkarni VM, Meaney PA, et al. Outcomes of in-hospital ventricular fibrillation in children. N Engl J Med 2006;354(22):2328–39.
11. Sutton RM, French B, Nishisaki A, et al. American Heart Association cardiopulmonary resuscitation quality targets are associated with improved arterial blood pressure during pediatric cardiac arrest. Resuscitation 2013;84(2):168–72.
12. Del Castillo J, Lopez-Herce J, Matamoros M, et al. Hyperoxia, hypocapnia and hypercapnia as outcome factors after cardiac arrest in children. Resuscitation 2012;83(12):1456–61.
13. Topjian AA, French B, Sutton RM, et al. Early postresuscitation hypotension is associated with increased mortality following pediatric cardiac arrest. Crit Care Med 2014;42(6):1518–23.
14. Brilli RJ, Gibson R, Luria JW, et al. Implementation of a medical emergency team in a large pediatric teaching hospital prevents respiratory and cardiopulmonary arrests outside the intensive care unit. Pediatr Crit Care Med 2007;8(3):236–46 [quiz: 247].
15. Berg RA, Sutton RM, Holubkov R, et al. Ratio of PICU versus ward cardiopulmonary resuscitation events is increasing. Crit Care Med 2013;41(10):2292–7.
16. Randolph AG, Gonzales CA, Cortellini L, et al. Growth of pediatric intensive care units in the United States from 1995 to 2001. J Pediatr 2004;144(6):792–8.
17. Willson DF, Dean JM, Newth C, et al. Collaborative Pediatric Critical Care Research Network (CPCCRN). Pediatr Crit Care Med 2006;7(4):301–7.
18. Peddy SB, Hazinski MF, Laussen PC, et al. Cardiopulmonary resuscitation: special considerations for infants and children with cardiac disease. Cardiol Young 2007;17(Suppl 2):116–26.
19. Parra DA, Totapally BR, Zahn E, et al. Outcome of cardiopulmonary resuscitation in a pediatric cardiac intensive care unit. Crit Care Med 2000;28(9):3296–300.
20. Rhodes JF, Blaufox AD, Seiden HS, et al. Cardiac arrest in infants after congenital heart surgery. Circulation 1999;100(19 Suppl):194–9.
21. Gupta P, Jacobs JP, Pasquali SK, et al. Epidemiology and outcomes after in-hospital cardiac arrest after pediatric cardiac surgery. Ann Thorac Surg 2014; 98(6):2138–43 [discussion: 2144].
22. Christenson J, Andrusiek D, Everson-Stewart S, et al. Chest compression fraction determines survival in patients with out-of-hospital ventricular fibrillation. Circulation 2009;120(13):1241–7.
23. Zuercher M, Hilwig RW, Ranger-Moore J, et al. Leaning during chest compressions impairs cardiac output and left ventricular myocardial blood flow in piglet cardiac arrest. Crit Care Med 2010;38(4):1141–6.
24. Aufderheide TP, Lurie KG. Death by hyperventilation: a common and life-threatening problem during cardiopulmonary resuscitation. Crit Care Med 2004;32(9 Suppl):S345–51.
25. Aase SO, Myklebust H. Compression depth estimation for CPR quality assessment using DSP on accelerometer signals. IEEE Trans Biomed Eng 2002;49(3):263–8.
26. Sutton RM, Niles D, Nysaether J, et al. Quantitative analysis of CPR quality during in-hospital resuscitation of older children and adolescents. Pediatrics 2009; 124(2):494–9.

27. Sutton RM, Maltese MR, Niles D, et al. Quantitative analysis of chest compression interruptions during in-hospital resuscitation of older children and adolescents. Resuscitation 2009;80(11):1259–63.
28. Niles D, Nysaether J, Nishisaki A, et al. Leaning is common during in-hospital pediatric CPR, and decreased with automated corrective feedback. Resuscitation 2009;80(5):553–7.
29. Wolfe H, Zebuhr C, Topjian AA, et al. Interdisciplinary ICU cardiac arrest debriefing improves survival outcomes*. Crit Care Med 2014;42(7):1688–95.
30. Kaye W, Mancini ME. Retention of cardiopulmonary resuscitation skills by physicians, registered nurses, and the general public. Crit Care Med 1986;14(7):620–2.
31. Sutton RM, Niles D, Meaney PA, et al. Low-dose, high-frequency CPR training improves skill retention of in-hospital pediatric providers. Pediatrics 2011;128(1):e145–51.
32. Sutton RM, Niles D, Meaney PA, et al. "Booster" training: evaluation of instructor-led bedside cardiopulmonary resuscitation skill training and automated corrective feedback to improve cardiopulmonary resuscitation compliance of pediatric basic life support providers during simulated cardiac arrest. Pediatr Crit Care Med 2011;12(3):e116–21.
33. Merchant RM, Yang L, Becker LB, et al. Incidence of treated cardiac arrest in hospitalized patients in the United States. Crit Care Med 2011;39(11):2401–6.
34. Meaney PA, Bobrow BJ, Mancini ME, et al. Cardiopulmonary resuscitation quality: [corrected] improving cardiac resuscitation outcomes both inside and outside the hospital: a consensus statement from the American Heart Association. Circulation 2013;128(4):417–35.
35. de Caen AR, Berg MD, Chameides L, et al. Part 12: pediatric advanced life support: 2015 American Heart Association guidelines update for cardiopulmonary resuscitation and emergency cardiovascular care. Circulation 2015;132(18 Suppl 2):S526–42.
36. Paradis NA, Martin GB, Rivers EP, et al. Coronary perfusion pressure and the return of spontaneous circulation in human cardiopulmonary resuscitation. JAMA 1990;263(8):1106–13.
37. Ornato JP, Garnett AR, Glauser FL. Relationship between cardiac output and the end-tidal carbon dioxide tension. Ann Emerg Med 1990;19(10):1104–6.
38. Sanders AB, Kern KB, Otto CW, et al. End-tidal carbon dioxide monitoring during cardiopulmonary resuscitation. A prognostic indicator for survival. JAMA 1989;262(10):1347–51.
39. Sheak KR, Wiebe DJ, Leary M, et al. Quantitative relationship between end-tidal carbon dioxide and CPR quality during both in-hospital and out-of-hospital cardiac arrest. Resuscitation 2015;89:149–54.
40. Hamrick JL, Hamrick JT, Lee JK, et al. Efficacy of chest compressions directed by end-tidal CO2 feedback in a pediatric resuscitation model of basic life support. J Am Heart Assoc 2014;3(2):e000450.
41. Sutton RM, French B, Meaney PA, et al. Physiologic monitoring of CPR quality during adult cardiac arrest: a propensity-matched cohort study. Resuscitation 2016;106:76–82.
42. Olasveengen TM, Sunde K, Brunborg C, et al. Intravenous drug administration during out-of-hospital cardiac arrest: a randomized trial. JAMA 2009;302(20):2222–9.
43. Paradis NA, Wenzel V, Southall J. Pressor drugs in the treatment of cardiac arrest. Cardiol Clin 2002;20(1):61–78.

44. Andersen LW, Berg KM, Saindon BZ, et al. Time to epinephrine and survival after pediatric in-hospital cardiac arrest. JAMA 2015;314(8):802–10.

45. Perondi MB, Reis AG, Paiva EF, et al. A comparison of high-dose and standard-dose epinephrine in children with cardiac arrest. N Engl J Med 2004;350(17): 1722–30.

46. Stiell IG, Hebert PC, Wells GA, et al. Vasopressin versus epinephrine for inhospital cardiac arrest: a randomised controlled trial. Lancet 2001;358(9276):105–9.

47. Duncan JM, Meaney P, Simpson P, et al. Vasopressin for in-hospital pediatric cardiac arrest: results from the American Heart Association National Registry of Cardiopulmonary Resuscitation. Pediatr Crit Care Med 2009;10(2):191–5.

48. Valdes SO, Donoghue AJ, Hoyme DB, et al. Outcomes associated with amiodarone and lidocaine in the treatment of in-hospital pediatric cardiac arrest with pulseless ventricular tachycardia or ventricular fibrillation. Resuscitation 2014; 85(3):381–6.

49. Shiima Y, Berg RA, Bogner HR, et al. Cardiac arrests associated with tracheal intubations in PICUs: a multicenter cohort study. Crit Care Med 2016;44(9): 1675–82.

50. Andersen LW, Granfeldt A, Callaway CW, et al. Association between tracheal intubation during adult in-hospital cardiac arrest and survival. JAMA 2017;317(5): 494–506.

51. Andersen LW, Raymond TT, Berg RA, et al. Association between tracheal intubation during pediatric in-hospital cardiac arrest and survival. JAMA 2016;316(17): 1786–97.

52. Conlon TW, Falkensammer CB, Hammond RS, et al. Association of left ventricular systolic function and vasopressor support with survival following pediatric out-of-hospital cardiac arrest. Pediatr Crit Care Med 2015;16(2):146–54.

53. Bembea MM, Nadkarni VM, Diener-West M, et al. Temperature patterns in the early postresuscitation period after pediatric inhospital cardiac arrest. Pediatr Crit Care Med 2010;11(6):723–30.

54. Moler FW, Silverstein FS, Holubkov R, et al. Therapeutic hypothermia after in-hospital cardiac arrest in children. N Engl J Med 2017;376(4):318–29.

55. Moler FW, Silverstein FS, Holubkov R, et al. Therapeutic hypothermia after out-of-hospital cardiac arrest in children. N Engl J Med 2015;372(20):1898–908.

56. Ferguson LP, Durward A, Tibby SM. Relationship between arterial partial oxygen pressure after resuscitation from cardiac arrest and mortality in children. Circulation 2012;126(3):335–42.

57. Beiser DG, Carr GE, Edelson DP, et al. Derangements in blood glucose following initial resuscitation from in-hospital cardiac arrest: a report from the national registry of cardiopulmonary resuscitation. Resuscitation 2009;80(6):624–30.

58. Abend NS, Topjian A, Ichord R, et al. Electroencephalographic monitoring during hypothermia after pediatric cardiac arrest. Neurology 2009;72(22):1931–40.

59. Topjian AA, Sanchez SM, Shults J, et al. Early electroencephalographic background features predict outcomes in children resuscitated from cardiac arrest. Pediatr Crit Care Med 2016;17(6):547–57.

60. Ortmann L, Prodhan P, Gossett J, et al. Outcomes after in-hospital cardiac arrest in children with cardiac disease: a report from get with the guidelines–resuscitation. Circulation 2011;124(21):2329–37.

61. Morris MC, Wernovsky G, Nadkarni VM. Survival outcomes after extracorporeal cardiopulmonary resuscitation instituted during active chest compressions following refractory in-hospital pediatric cardiac arrest. Pediatr Crit Care Med 2004;5(5):440–6.

62. Lasa JJ, Rogers RS, Localio R, et al. Extracorporeal cardiopulmonary resuscitation (E-CPR) during pediatric in-hospital cardiopulmonary arrest is associated with improved survival to discharge: a report from the american heart association's get with the guidelines-resuscitation (GWTG-R) registry. Circulation 2016; 133(2):165–76.

63. Meaney PA, Nadkarni VM, Cook EF, et al. American Heart Association National Registry of Cardiopulmonary Resuscitation Investigators. Higher survival rates among younger patients after pediatric intensive care unit cardiac arrests. Pediatrics 2006;118(6):2424–33.

Management Issues in Critically Ill Pediatric Patients with Trauma

Omar Z. Ahmed, MD*, Randall S. Burd, MD, PhD

KEYWORDS

- Pediatric trauma • Deep venous thrombosis • Blunt cardiac injury
- Delayed diagnosis of injury • Solid organ injury • Blunt cerebrovascular injury
- Component therapy • Chest wall trauma

KEY POINTS

- The use of component therapy during massive transfusion can help reverse the effects of coagulopathy during trauma resuscitation.
- Isolated solid organ injury in hemodynamically stable patients can be observed outside of an intensive care setting.
- Pulmonary contusions are more common than rib fractures after pediatric injury and can increase morbidity during recovery from other injuries.
- In the absence of a contraindication, aspirin should be used in the management of grade I blunt cerebrovascular injury.
- Postpubertal and severely injured adolescent traumas should be considered for thromboembolism prophylaxis.

INTRODUCTION

The management of pediatric patients with trauma poses many unique challenges. Severe injuries in pediatric trauma are rare, making it difficult to obtain sufficient data to develop evidence-based treatment algorithms for many injuries. This lack of data results in the need to rely on either guidelines developed for adults that may not be directly applicable to children or to rely only on clinical judgment. This article provides an overview of the treatment of critically injured children and highlights several areas of management that require an integrated approach between trauma surgeons and critical care physicians.

Disclosure: The investigators have nothing to disclose.
Department of General and Thoracic Surgery, Division of Trauma and Burn Surgery, Children's National Medical Center, 111 Michigan Avenue Northwest, Washington, DC 20010, USA
* Corresponding author.
E-mail address: rburd@childrensnational.org

Pediatr Clin N Am 64 (2017) 973–990
http://dx.doi.org/10.1016/j.pcl.2017.06.002

OVERVIEW

Data obtained from the National Trauma Databank in 2014 show that 42% of injured children (n = 29,725) seen at trauma centers are admitted to an intensive care unit during their hospitalizations (**Fig. 1**). The average age of injured children admitted to an intensive care unit is 8 years old and these children spend 5 days on average in the intensive care unit. Most children who are admitted to an intensive care unit have sustained blunt trauma (91%). Children with either a head or neck injury represent the most common injuries requiring admission to the intensive care unit (57%). Among children with a head or neck injury, most had injuries classified as at least moderate (**Fig. 2**). Excluding patients who went to the operating room and those who died in the emergency department, only 19% of patients (172 out of 908) who died during their hospitalizations were treated in the intensive care unit. More than 50% of injured children in intensive care units have an injury severity score (ISS) greater than 15, showing the complexity of these patients (**Fig. 3**). Injured children admitted to an intensive care unit at any time during their hospitalizations have as much as a 3-fold greater risk of hospital readmission than do injured children who do not require intensive monitoring.[1] Although care should be improved in all settings, several studies have suggested that critically injured children have lower mortality and lower hospital length of stay when treated in a pediatric hospital compared with treatment in an adult hospital.[2] The better outcomes in these patients support the selective triage of seriously injured children to trauma centers with pediatric intensive care units when this is an available option.[3]

FLUID RESUSCITATION

Fluid resuscitation is a critical component of the early management of many injured children. Over-resuscitation and under-resuscitation can each have adverse effects. Inadequate resuscitation can worsen the shock state, whereas the administration of excess fluid can trigger a cascade of adverse events, including oxygen desaturation, prolongation of intubation, and edema. For hemodynamically unstable children, standard recommendations for initial resuscitation are to administer a crystalloid fluid bolus of 20 mL/kg, to repeat this bolus if needed, and to then begin transfusion of

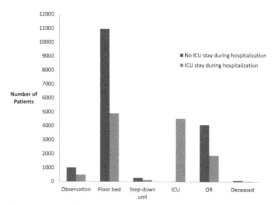

Fig. 1. Emergency department disposition of pediatric patients with trauma. ICU, intensive care unit; OR, operating room. (*Data from* National Trauma Data Bank. 2014. Available at: https://www.facs.org/~/media/files/quality%20programs/trauma/ntdb/ntdb%20pediatric%20annual%20report%202014.ashx.)

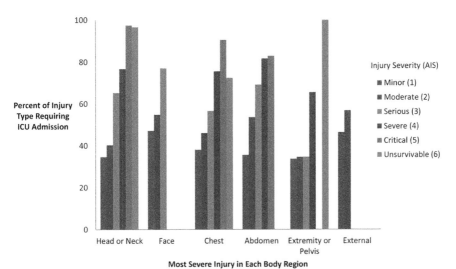

Fig. 2. Percentage of body region injury severity admitted to the ICU. AIS, Abbreviated Injury Scale. (*Data from* National Trauma Data Bank. 2014. Available at: https://www.facs.org/~/media/files/quality%20programs/trauma/ntdb/ntdb%20pediatric%20annual%20report%202014.ashx.)

packed red blood cells (PRBCs) with an initial bolus volume of 10 mL/kg.[4] An assessment of the patient's signs and symptoms should direct fluid resuscitation, which includes the patient's vital signs, the patient's mental status, and a physical examination assessing peripheral perfusion. Although most children are resuscitated initially with crystalloid, initial resuscitation with blood components is preferred in some settings. Blood transfusion is preferred to crystalloid administration in the setting of blood loss after injury when the initial hemoglobin level is less than 7 g/dL. Although this scenario is typically not seen in the emergency department, it may be observed after

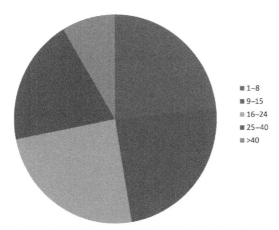

Fig. 3. ISS of ICU patients. (*Data from* National Trauma Data Bank. 2014. Available at: https://www.facs.org/~/media/files/quality%20programs/trauma/ntdb/ntdb%20pediatric%20annual%20report%202014.ashx.)

admission to an inpatient setting. Because the initial administration of crystalloid may lead to hemodilution and new or worsened symptoms related to blood loss, blood products should be given even in the absence of signs or symptoms of anemia.[5]

Controlled resuscitation, also known as permissive hypotension, has been increasingly adopted as a strategy for fluid management among adult patients with hemorrhagic shock. Controlled resuscitation is a nonaggressive approach to fluid administration in patients who are volume depleted because of hemorrhage. When using this strategy, normal vital sign values are not the main target of therapy. The goal of controlled resuscitation instead is to stabilize the patient's hemodynamic status but at a lower blood pressure than normal. Several explanations have been proposed to account for the potential benefits of permissive hypotension, which include the minimization of hydrostatic pressure for stabilizing clot and reduction of the dilutional effects of coagulopathy.[6–8] Animal studies have shown that fluid resuscitation reduces mortality when used for treatment of large-volume blood loss and increases mortality when used for less severe hemorrhage compared with no fluid resuscitation.[9] These findings suggest that the benefits of fluid resuscitation do not always justify its risks and that the approach to fluid resuscitation should be tailored to the clinical setting. For example, hemodynamically stable patients who have bled from a solid organ injury without evidence of ongoing bleeding should be treated with controlled resuscitation rather than with aggressive fluid resuscitation. Findings from animal studies also show that the use of controlled resuscitation decreases mortality for injuries associated with hemorrhage, regardless of blood volume lost.[9] Several reasons may account for the decreased mortality associated with controlled resuscitation, including fewer complications related to fluid overload (pulmonary congestion, edema, electrolyte derangements) and decreased dilutional coagulopathy.

Because of differences between adult and pediatric physiology, extrapolating findings from adult studies to make recommendations for treating injured children with hemorrhagic shock may not be appropriate. Compared with adults, children can maintain a normal blood pressure even in the setting of significant blood loss and ongoing hemorrhage. Hypotension may also not develop in children until the proportion of lost blood volume is as high as 45%, a volume requiring intervention in most patients.[4] Despite evidence of the benefits of permissive hypotension in adults and data obtained from animal studies, its role in managing hemorrhagic shock after pediatric injury is uncertain. Limitation of fluid resuscitation may not be optimal because of the child's delayed presentation of hypotension in hemorrhagic shock, decreasing the value of blood pressure as an end point for controlled resuscitation in children. The applicability of controlled resuscitation in children may then depend on approaches that can identify the shock state sooner than standard vital sign measurements and other physical examination adjuncts.

Successful resuscitation requires coordination of prehospital and initial hospital care. When provided with details of the injury, the hospital team can anticipate future blood loss when given initial estimates of the blood volume already lost. Early notification of the patient's volume status can increase the timeliness of treatment in the trauma bay and intensive care unit, just as early notification by emergency medical services improves treatment of other medical conditions.[10] With early knowledge of the patient's volume status, initial hospital management can quickly begin, before patient arrival if needed, including the release of blood products, setting up central venous or arterial lines, or preparing the operating room. Because initiating these interventions can be time consuming, early preparation for lifesaving treatments allows for more rapid treatment and can have a major effect on patients for whom minutes and seconds matter.[10]

Acid-base status based on arterial blood gas measurement can be useful for managing critically injured pediatric patients with trauma. Injured children who have undergone an arterial blood gas test can be classified as having a mild base deficit (greater than −5) or severe base deficit (less than or equal to −5). A severe base deficit is associated with a high risk of mortality (35%), whereas a mild base deficit is associated with survival. Among survivors of pediatric injury, most (75%) have their base deficits corrected within 48 hours. These results highlight the importance of early resuscitation and correction of acidosis on survival after pediatric injury.[11] An admission base deficit also correlates with mortality. A higher mortality is observed in children with an admission base deficit less than −8. Injured children with an admission base deficit between −4 and −8 have a 12% mortality compared with those with base deficits between −8 and −12, who have a mortality of 32%.[12] Injured children found to have a severe base deficit require rapid identification of the source of acidosis (eg, hemorrhage, intra-abdominal sepsis related to intestinal injury, or decreased respiratory efforts related to chest injury) and prompt intervention to reverse its effects.

Lethal triad is a term used to describe the cycle of acidosis, coagulopathy, and hypothermia that can occur during hemorrhagic shock. Each factor negatively affects the others, amplifying the deleterious effects of each. Even in the absence of significant blood loss, injured patients have an increased risk of bleeding if they have a severe injury.[13–18] This bleeding diathesis is known as acute coagulopathy of trauma. It may not be related to the dilution of clotting factors associated with crystalloid fluid administration but may be the result of tissue injury and subsequent triggering of inflammatory changes. Estimates of the prevalence of acute coagulopathy of trauma vary in injured children, but it may exceed 25%.[13–19] Children with blood loss large enough to require blood transfusion need monitoring of their coagulation profile early on during their admission to correct their coagulopathy.

Damage control laparotomy is a strategy used when patients with hemoperitoneum secondary to trauma, cannot undergo extensive surgical procedures because of evidence of the lethal triad. The major goals of damage control laparotomy are to control active hemorrhage from major vascular injuries as quickly as possible and to limit abdominal contamination, rather than proceeding with more time-consuming definitive surgical treatments.[20] Active bleeding from a solid organ or compressible vessel may be controlled by tightly packing the affected abdominal region with gauze. To control intra-abdominal contamination, injured bowel is stapled off at the site of injury rather than repaired using a more time-consuming intestinal anastomosis. The abdomen is temporarily covered with an occlusive dressing and return to the operating room is planned within the next 48 hours. By reducing or stopping ongoing hemorrhage and intra-abdominal contamination, the lethal triad can be corrected or avoided better than with definitive surgery. The added time in the operating room for definitive surgical treatment can lead to continued metabolic stress, further heat loss, and worsened coagulopathy.[21,22] Critically injured patients with the lethal triad treated with damage control laparotomy have a lower mortality than those undergoing definitive surgery, supporting the conceptual benefits of this approach.[22]

The continued use of crystalloid and PRBCs without the use of other blood products in patients with the lethal triad may worsen hypothermia and coagulopathy.[23] This understanding has led to the development of component therapy. Component therapy is the use of other blood products in addition to PRBCs (eg, fresh frozen plasma [FFP], platelets, and cryoprecipitate) during initial resuscitation. The use of all blood components is essential for the treatment of patients receiving massive transfusion to counter the effects of dilutional coagulopathy. With the administration of only PRBCs, dilution of platelets and clotting factors may occur and inhibit the contribution of each in clot formation and hemorrhage control. The goal of component therapy is to return the clotting cascade to its normal balance by replenishing all the components necessary for coagulation rather than providing only fluid replacement, which improves blood pressure and oxygen delivery.

Massive blood transfusion protocols (MBTPs) are now used at most pediatric and adult trauma centers in the United States.[24] Although clinical judgment usually directs the activation of these protocols, several guidelines can be used to determine the need to activate the protocol, including the loss of 1 blood volume within 24 hours or the loss of half of a blood volume within 2 hours.[25] An estimate of blood volume can be made from previously published data based on age and weight (**Table 1**).[26] Most centers with a massive transfusion protocol have adopted a 1:1:1 of PRBC/FFP/platelet administration. However, the ratio used at different centers varies, and the most appropriate ratio for transfusion of products in children remains controversial. Several guidelines have been established at pediatric and adult hospitals that can guide the initial implementation of component replacement (**Fig. 4**, **Table 2**).[27,28]

Reports from emergency medical services may indicate that several rounds of blood product administration may be necessary to stabilize a patient in the emergency department. Activation of an MBTP can then be based on prehospital reports or reports from referral hospitals. Some injured children do not require activation of the MBTP initially but may then need this additional access to blood products after reaching an inpatient unit. This delay in needed transfusion may occur because of a delayed diagnosis of injury. In this scenario, activation of the MBTP should be viewed as a bridge to more definitive therapy, such as surgery or treatment in the interventional radiology suite. It is preferred to have a low threshold when deciding whether to activate the MBTP. Returning unused items to the blood bank is preferable to the potential consequences of delayed administration of blood products.

SOLID ORGAN INJURY

Solid organ injury after blunt trauma includes injuries to the liver, spleen, and kidney. Solid organ injuries can be suspected based on a history of blunt torso trauma and signs and symptoms of injury. Intra-abdominal injury requiring intervention can be excluded (likelihood of injury <0.1%) based on the initial clinical presentation: the absence of abdominal pain, the absence of tenderness or external evidence of abdominal wall trauma (seat belt sign), no external evidence of chest wall injury, the absence of vomiting, and the absence of significant head injury.[29] Except for hemodynamically unstable patients who require immediate laparotomy, solid organ injuries are usually identified by computed tomography in at-risk patients. Although focused

Table 1	
Estimated circulating blood volume versus age or weight	
Age	**Estimated Blood Volume (mL/kg)**
Premature infant	90–100
Term infant - 3 months	80–90
Children older than 3 months	70
Very obese children	65

From Barcelona SL, Thompson AA, Coté CJ. Intraoperative pediatric blood transfusion therapy: a review of common issues. Part II: transfusion therapy, special considerations, and reduction of allogenic blood transfusions. Paediatr Anaesth 2005;15(10):814–30.

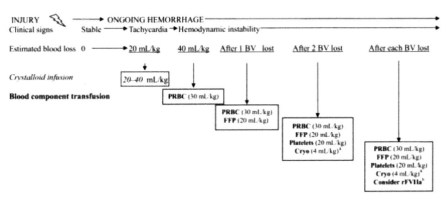

Fig. 4. A 30:20:20 massive transfusion protocol for treatment of hemorrhagic shock in pediatric trauma (for patients with estimated weight <30 kg). For patients who weigh more than 30 kg, a 1:1:1 algorithm should be followed. Transfuse blood component volumes of 1 unit of PRBCs to 1 unit of FFP to 1 unit of pooled platelets, as in adult protocols (see text). [a] Cryoprecipitate (Cryo) at a volume of 4 mL/kg may be given after administration of all 3 components (after estimated loss of 2 blood volumes) or if fibrinogen levels decrease to less than 1 to 1.5 g/L. [b] Consider off-label use of recombinant factor VIIa (rFVIIa), 90 μg/kg, if ongoing bleeding persists after loss of 3 blood volumes. BV, estimated blood volume (generally 70–90 mL/kg based on weight of child, as shown in **Table 1**).[2] (*From* Dehmer JJ, Adamson WT. Massive transfusion and blood product use in the pediatric trauma patient. Semin Pediatr Surg 2010;19(4):286–91; and *Adapted from* Paterson NA. Validation of a theoretically derived model for the management of massive blood loss in pediatric patients—a case report. Paediatr Anaesth 2009;19(5):535–40.)

assessment with sonography for trauma (FAST) has seen wide adoption in trauma centers worldwide, its low sensitivity and specificity for diagnosing abdominal injuries in children may limit its utility as a screening test in children.[30] Grading scales are available based on computed tomography findings to standardize reporting of the severity of solid organ injuries (**Table 3**). As recently as 50 years ago, it was common belief that splenic injuries were almost always fatal because of the potential for continued bleeding unless a splenectomy was performed, and that splenorrhaphy was not safe, even for minor injuries.[31] Studies in the 1960s and 1970s showed that nonoperative management of splenic injuries was a safe option after blunt trauma.[31,32] In the presence of hemodynamic stability, nonoperative management has also been shown to be appropriate for managing blunt splenic injury, even when active bleeding is identified by contrast extravasation.[33] Angioembolization may be a lower risk alternative to surgery for solid organ injury but has yet to be established as an effective strategy in hemodynamically stable patients, even in the presence of contrast extravasation.[32] Although nonoperative management of blunt splenic injuries has been standard practice for more than a few decades, this approach continues to be adopted, as suggested by a decline in the percentage of children undergoing splenectomy after blunt trauma (11% to 3%) over the last 2 decades.[34]

Nonoperative management has also become standard management for most hemodynamically stable injured children with blunt liver or renal injuries.[35–37] Blunt renal injury is associated with mechanisms of injury involving sudden deceleration. Children are more susceptible to major renal injuries (grade IV or V) after blunt abdominal trauma than are adults, likely because of a less protective musculoskeletal system and decreased perinephric fat.[38] The likelihood of requiring blood transfusion for blunt

Table 2
Children's National Medical Center Pediatric Massive Transfusion Protocol

Order of Packages to Transfuse[a]	Neonate 0–4 kg	Infant 5–9 kg	Young Child 10–24 kg	Older Child 25–49 kg	Teen/Adult ≥50 kg
Emergency release (A)	0.5 RBC	1 RBC	2 RBC	3 RBC	5 RBC
B	0.5 RBC	1 RBC	2 RBC	3 RBC	5 RBC
	0.5 FFP	1 FFP	2 FFP	3 FFP	5 FFP
	2 eu Plt	3 eu Plt	4 eu Plt	6 eu Plt	6 eu Plt
C	0.5 RBC	1 RBC	2 RBC	3 RBC	5 RBC
	0.5 FFP	1 FFP	2 FFP	3 FFP	5 FFP
	2 Cryo	3 Cryo	4 Cryo	6 Cryo	8 Cryo
B	0.5 RBC	1 RBC	2 RBC	3 RBC	5 RBC
	0.5 FFP	1 FFP	2 FFP	3 FFP	5 FFP
	2 eu Plt	3 eu Plt	4 eu Plt	6 eu Plt	6 eu Plt
C	0.5 RBC	1 RBC	2 RBC	3 RBC	5 RBC
	0.5 FFP	1 FFP	2 FFP	3 FFP	5 FFP
	2 Cryo	3 Cryo	4 Cryo	6 eu Plt	8 Cryo
B	0.5 RBC	1 RBC	2 RBC	3 RBC	5 RBC
	0.5 FFP	1 FFP	2 FFP	3 FFP	5 FFP
	2 eu Plt	3 eu Plt	4 eu Plt	6 eu Plt	6 eu Plt
C	0.5 RBC	1 RBC	2 RBC	3 RBC	5 RBC
	0.5 FFP	1 FFP	2 FFP	3 FFP	5 FFP
	2 Cryo	3 Cryo	4 Cryo	6 eu Plt	8 Cryo

Abbreviations: Cryo, cryoprecipitate (in units); eu Plt, platelet concentrate (in equivalent units) FFP, fresh frozen plasma (in units); RBC, red blood cells (in units).
[a] Letters denote package type to be released correlating with weight-associated package contents.
Courtesy of Children's National Medical Center, Division of Laboratory Medicine, Transfusion Medicine.

Table 3
Summary of grade of solid organ injury by laceration

	Liver	Spleen	Kidney
Grade I	<1 cm of parenchymal depth injury	<1 cm of parenchymal depth injury	Subcapsular hematoma without parenchymal injury
Grade II	1–3 cm of parenchymal depth injury	1–3 cm of parenchymal depth injury	<1 cm parenchymal depth of renal cortex without urinary extravasation
Grade III	>3 cm of parenchymal depth injury	>3 cm of parenchymal depth injury or trabecular vessel involvement	>1 cm parenchymal depth of renal cortex without collecting system rupture or urinary extravasation
Grade IV	Injury of 25%–75% of hepatic lobe	Vessel involvement with >25% splenic devascularization	Parenchymal laceration extending through renal cortex, medulla, and collecting system
Grade V	Injury to >75% of hepatic lobe	Shattered spleen or complete splenic devascularization	Completely shattered kidney

Adapted from Tinkoff G, Esposito TJ, Reed J, et al. American Association for the Surgery of Trauma Organ Injury Scale I: spleen, liver, and kidney, validation based on the National Trauma Data Bank. Am Coll Surg 2008;207(5):646–55.

renal injury is associated with increasing grade of injury.[39] Despite imaging and gross hematuria suggesting serious injury to the kidney, the kidney continues to function well after blunt injury in children.[37]

Blunt hepatic and splenic injuries can be observed outside of an intensive care unit setting, with the level of monitoring dependent on the physiologic sequelae of the injury rather than the grade of injury. An analysis of 832 children with isolated splenic or hepatic injuries showed that the need for blood transfusion and for surgery increased with higher grade. The frequency of needing transfusion was as high as 26% among children with grade IV injuries (**Table 4**).[40] A difference in hospital length of stay between different grades of splenic and hepatic injury has also been observed (**Table 5**), showing the resource needs of higher grade injuries. The increased likelihood that grade IV injuries require intervention has prompted the recommendation that children with these injuries should be admitted to an intensive care unit. Because of the force required to cause a grade V hepatic or splenic injury, these injuries rarely occur in isolation. Patients with grade V hepatic or splenic injury usually have injuries affecting other body regions rather than an isolated solid organ injury.[40] When no other injuries are present, isolated grade V hepatic and splenic injuries can also be managed nonoperatively in the presence of hemodynamic stability.[41]

Postinjury imaging with either ultrasonography or computed tomography has previously been performed before discharge, before follow-up, or at both times for monitoring the healing process of solid organ injuries. Although once common, follow-up imaging is now not routinely performed and is not needed for most hepatic, splenic, or uncomplicated renal injuries after hemodynamic stability has been established and symptoms have resolved.[40,42,43] Changes in management for blunt hepatic or splenic injuries (eg, surgery, embolization in the interventional radiology suite, or blood transfusion) are now made mostly on clinical criteria, with imaging contributing little to the decision to pursue operative treatment. Evidence of worsening clinical status, including tachycardia, abdominal distension, and worsening anemia, is more reliable for determining the need for operative treatment than findings on imaging.[40,42] However, patients with a complicated blunt renal injury with contrast extravasation should undergo follow-up imaging. These patients are at an increased risk for developing a urinoma and further imaging is needed to identify this potential complication.[43,44]

Table 4
Resource use and activity restriction in 832 children with isolated spleen or liver injury

	CT Grade			
	I	II	III	IV
Admitted to ICU (%)	55.0	54.3	72.3	85.4
Number of Hospital Days (mean)	4.3	5.3	7.1	7.6
Transfused (%)	1.8	5.2	10.1[a]	26.6[a]
Laparotomy (%)	None	1.0	2.7[b]	12.6[b]
Activity restriction weeks (mean)	5.1	6.2	7.5	9.2

Abbreviations: CT, computed tomography; ICU, intensive care unit.
[a] Grade III versus grade IV; $P<.014$.
[b] Grade III versus grade IV; $P<.0001$.
Adapted from Stylianos S. Evidence-based guidelines for resource utilization in children with isolated spleen or liver injury. The APSA Trauma Committee. J Pediatr Surg 2000;35(2):164–7; [discussion: 167–9].

	CT Grade			
	I	II	III	IV
ICU stay (d)	None	None	None	1
Hospital stay (d)	2	3	4	5
Predischarge imaging	None	None	None	None
Postdischarge imaging	None	None	None	None
Return to full-contact sports (wk)	3	4	5	6

Table 5
Proposed guidelines for resource use in children with isolated spleen or liver injury

Adapted from Stylianos S. Evidence-based guidelines for resource utilization in children with isolated spleen or liver injury. The APSA Trauma Committee. J Pediatr Surg 2000;35(2):164–7; [discussion: 167–9].

CHEST WALL INJURIES

Injury to the thoracic cavity can be life-threatening, related to a variety of sequelae, including pneumothorax, flail chest, and tachyarrhythmias caused by blunt cardiac injury. Although injury to the thorax occurs in only about 10% of admitted injured children, its presence can signify the existence of severe injury within the chest, as well as within other body regions.[45] Because of potentially lethal complications associated with chest wall injuries, assessment of children who have sustained severe chest trauma should also focus on identifying these associated injuries. Adjunct tools that are rapidly available include electrocardiograms and FAST examination. For example, any patient presenting with blunt thoracic trauma severe enough to cause a sternal fracture should undergo an electrocardiogram to evaluate for abnormal findings (arrhythmia, ectopy) and to determine whether echocardiography is needed. A FAST can be used to look for pericardial fluid or obvious abnormalities in heart function.[46] Evaluating patients with chest wall injuries requires an understanding of their associated injuries and recognition of their clinical presentations.

Pulmonary contusion is common after blunt trauma to the chest, occurring in slightly more than half of patients sustaining significant chest trauma.[47] Chest radiograph can be used to diagnose pulmonary contusion but this injury is often missed if a radiograph is performed early after injury. A contusion on chest radiograph is often better seen 24 hours after injury than at the time of admission (92% vs 47%). Computed tomography is superior to chest radiograph for detecting pulmonary contusions, with sensitivity reported up to 100% and a specificity of 60%.[48,49] A chest radiograph can be used to evaluate for worsening of pulmonary contusions if a patient's clinical status is not improving. Pulmonary contusions can result in a restrictive pattern of breathing, an effect on respiratory dynamics that can lead to hypercarbia and difficulty weaning intubated patients. The associated musculoskeletal pain that accompanies pulmonary contusions can also lead to splinting, which may restrict ventilation. After sustaining chest injury, children are more prone to develop hypoxemia caused by restricted respiratory dynamics than adults. Younger children have a lower functional residual capacity and higher oxygen demand. For this reason, infants and toddlers have a higher need for oxygen and decreased ability to improve oxygenation through ventilation.[45] These differences in respiratory dynamics explain why children are more susceptible to hypoxemia than adults and explain the need for early detection of labored breathing such as tachypnea, use of accessory muscles of breathing, or declining oxygen saturation among children with chest wall injuries.

The causes of and forces required to cause skeletal injuries differ in younger and older children. As an example, rib fractures need to be evaluated from different perspectives depending on the age of the patient. Because of the pliability of infants' bones, rib fractures in infants are not common and are associated with a significant amount of chest wall force. When these fractures are identified in an infant, nonaccidental trauma should be suspected, prompting a work-up to identify other injuries related to this mechanism of injury.[50] Although still uncommon, rib fractures are more often observed in older children than in infants, with an overall 2% incidence. Because rib fractures are caused by significant blunt force, older children should also be evaluated for other injuries.[50,51] The types of associated injuries depend on the location of the rib fractures. Upper rib fractures are associated with concomitant pulmonary contusions or injury to the great vessels. Because lower ribs overlie the abdomen, fractures in this location are more likely to be associated with intraabdominal solid organ injuries.[52,53]

Blunt cardiac injury is uncommon, occurring in less than 5% of children with blunt thoracic trauma. Motor vehicle collisions and being struck by motor vehicles (84%) are the major mechanisms associated with blunt cardiac injury among injured children. Although encompassing a range of injuries, including myocardial laceration and papillary muscle dysfunction or disruption, the most common type of blunt cardiac injury is contusion (95%).[54] The presentation of blunt cardiac injury in children can vary from chest pain to dysrhythmias to cardiac arrest, sometimes occurring with minimal external indication of injury. Signs and symptoms suggesting cardiac injury include chest pain, ecchymosis of the chest, arrhythmias, hypotension, or signs of tamponade.[55] Because of the potential for arrhythmias and the development of a hemopericardium caused by cardiac contusion, blunt cardiac injury should be considered even in the absence of symptoms after major chest trauma.[54]

When blunt cardiac injury is suspected or confirmed, concomitant injuries often occur, including rib fractures and pulmonary contusions.[54] The absence of rib fractures does not rule out a cardiac contusion after blunt thoracic injury. Children presenting with signs or symptoms of blunt cardiac injury need to be evaluated with an electrocardiogram. Any child with blunt thoracic trauma with hemodynamic instability should be evaluated with a FAST examination focusing on the pericardium to identify hemopericardium. Concerns for blunt cardiac injury caused by unstable hemodynamics need to be addressed with the performance of a transthoracic echocardiogram, even in the absence of findings on FAST examination of the pericardium.[54]

Controlling pain and maintaining oxygenation are essential components of the management of children with chest wall injury. Pain management is needed for ensuring adequate respiratory dynamics and oxygenation. Minimizing pain reduces splinting, decreasing atelectasis and associated hypoxemia or pneumonia. Patients with rib fractures may require additional pain management measures, including epidural anesthesia, rib blocks, or patient-controlled analgesia pumps.[45] However, respiratory depression and lethargy associated with opioid drugs can worsen hypoxemia and hypercarbia. Although the use of adjunctive pain management measures for severe chest injury has not been reported in children, findings from adult studies have favored the use of epidural anesthesia for significant thoracic trauma.[56–58] A patient's age and ability to cooperate during minimally invasive procedures (epidural, rib block) are factors in determining the best management. Infants and children may be better candidates for intravenous, oral, and transcutaneous pain control, whereas adolescents may be more likely to tolerate epidural and rib block procedures.

BLUNT CEREBROVASCULAR INJURY

Intracranial or extracranial injuries to the carotid or vertebral arteries resulting from blunt trauma are collectively known as blunt cerebrovascular injuries (BCVIs). These injuries are classified using a scale from grade I (<25% narrowing of the lumen caused by intimal injury) to grade V (vessel transection) (**Table 6**). Variability in screening practices makes it difficult to determine the incidence of BCVI after pediatric injury but this injury has been identified in up to 8% of injured children who underwent screening imaging.[59] The most frequently involved vessel in BCVI is the carotid artery, with the intracranial carotid artery affected more often than the extracranial carotid artery (69% vs 23%, respectively).[59] Although the incidence is likely low after pediatric injury, the impact of BCVI can be significant and includes stroke and permanent neurologic deficits.

BCVI can be suspected based on other injuries (Le Fort II or III fractures, cervical spine fracture) or patient signs (cervical bruit, ischemic stroke), but establishing the diagnosis requires imaging. Computed tomography of the head and neck is most commonly recommended. Level III evidence based on adult data supports screening for BCVI in patients with neurologic deficits that cannot be explained with already identified injuries.[60] Despite being a prior recommendation, a cervical seatbelt sign (ecchymosis of the neck secondary to a seatbelt) is no longer considered an indication to screen for BCVI in the absence of other findings suggestive of cervical vasculature injury, such as neurologic deficits or first rib fracture. Patients with BCVI typically are more severely injured, often with a moderate to severe head injury.[61] Because of the need for prompt imaging, a high index of suspicion is needed to identify these injuries in injured children who sustain severe blunt force to the head or neck.

Many treatment options can be used to manage BCVI, including antiplatelet therapy, anticoagulation, endovascular or open surgery, or observation with serial examination. Because of the rarity of this injury, few studies have described BCVI and its management in children. In a recent study, 645 injured children with suspected BCVI were evaluated using computed tomography angiography. However, the treatment chosen for 52 patients with BCVI had no effect on progression of injury or mortality.[59] Because of the low incidence of BCVI, only the recommendation of using aspirin for grade I injuries has been made. A recommendation for 3 months of

Table 6
Blunt carotid arterial injury grading scale

Injury Grade	Description of Injury	ICD-9	AIS 90 Score Intracranial	Cervical[a]
I	Luminal irregularity or vessel dissection resulting in <25% luminal narrowing	900.03[b]	3	3
II	Vessel dissection causing ≥25% luminal narrowing, intraluminal thrombus, or a raised intimal flap	900.03	3	3
III	Pseudoaneurysm	900.03	3	3
IV	Occlusion of vessel	900.03	4	3
V	Vessel transection with free extravasation	900.03	5	4

Abbreviations: AIS, Abbreviated Injury Scale; ICD-9, International Classification of Diseases, Ninth Revision.
[a] Add 1 point if neurologic deficit (stroke) is not head-injury related.
[b] Internal carotid artery injury; ICD-9 code for common carotid artery injury is 900.01.
From Biffl WL, Moore EE, Offner PJ, et al. Blunt carotid arterial injuries: implications of a new grading scale. The Journal of trauma. Nov 1999;47(5):845–853; with permission.

treatment with follow-up imaging to monitor for evidence of radiographic stabilization of injury is only based on expert opinion.[59] Insufficient evidence exists for guiding the management of higher grade injuries with anticoagulants (eg, with heparin) or antiplatelets (eg, with aspirin or clopidogrel), medications that increase the risk of bleeding at the site of injury and other locations.

DELAYED DIAGNOSIS OF INJURY

Injuries can be missed during the initial evaluation of children. Transfer of the patient from the trauma bay to the next level of care can serve as a checkpoint to identify previously missed injuries. Providers can use this transition to reassess the patient and review initial management. Missed injuries are more common when children present with severe injuries or are hemodynamically unstable.[62] The Advanced Trauma Life Support protocol includes a head to toe examination to evaluate for all injuries, but deviations from this protocol often occur, even at experienced centers.[63] Medical team members receiving patients with trauma after initial management in the trauma bay should not only reassess the initial findings but be aware that many injuries are discovered even days after admission. Although most missed injuries have minimal effect on outcome, delayed recognition of injuries such as missed small bowel injuries have been associated with mortality.[64]

Diagnoses made more than 12 hours after hospital admission are defined as delays in the diagnosis of injury. These delays in diagnosis can be a source of major morbidity, such as a delay in the stabilization of a cervical spine injury, fixation of fractures, or recognition of abdominal injury requiring surgery. The most common injuries associated with a delayed diagnosis of injury in children are fractures (71%).[62] Changes in management related to delayed recognition of injuries can vary from minor interventions, such as sling placement after identification of an extremity fracture, to major interventions, such as the placement of a cervical collar to protect against sequelae of spinal cord injury after identification of a cervical fracture. Changes in patient management also can extend past hospital discharge. For example, a delay in identifying children subjected to nonaccidental trauma delays notification of child protective services and prolongs the exposure of these children to an unsafe environment in the home.[62]

Several factors have been identified that are associated with delayed diagnosis of injury. Included among these risk factors are an altered level of consciousness of the patient, barriers of communication between the patient and providers, the presence of multiple injuries, blunt mechanisms of injury, and admission to services other than the trauma surgery service.[62,65,66] A delayed diagnosis of injury is most commonly associated with factors that prevent communication between the patient and the medical team. These factors are relevant in intubated patients, patients who are not alert, and preverbal patients.[62] Difference in language preference between the medical team and the patient or the family can also contribute to poor communication. A thorough head to toe reevaluation, again looking for injuries (tertiary survey), should be performed on all injured children to minimize the number of delayed diagnoses of injury and the effects they can have on the child.[62]

THROMBOEMBOLISM PROPHYLAXIS MANAGEMENT

Trauma is a risk factor for the development of thromboembolism.[67] Despite the hypercoagulable risk associated with trauma, the prevalence of a symptomatic thromboembolism after pediatric injury is low (<0.1%).[68,69] Few studies have focused on screening for the development of thromboembolism in pediatric trauma because of its low incidence. Despite its infrequent occurrence, guidelines are needed to aid in the management of children who have an increased risk of thromboembolism. An increasing risk for thromboembolism is associated with increasing injury severity Older age is also associated with an increased risk of thromboembolism formation with children more than 10 years old having the greatest risk. Other risk factors have also been identified, including major vascular injury, central venous line placement, craniotomy, and severe spine injury.[68] These injuries and procedures are associated with the Virchow triad: venous stasis, endothelial cell injury, and hypercoagulability.[70] The elements of the Virchow triad encompass the endovascular changes needed to promote venous thrombosis.

An additional challenge to appropriately screening injured children who have a thromboembolism is identifying these patients in a cost-effective manner. The incidence of symptomatic venous thromboembolism is higher for children older than 17 years (0.5%) compared with children of all ages. Screening is not routinely used because of this low incidence.[71] Symptomatic and asymptomatic injured children requiring at least a 24-hour intensive care unit length of stay have a minimal risk of thromboembolism. An increase in risk is noted as age increases after 14 years old (from 0.6% in children 14–17 years old to 1.0% in those 18–21 years old). The risk is also higher for patients who spend 4 or more days in the intensive care unit (1.6%) and those who spend 4 or more days on the ventilator (2.2%).[72]

Recent guidelines for venous thromboembolism prophylaxis in the pediatric trauma population have been developed that include age and injury severity as factors for guiding management. Pediatric patients with trauma who are more than 15 years old and those with severe injury (ISS >25) have been identified as having a higher risk for the development of a thromboembolism. Pharmacologic venous thromboembolism prophylaxis has been recommended for patients with trauma with a low risk of bleeding who are older than 15 years and for postpubertal patients with an ISS greater than 25. The recommendation of mechanical prophylaxis has also been made for those older than 15 years with a low risk of bleeding and postpubertal patients with severe injuries (ISS >25). Mechanical prophylaxis should be used in addition to pharmacologic prophylaxis and when pharmacologic prophylaxis is contraindicated in at-risk injured children. Pharmacologic prophylaxis has not been recommended for prepubertal patients, regardless of injury severity. Patients should be screened for venous thromboembolism with daily physical examinations rather than with ultrasonography surveillance, looking for extremity edema and pain, tachycardia, and low oxygen saturation that does not improve with supplemental oxygen.[73] Children who receive pharmacologic prophylaxis should be preferentially treated with low-molecular-weight heparin given its safety profile in children.[74]

SUMMARY

The presentation and physiologic response to injury in children are very different from those in adults. Injured children can maintain normal vital signs even after significant volume depletion before sudden clinical decline. For these reasons, early fluid resuscitation and correction of acidosis is central to the treatment of injured children in hemorrhagic shock. In addition, large-volume, ongoing hemorrhage is best managed with initiation of an MBTP. Resuscitation and correction of coagulopathy in these volume-depleted patients are more important than definitive treatment of their injuries. Reevaluation is critical in caring for these patients because many injuries are managed nonoperatively, such as in solid organ injuries in hemodynamically stable children. Differences in injured children also include the relative low risk of certain injuries such as rib fractures and a lower incidence of complications of injury, such as thromboembolism. Caregivers treating injured children have to be able to not only diagnose injuries in children but be able to recognize injury patterns to find associated injuries.

REFERENCES

1. Naseem HU, Dorman RM, Bass KD, et al. Intensive care unit admission predicts hospital readmission in pediatric trauma. J Surg Res 2016;205(2):456–63.
2. Densmore JC, Lim HJ, Oldham KT, et al. Outcomes and delivery of care in pediatric injury. J Pediatr Surg 2006;41(1):92–8 [discussion: 92–8].
3. Farrell LS, Hannan EL, Cooper A. Severity of injury and mortality associated with pediatric blunt injuries: hospitals with pediatric intensive care units versus other hospitals. Pediatr Crit Care Med 2004;5(1):5–9.
4. Advanced trauma life support: student course manual. Chicago: American College of Surgeons; 2012.
5. Lacroix J, Hébert PC, Hutchison JS, et al. Transfusion strategies for patients in pediatric intensive care units. N Engl J Med 2007;356(16):1609–19.
6. Sondeen JL, Coppes VG, Holcomb JB. Blood pressure at which rebleeding occurs after resuscitation in swine with aortic injury. J Trauma 2003;54(5 Suppl): S110–7.
7. Brohi K, Singh J, Heron M, et al. Acute traumatic coagulopathy. J Trauma 2003; 54(6):1127–30.
8. Cotton BA, Guy JS, Morris JA Jr, et al. The cellular, metabolic, and systemic consequences of aggressive fluid resuscitation strategies. Shock 2006;26(2): 115–21.
9. Mapstone J, Roberts I, Evans P. Fluid resuscitation strategies: a systematic review of animal trials. J Trauma 2003;55(3):571–89.
10. Abdullah AR, Smith EE, Biddinger PD, et al. Advance hospital notification by EMS in acute stroke is associated with shorter door-to-computed tomography time and increased likelihood of administration of tissue-plasminogen activator. Prehosp Emerg Care 2008;12(4):426–31.
11. Randolph LC, Takacs M, Davis KA. Resuscitation in the pediatric trauma population: admission base deficit remains an important prognostic indicator. J Trauma 2002;53(5):838–42.
12. Kincaid EH, Chang MC, Letton RW, et al. Admission base deficit in pediatric trauma: a study using the National Trauma Data Bank. J Trauma 2001;51(2): 332–5.
13. Hendrickson JE, Shaz BH, Pereira G, et al. Coagulopathy is prevalent and associated with adverse outcomes in transfused pediatric trauma patients. J Pediatr 2012;160(2):204–9.e3.
14. Talving P, Benfield R, Hadjizacharia P, et al. Coagulopathy in severe traumatic brain injury: a prospective study. J Trauma 2009;66(1):55–61 [discussion: 61–2].
15. Holmes JF, Goodwin HC, Land C, et al. Coagulation testing in pediatric blunt trauma patients. Pediatr Emerg Care 2001;17(5):324–8.
16. Hymel KP, Abshire TC, Luckey DW, et al. Coagulopathy in pediatric abusive head trauma. Pediatrics 1997;99(3):371–5.
17. Miner ME, Kaufman HH, Graham SH, et al. Disseminated intravascular coagulation fibrinolytic syndrome following head injury in children: frequency and prognostic implications. J Pediatr 1982;100(5):687–91.

18. Hughes NT, Burd RS, Teach SJ. Damage control resuscitation: permissive hypotension and massive transfusion protocols. Pediatr Emerg Care 2014;30(9):651–6 [quiz: 657–8].

19. Hess JR, Brohi K, Dutton RP, et al. The coagulopathy of trauma: a review of mechanisms. J Trauma 2008;65(4):748–54.

20. Rotondo MF, Schwab CW, McGonigal MD, et al. 'Damage control': an approach for improved survival in exsanguinating penetrating abdominal injury. J Trauma 1993;35(3):375–82 [discussion: 382–3].

21. Scalea T. What's new in trauma in the past 10 years. Int Anesthesiol Clin 2002; 40(3):1–17.

22. Lee JC, Peitzman AB. Damage-control laparotomy. Curr Opin Crit Care 2006; 12(4):346–50.

23. MacLeod JB. Trauma and coagulopathy: a new paradigm to consider. Arch Surg 2008;143(8):797–801.

24. Schuster KM, Davis KA, Lui FY, et al. The status of massive transfusion protocols in United States trauma centers: massive transfusion or massive confusion? Transfusion 2010;50(7):1545–51.

25. Rossaint R, Bouillon B, Cerny V, et al. Management of bleeding following major trauma: an updated European guideline. Crit Care 2010;14(2):R52. Massive transfusion from CNMC.

26. Barcelona SL, Thompson AA, Coté CJ. Intraoperative pediatric blood transfusion therapy: a review of common issues. Part II: transfusion therapy, special considerations, and reduction of allogenic blood transfusions. Paediatr Anaesth 2005; 15(10):814–30.

27. Paterson NA. Validation of a theoretically derived model for the management of massive blood loss in pediatric patients - a case report. Paediatr Anaesth 2009;19(5):535–40.

28. Dehmer JJ, Adamson WT. Massive transfusion and blood product use in the pediatric trauma patient. Semin Pediatr Surg 2010;19(4):286–91.

29. Holmes JF, Lillis K, Monroe D, et al. Identifying children at very low risk of clinically important blunt abdominal injuries. Ann Emerg Med 2013;62(2):107–16.e2.

30. Coley BD, Mutabagani KH, Martin LC, et al. Focused abdominal sonography for trauma (FAST) in children with blunt abdominal trauma. J Trauma 2000;48(5): 902–6.

31. Upadhyaya P. Conservative management of splenic trauma: history and current trends. Pediatr Surg Int 2003;19(9–10):617–27.

32. Bansal S, Karrer FM, Hansen K, et al. Contrast blush in pediatric blunt splenic trauma does not warrant the routine use of angiography and embolization. Am J Surg 2015;210(2):345–50.

33. Davies DA, Ein SH, Pearl R, et al. What is the significance of contrast "blush" in pediatric blunt splenic trauma? J Pediatr Surg 2010;45(5):916–20.

34. Murphy EE, Murphy SG, Cipolle MD, et al. The pediatric trauma center and the inclusive trauma system: impact on splenectomy rates. J Trauma Acute Care Surg 2015;78(5):930–3 [discussion: 933–4].

35. Grisoni ER, Gauderer MW, Ferron J, et al. Nonoperative management of liver injuries following blunt abdominal trauma in children. J Pediatr Surg 1984;19(5): 515–8.

36. Gross M, Lynch F, Canty T Sr, et al. Management of pediatric liver injuries: a 13-year experience at a pediatric trauma center. J Pediatr Surg 1999;34(5): 811–6 [discussion: 816–7].

37. Margenthaler JA, Weber TR, Keller MS. Blunt renal trauma in children: experience with conservative management at a pediatric trauma center. J Trauma 2002; 52(5):928–32.
38. Brown SL, Elder JS, Spirnak JP. Are pediatric patients more susceptible to major renal injury from blunt trauma? A comparative study. J Urol 1998;160(1):138–40.
39. Nance ML, Lutz N, Carr MC, et al. Blunt renal injuries in children can be managed nonoperatively: outcome in a consecutive series of patients. J Trauma 2004; 57(3):474–8 [discussion: 478].
40. Stylianos S. Evidence-based guidelines for resource utilization in children with isolated spleen or liver injury. The APSA Trauma Committee. J Pediatr Surg 2000;35(2):164–7 [discussion: 167–9].
41. McVay MR, Kokoska ER, Jackson RJ, et al. Throwing out the "grade" book: management of isolated spleen and liver injury based on hemodynamic status. J Pediatr Surg 2008;43(6):1072–6.
42. Navarro O, Babyn PS, Pearl RH. The value of routine follow-up imaging in pediatric blunt liver trauma. Pediatr Radiol 2000;30(8):546–50.
43. Mizzi A, Shabani A, Watt A. The role of follow-up imaging in paediatric blunt abdominal trauma. Clin Radiol 2002;57(10):908–12.
44. Malcolm JB, Derweesh IH, Mehrazin R, et al. Nonoperative management of blunt renal trauma: is routine early follow-up imaging necessary? BMC Urol 2008;8:11.
45. Bliss D, Silen M. Pediatric thoracic trauma. Crit Care Med 2002;30(11 Suppl): S409–15.
46. Chiu WC, D'Amelio LF, Hammond JS. Sternal fractures in blunt chest trauma: a practical algorithm for management. Am J Emerg Med 1997;15(3):252–5.
47. Nakayama DK, Ramenofsky ML, Rowe MI. Chest injuries in childhood. Ann Surg 1989;210(6):770–5.
48. Cohn SM, Dubose JJ. Pulmonary contusion: an update on recent advances in clinical management. World J Surg 2010;34(8):1959–70.
49. Aghayev E, Christe A, Sonnenschein M, et al. Postmortem imaging of blunt chest trauma using CT and MRI: comparison with autopsy. J Thorac Imaging 2008; 23(1):20–7.
50. Cadzow SP, Armstrong KL. Rib fractures in infants: red alert! The clinical features, investigations and child protection outcomes. J Paediatr Child Health 2000; 36(4):322–6.
51. Garcia VF, Gotschall CS, Eichelberger MR, et al. Rib fractures in children: a marker of severe trauma. J Trauma 1990;30(6):695–700.
52. Al-Hassani A, Abdulrahman H, Afifi I, et al. Rib fracture patterns predict thoracic chest wall and abdominal solid organ injury. Am Surg 2010;76(8):888–91.
53. Harris GJ, Soper RT. Pediatric first rib fractures. J Trauma 1990;30(3):343–5.
54. Dowd MD, Krug S. Pediatric blunt cardiac injury: epidemiology, clinical features, and diagnosis. Pediatric emergency medicine collaborative research committee: working group on blunt cardiac injury. J Trauma 1996;40(1):61–7.
55. Milligan J, Potts JE, Human DG, et al. The protean manifestations of blunt cardiac trauma in children. Pediatr Emerg Care 2005;21(5):312–7.
56. Mackersie RC, Karagianes TG, Hoyt DB, et al. Prospective evaluation of epidural and intravenous administration of fentanyl for pain control and restoration of ventilatory function following multiple rib fractures. J Trauma 1991;31(4):443–9 [discussion: 449–51].
57. Moon MR, Luchette FA, Gibson SW, et al. Prospective, randomized comparison of epidural versus parenteral opioid analgesia in thoracic trauma. Ann Surg 1999;229(5):684–91 [discussion: 691–2].

58. Sirmali M, Turut H, Topcu S, et al. A comprehensive analysis of traumatic rib fractures: morbidity, mortality and management. Eur J Cardiothorac Surg 2003;24(1): 133–8.

59. Dewan MC, Ravindra VM, Gannon S, et al. Treatment practices and outcomes after blunt cerebrovascular injury in children. Neurosurgery 2016;79(6):872–8.

60. Bromberg WJ, Collier BC, Diebel LN, et al. Blunt cerebrovascular injury practice management guidelines: the Eastern Association for the Surgery of Trauma. J Trauma 2010;68(2):471–7.

61. Desai NK, Kang J, Chokshi FH. Screening CT angiography for pediatric blunt cerebrovascular injury with emphasis on the cervical "seatbelt sign". AJNR Am J Neuroradiol 2014;35(9):1836–40.

62. Furnival RA, Woodward GA, Schunk JE. Delayed diagnosis of injury in pediatric trauma. Pediatrics 1996;98(1):56–62.

63. Webman RB, Fritzeen JL, Yang J, et al. Classification and team response to nonroutine events occurring during pediatric trauma resuscitation. J Trauma Acute Care Surg 2016;81(4):666–73.

64. Fakhry SM, Brownstein M, Watts DD, et al. Relatively short diagnostic delays (<8 hours) produce morbidity and mortality in blunt small bowel injury: an analysis of time to operative intervention in 198 patients from a multicenter experience. J Trauma 2000;48(3):408–14 [discussion: 414–5].

65. Orenstein JB, Klein BL, Ochsenschlager DW. Delayed diagnosis of pediatric cervical spine injury. Pediatrics 1992;89(6 Pt 2):1185–8.

66. Enderson BL, Maull KI. Missed injuries. The trauma surgeon's nemesis. Surg Clin North Am 1991;71(2):399–418.

67. Heit JA, Silverstein MD, Mohr DN, et al. Risk factors for deep vein thrombosis and pulmonary embolism: a population-based case-control study. Arch Intern Med 2000;160(6):809–15.

68. Vavilala MS, Nathens AB, Jurkovich GJ, et al. Risk factors for venous thromboembolism in pediatric trauma. J Trauma 2002;52(5):922–7.

69. Grandas OH, Klar M, Goldman MH, et al. Deep venous thrombosis in the pediatric trauma population: an unusual event: report of three cases. Am Surg 2000; 66(3):273–6.

70. Dickson BC. Venous thrombosis: on the history of Virchow's triad. Univ Toronto Med J 2004;81(3):166–71.

71. Azu MC, McCormack JE, Scriven RJ, et al. Venous thromboembolic events in pediatric trauma patients: is prophylaxis necessary? J Trauma 2005;59(6):1345–9.

72. O'Brien SH, Candrilli SD. In the absence of a central venous catheter, risk of venous thromboembolism is low in critically injured children, adolescents, and young adults: evidence from the National Trauma Data Bank. Pediatr Crit Care Med 2011;12(3):251–6.

73. Mahajerin A, Petty JK, Hanson SJ, et al. Prophylaxis against venous thromboembolism in pediatric trauma: a practice management guideline from the Eastern Association for the Surgery of Trauma and the Pediatric Trauma Society. J Trauma Acute Care Surg 2017;82(3):627–36.

74. Bidlingmaier C, Kenet G, Kurnik K, et al. Safety and efficacy of low molecular weight heparins in children: a systematic review of the literature and meta-analysis of single-arm studies. Semin Thromb Hemost 2011;37(7):814–25.

Transfusion Decision Making in Pediatric Critical Illness

Chris Markham, MD[a], Peter Hovmand, PhD[b], Allan Doctor, MD[a],*

KEYWORDS

- Anemia • Transfusion decision making • Systems dynamics • Precision medicine

KEY POINTS

- A transfusion is indicated when O_2 delivery fails to meet metabolic need (or failure is impending).
- Additionally, the risk and impact of O_2 delivery failure should exceed the risk and impact of harm anticipated from transfusion.
- Transfusion should be appropriately sequenced with other interventions (based on principles of integrative physiology, potential morbidity, likelihood to optimize O_2 delivery, and context specific to individual patient trajectories).
- Once the decision to transfuse has been made, clinicians should use a titrated approach to administering red blood cells to maintain the risk of transfusion as low as is reasonably achievable while monitoring for resolution of anemia intolerance and improvement in O_2 delivery.

INTRODUCTION

Patients in the intensive care unit are frequently found to be anemic.[1] It is reasonable to consider that, in the setting of anemia, transfusion should maintain hemoglobin concentration ([Hb]) above thresholds that impair oxygen delivery, for which, historically, normal [Hb] values were presumed necessary during stress.[2] We now understand three key issues relating anemia and transfusion: (1) anemia may be well tolerated by patients with sufficient physiologic reserve (ability to increase blood flow to tissue in the setting of decreased blood oxygen content),[3–9] (2) donor red blood cell (RBC) physiology is impaired compared with that for native

Conflicts of Interest: The authors have no relevant conflicts to disclose.
[a] Division of Critical Care Medicine, Department of Pediatrics, Washington University School of Medicine, McDonnell Pediatric Research Building, Campus Box 8208, 660 South Euclid Avenue, St Louis, MO 63110-1093, USA; [b] Social Systems Design Laboratory, Brown School of Social Work, Washington University, Campus Box 1196, 1 Brookings Drive, St Louis, MO 63130, USA
* Corresponding author.
E-mail address: Doctor@wustl.edu

Pediatr Clin N Am 64 (2017) 991–1015
http://dx.doi.org/10.1016/j.pcl.2017.06.003
0031-3955/17/© 2017 Elsevier Inc. All rights reserved.
pediatric.theclinics.com

red blood cells (known as the storage lesion),[10,11] and (3) patients transfused for indications other than anemia-attributable oxygen delivery failure have worse outcomes than those (with similar anemia) who are not transfused.[12,13] Despite this understanding, there is a lack of approaches to transfusion decision making (TDM) that (1) differentiate between patients who require transfusions and those who do not, and (2) guide transfusion timing and amount based on oxygen delivery–based targets. This article explores such approaches to TDM by examining advances from historical perspectives to the currently accepted practice standards. We further illustrate continued advances are leading to a fundamental paradigm shift transfusion medicine.

GENERAL BASIS FOR TRANSFUSION DECISIONS

Acute RBC transfusion is indicated to improve O_2 delivery, or to relieve the physiologic stress imposed by compensated anemia. The former indication includes situations in which blood O_2 content (often in combination with diminished blood volume) is rate limiting in transfer of O_2 from lung to tissue (eg, hemorrhagic shock or normovolemic anemia sufficient to cause anaerobic metabolism); such diminished O_2 delivery may either be global or specific to compromised vital organs, (eg, during stroke or myocardial infarction). The latter indication includes situations in which (1) anemia complicates other disorders, and (2) the compensation for anemia (rather than anemia, itself) comprises the threat to health status (eg, nonhemorrhagic shock states, hypermetabolic states) or situations in which the ability to compensate for anemia is limited by other disorders (eg, respiratory disease, heart failure). In this context, the benefit anticipated from improving O_2 carrying capacity (to relieve the physiologic stress of compensated anemia) must be balanced against potential adverse influence of transfusion on recipient O_2 delivery homeostasis.

RED BLOOD CELLS ARE ALTERED BY PROCESSING AND STORAGE

Mounting evidence suggests that stored RBCs (and RBC unit supernatants) may, paradoxically, impair physiologic reflexes fundamental to O_2 delivery homeostasis. This consideration is relevant not only to prudent bedside decision making but also to clinical trial design as well as to robust evaluation of RBC processing and storage. Many recent reports summarize the changes that occur with RBC storage[14–19] (Fig. 1). These reports document increased potassium and lactate levels and free [Hb] with increased RBC storage time.[10,20] In addition, RBCs lose deformability with increased duration of storage,[10] limiting passage through the microcirculation, which is further impaired by increased RBC aggregation and adhesion to endothelium.[10,21–23] As noted earlier, the concentration of 2,3-diphosphoglycerate decreases with storage time,[10] and the resultant increase in oxygen affinity limits oxygen unloading from hemoglobin during systemic perfusion.[24] RBC storage also affects recipient immune function. Stored RBCs induce alterations in multiple cytokines after incubation with plasma or whole blood, including increased levels of interleukin (IL)-6, IL-8, phospholipase A2, and superoxide anions, and decreased tumor necrosis factor-alpha concentrations.[20,25] The clinical consequences of this phenomenon was first recognized in the 1970s when Opelz and Terasaki[26] reported improved renal allograft success in patients transfused before transplant. Subsequently, additional reports indicating an immune-suppressive effect of RBC transfusions have documented an association with increased cancer reoccurrence, live

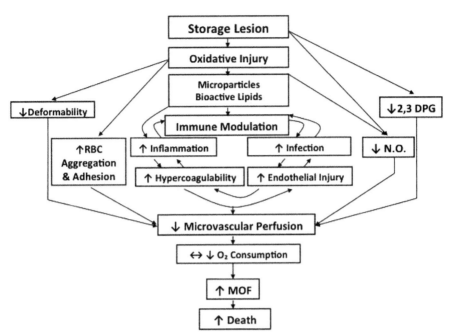

Fig. 1. The contributing factors and results of the RBC storage lesion. DPG, diphosphoglycerate; N.O, Nitric oxide; MOF, multiple organ failure.

births in women with a history of spontaneous abortions, and increased postoperative infection rates.[27,28]

Additionally RBC microparticles released during RBC storage may also account for the influence of transfusion on donor immune and coagulation systems.[29,30] The oxidative injury that occurs during storage leads to formation of RBC membrane microparticles and release of bioactive lipids from its membrane.[31] Such RBC microparticles contain CD47 antigens associated with macrophage inhibition.[31] Other data suggest that increased generation of procoagulant phospholipids occurs during RBC storage.[32,33] These bioactive lipids, such as lysophosphatidylcholine, have also been shown to be proinflammatory and are associated with an increased risk of acute lung injury.[34] The immune dysfunction secondary to transfusion has been termed transfusion-related immune modulation and has been well described.[35,36] The transfusion of RBCs of increased storage duration has also been associated with transfusion-related acute lung injury via proinflammatory mechanisms.[28]

Overall, the spectrum and prevalence of noninfectious serious hazards of transfusion (NISHOT) continues to grow over time, and to date it seems that RBC transfusion may be associated with acute lung injury, circulatory overload, gut injury, immunomodulation, and worsening of sepsis.[37] In addition, it is now appreciated that red cells are a key driver in blood flow distribution through their effects on local vasomotor tone via a nitric oxide transport shuttle.[38] Under normal physiologic stress, O_2 delivery to tissues is more dependent on blood flow than on blood O_2 content,[39] which suggests that the quality of RBCs is more important than the quantity of RBCs in effecting O_2 delivery at the tissue level. However, donor RBCs lose these control mechanisms during storage.[10]

CURRENT STRATEGIES AND FUTURE DIRECTIONS IN TRANSFUSION DECISION MAKING

As indicated earlier, with improved understanding of vascular signaling and gas transport by RBCs[38,40,41] and of the full array of defects comprising the RBC storage lesion,[10,11] it is now appreciated that (1) donor and recipient RBCs do not have similar physiology; and (2) RBC transfusion may cause harm (beyond transfusion reactions and transmission of infection), and that this harm seems to be progressive with transfusion volume, frequency, and donor exposure. As such, newer so-called restrictive [Hb] thresholds for transfusion (~ 7 g/dL) are now appreciated to be at least noninferior (and in many cases, superior) to more liberal [Hb] thresholds (~ 9 g/dL) for a broad array of conditions,[42–48] even in actively bleeding patients.[49] Although traditional transfusion thresholds are currently undergoing a broad reset, a comprehensive paradigm shift is emerging in approach to the critically ill, with reconsideration of the so-called [Hb] trigger strategy. Clearly, it is not feasible to define specific [Hb] boundaries across the complex interaction of developmental-specific, condition-specific, and stress-specific situations in ICUs. Ideally, the decision to transfuse should be based on individual and context-specific consideration of the degree to which anemia contributes to lack of tissue O_2 delivery (and/or reserve).[50–53] This distinction is exemplified by using physiologic transfusion triggers (eg, transfusing only to rectify abnormal measures of perfusion sufficiency (or reserve), rather than to maintain a specific [Hb], irrespective of context).[54,55]

Given that the transfusion goal (end point) is to maintain O_2 delivery and O_2 consumption, and because these metrics are not easily measured directly, surrogate end points for transfusion must be selected (as for any intervention). The end point in current use, and for which outcome data exist, is [Hb]. Formal criteria have been developed to determine suitability of therapeutic end-points (Prentice Criteria), which specify that end points (1) be in direct relationship to the causal path between disease (in this case, anemia) and outcome (in this case, adequate O_2 delivery), and (2) show time-sensitive response to therapy in a fashion that (3) reliably predicts the effect of treatment on outcome.[56–61] [Hb] overtly fails these criteria (most notably criterion 3) and is suboptimal as a sole, context-free trigger for transfusion.

The [Hb] threshold strategy informs clinicians principally about those patients who do not require transfusion (eg, evidence indicates that permissive anemia is safe above specific [Hb] thresholds). Because it is not feasible to define specific [Hb] boundaries across the complex interaction of developmental-specific, condition-specific, and stress-specific situations encountered in the pediatric intensive care unit (PICU), this strategy cannot identify patients for whom permissive anemia is unsafe and nor are these data sufficient to guide transfusion timing/amount.

Ideally, the decision to transfuse might be based on physiologic metrics and/or biomarkers that enable individual-specific and context-specific assessment of the degree to which anemia specifically contributes to tissue O_2 delivery constraint. Current PICU monitoring reports (with varying accuracy and precision) isolated components of the O_2 delivery system and related failure signals from which bedside clinicians infer adequacy of O_2 content; importantly, clinicians lack an evidence base and decision-making structure that (1) identifies specific individuals for whom permissive anemia is unsafe, and (2) can guide transfusion timing/amount in such patients.

There are four critical components to personalized decision making regarding indication for RBC transfusions: individual tolerance of anemia, likelihood of harm from persistent anemia, likelihood of harm from compensatory physiology, and degree of harm from transfusion. Providers face two major barriers in measuring and evaluating these factors.

The first of these barriers is that individual tolerance to anemia is variable, and there is a lack of markers that clearly identify prefailure states, as compensatory physiology is exhausted. It is known that, by increasing cardiac output, healthy individuals can tolerate extrem anemia for short periods without any negative effects[5] (**Table 1**). Moreover, where documented, thresholds for O_2 supply dependency are substantially lower than originally thought, even in the setting of critical illness and sepsis.[9] Note that there is significant individual variation in anemia tolerance is related to ability to increase cardiac output (eg, heart block or heart failure), impaired ability to regulate vascular tone (eg, sepsis, spinal shock), or impaired red cell function (eg, sickle cell disease).[8] Moreover, anemia tolerance is difficult to measure at the level of the individual because of poor surrogate outcomes for the balance of O_2 delivery and consumption.[54,62,63]

The second barrier to precision TDM is difficulty measuring the likelihood of harm from anemia and the likelihood of harm from compensatory physiology. Much of the uncertainty in RBC transfusion stems from our inability to quantify anemia risk and to balance that against risk of harm from the transfusion, itself. Moreover, to date there are no individual biomarkers that fulfill the Prentice criteria as surrogate end-points for transfusion indication or therapeutic efficacy.[9,64–66] As such, clinicians operate with a plurality of perspectives and approaches to practice regarding RBC transfusion.[53,63] Advancing the understanding of O_2 delivery remains a complex challenge that will require continued research collaboration, transdisciplinary research, and integration of knowledge between multiple disciplines. Systems science is the perfect tool to realize these multidisciplinary goals.[67,68]

ON SYSTEMS DYNAMICS AND GROUP MODEL BUILDING

Broadly, systems dynamics is a framework for understanding complex systems and their behavior over time. To date, systems dynamics methods have been used in

Table 1
Response to acute isovolemic anemia. All variables except for plasma lactate level were statistically significantly different with anemia

Variable	Hemoglobin Range (Before) 125–134 g/L (n = 23)	Hemoglobin Range (After) 45–54 g/L (n = 28)
SVRI (dyne/s/cm^{-5}/m^2)	2372 (541)	1001 (176)
HR (beats/min)	58 (11)	92 (12)
SVI (mL/m^2)	52 (9)	62 (8)
CI (L/m^2)	3.05 (0.69)	5.71 (0.87)
TO$_2$ (mL O$_2$/kg/min)	13.5 (2.7)	10.7 (2.0)
S$_v$O$_2$ (%)	77.1 (3.3)	69.6 (5.6)
Vo$_2$ (mL O$_2$/kg/min)	3.01 (0.42)	3.42 (0.54)
Plasma lactate (mmol/L)	0.77 (0.40)	0.62 (0.19)
Arterial blood pH	7.395 (0.016)	7.445 (0.025)
Base-excess (mEq/L)	1.3 (1.5)	4.2 (2.2)
Vo$_2$/To$_2$	0.23 (0.03)	0.32 (0.04)

Abbreviations: CI, cardiac index; HR, heart rate; SVI stroke volume index; S$_v$O$_2$, mixed venous oxyhemoglobin saturation; SVRI, systemic vascular resistance index; To$_2$, oxygen transport; Vo$_2$, oxygen consumption.

From Weiskopf RB, Viele MK, Feiner J, et al. Human cardiovascular and metabolic response to acute, severe isovolemic anemia. JAMA 1998;279(3):217–21.

medicine as a tool for public health policy makers to inform decisions in the areas of tobacco control and prevention, cancer prevention and treatment, infectious diseases, obesity, domestic violence, and infant mortality.[69–72] The principal strength of systems dynamics is the incorporation of complex interactions of multiple variables with emergent behaviors (the output of the interactions is greater than the sum of the parts). Specifically, systems dynamics methodologies identify interventions on a discrete system component may lead to unintended adverse effects in remote system components and explain paradoxic effects.[67] In contrast, these methods may also help identify key variables and their interactions that form leverage points at which interventions generate exponential effects. In general, this approach represents systems with formal mathematical models that assimilate the knowledge of multiple individuals across a variety of domains.

System dynamics uses causal maps with specific diagramming customs that pair visual representation of the system with the mathematical model used to simulate the system. Specific examples include causal maps, causal loop diagrams, and stock-and-flow diagrams. **Fig. 2** is a simplified causal loop diagram highlighting the interplay between general health, medical complications, diagnosis, and treatment. The arcs represent hypothesized causal relationships, with a positive sign indicating a direct correlation between the variables and a negative sign indicating an inverse correlation between the variables. For example, the healthier an individual is, the less likely that individual is to have medical complications (assuming all other variables do not change); conversely, an individual affected by illness is more likely to have complications.

There are 2 principal feedback loop categories: reinforcing feedback loops, in which a perturbation in one direction is magnified by the direct relationship of all of the variables connected in that loop; and balancing feedback loops, in which a perturbation is mitigated by 1 or more of the inverse relationships of the variables in that loop. Reinforcing feedback loops can be virtuous (ie, a person is healthy and so has fewer complications over time, which increases that person's overall health) or vicious (ie, a person is unhealthy and subject to complications that further decrease that person's health, which again subjects them to further complications).[71] In stable systems, reinforcing feedback loops are damped by balancing feedback loops. In our example, as a patient's health decreases, they are subject to tests that may lead to a diagnosis, which leads to treatment that can increase overall health. In this simplified example, the overall health of the individual depends on which of the feedback loops is contributing more to the person's health. For variables in which there is a time delay between one variable's effect on another, the connecting arrow is conventionally modeled with

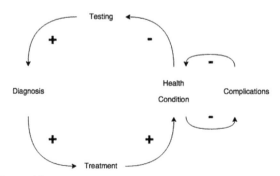

Fig. 2. Simplified causal loop.

two vertical lines to indicate the delayed effect. It is easy to imagine how the complexity of these models increases as more variables are incorporated.

The process of group model building (GMB) was developed to enable robust creation of causal loop diagrams and related quantitative systems dynamics models. GMB is a method of engaging stakeholders and/or content experts to collectively reveal their mental maps and compose the structure of a system under study, and, likewise, to participate in the analysis and implementation of solutions to related questions. Importantly, GMB offers a replicable method to address complex problems involving multiple stakeholders with diverse viewpoints. In particular, GMB can inform the identification, sequencing, implementation, and evaluation of translational strategies involving the establishment and scaling up of new clinical practices and practice guidelines.[71]

APPLYING GROUP MODEL BUILDING TO TRANSFUSION DECISION MAKING

The authors recently engaged intensivists from around the globe in an iterative GMB process to map TDM. The process resulted in a causal loop diagram of key features that might inform TDM, which is presented in **Fig. 3** with explanations of the concepts and relationships. This diagram was nucleated by a single loop comprising the relationship between general health and complications, and then was elaborated to include the complex reciprocal relationships between O_2 delivery and consumption, on which TDM context was focused. The next layer of the model indicates the compensatory physiology that comprises O_2 delivery homeostasis as well as the consequences that emerge in the setting of O_2 delivery failure. Subsequently, the group layered the process of diagnostic testing and therapeutic intervention. Through proctored discussion, the concept of individual anemia tolerance was then incorporated into the model. Importantly, the issue of temporal evolution (of either disease

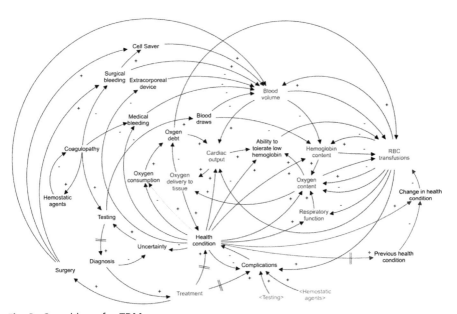

Fig. 3. Causal loop for TDM.

progression or resolution) and anticipated physiologic states (patient trajectories) were added. As shown in **Table 2** and **Fig. 3**, there are 26 factors influencing TDM that form several linked balancing and reinforcing feedback loops that may comprise an individual's physiology related to the following key variables: O_2 content, cardiac output, blood loss, O_2 debt, and illness trajectory. All are modified by one central variable: an individual's anemia tolerance. Most of the feedback loops in this causal loop diagram are balancing loops; the principal 2 are highlighted in **Fig. 4A**. Although most of the loops are balancing loops, the model does include a few reinforcing loops, and **Fig. 4B** highlights the most central of these reinforcing loops.

The most striking feature of this causal loop diagram is its complexity; it seems unlikely that a clinician making the decision to transfuse is able to carefully weigh each of the variables presented in this model. Such complexity may account for the extreme variation in transfusion practices for critically ill patients. However, focused analysis reveals that the model's components can be distilled to five key groups (O_2 content, cardiac output, blood loss, O_2 debt, and illness trajectory).

Further review identified the greater abundance of balancing feedback loops than of reinforcing feedback loops; this reflects the common propensity of a system structure favoring homeostasis. As such most preturbations that disrupt the system away from equilibrium is balanced by regulatory mechanisms that return the system toward equilibrium. It is important to remember that these loops balance up to the point at which a variable is maximally perturbed, after which a loop that initially acts as a balancing loop may transition into a reinforcing loop. For example, in **Fig. 4A**, if O_2 delivery to tissues is decreased then O_2 debt is increased, and cardiac output should naturally increase, but there is a maximum amount that cardiac output can increase for any individual.[73] Past this point, this balancing loop becomes a reinforcing loop.

Recall that, in this model, reinforcing loops demand more attention because of the potential for unchecked harm to an individual with even a slight decline in any of the variables in the loop. Consider one of the key reinforcing loops in **Fig. 4B**: if an individual's cardiac output decreases, then O_2 delivery to tissues will decrease (all other variables being equal), which will decrease the individual's overall health condition and cause further depression of cardiac output. Similarly, these loops highlight areas requiring vigilance and that may serve as a focus for intervention, because of the opportunity for amplifying benefits for any given intervention.

Table 2
Causal loop diagram variables grouped by associated physiologic theme

Oxygen Content	Cardiac Output	Blood Loss	Oxygen Debt	Illness Trajectory
Hemoglobin content	Health condition	Medical bleeding	Oxygen delivery to tissue	Previous health condition
Respiratory function	Blood volume	Testing	Oxygen consumption	Change in health condition
Health condition	RBC transfusions	Surgical bleeding	Oxygen content	Ability to tolerate low hemoglobin level
RBC transfusions		Blood draws	RBC transfusions	
		Cell saver		Diagnosis
		Extracorporeal device		Uncertainty
		Coagulopathy		Treatment
		Hemostatic agents		Complications
		Surgery		

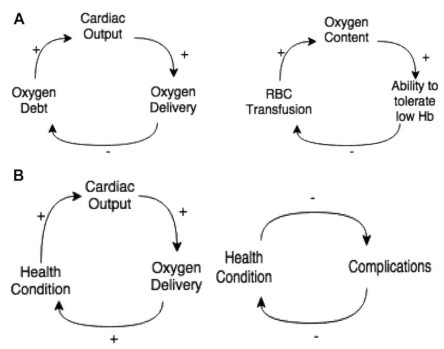

Fig. 4. (A) Key balancing loops. (B) Key reinforcing loops.

DECISION PATHS FOR TRANSFUSION DECISION MAKING

As a consequence of implicit synergy, reinforcing feedback loops identify opportunities for intervention in decompensating patients. For example, before RBC transfusion, clinicians may consider the opportunity to optimize components that comprise positive feedback loops. In this model, there are only four variables in the two reinforcing feedback loops: health condition, complications, cardiac output, and O_2 delivery. Cardiac output and O_2 delivery are uniquely important variables because they are elements in both balancing and reinforcing loops. With this in mind, a decision path emerges for individualized TDM based on physiologic goals. Initially, once anemia is identified, clinicians may consider that RBC transfusion is not necessary until O_2 delivery fails to meet metabolic need significantly enough to injure or threaten injury. If this is the case for a patient, then a transfusion is indicated if the risk and impact of this injury exceed the risk and impact of harm anticipated from an RBC transfusion.[54] Of note, the choice to transfuse should be appropriately sequenced with other interventions based on principles of integrative physiology, potential morbidity, and likelihood to optimize O_2 delivery.[53] Notably, this decision path should also be conditioned by patient trajectory (continued decompensation vs stabilization or recovery). The threshold for transfusion may be lower in decompensating patients (future state is anticipated to worsen) and, conversely, the threshold may be higher in recovering patients (future state is anticipated to be better).

SYSTEMS-PHYSIOLOGY APPROACH TO TRANSFUSION DECISION MAKING

One approach to implementing such a systems-physiology perspective to TDM is to consider the decision in the context of three possible patient states. First, patients who are in a state of supply dependency in which O_2 carrying capacity, specifically, is principally responsible for inadequate oxygen delivery; such patients merit urgent transfusion. In contrast, if a different component of the oxygen delivery system is principally responsible for inadequate oxygen delivery, transfusion to rectify anemia will not improve oxygen delivery (eg, if dough does not rise, and yeast is rate limiting, adding flour, even if less is present than desired, will not cause the dough to rise). Second, patients with anemia, who are in a compensated state; for example, O_2 delivery is still adequate to meet demands of respiring tissue and, notably, by inference, the magnitude of the physiologic threat imposed by anemia is identifiable by the degree to which features of the O_2 delivery homeostatic system are activated to balance the loss in O_2 content attributable to anemia. This fundamental insight provides the context (to specific [Hb] measurements) needed to assess anemia tolerance (1) on an individual level and (2) within individual disease/recovery trajectories. Third, patients with anemia who are in a globally compensated state but show organ-specific evidence of anemia intolerance (eg, to brain, heart, liver/bowel, kidney, or limb). Examples of conditions in this category include stroke, coronary insufficiency, necrotizing enterocolitis, intra-abdominal hypertension, and crushed limb. In such settings, transfusion may be appropriate, despite the absence of indications in the first or second categories.

This process (and potentially suitable biomarkers) is shown in **Fig. 5** and **Tables 3–5**. Of note, in applying this approach, no single metric or biomarker (in isolation) should be expected to adequately report patient status with regard to categories 1 to 3 (as discussed earlier). Moreover, metric and/or biomarker trajectory (direction of change, rate of change, or minimum change over time) is likely to be as important in

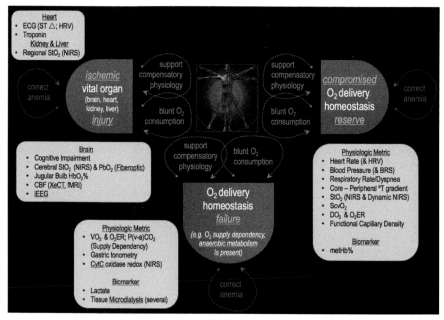

Fig. 5. Systems-physiology approach to TDM. CBF, cerebral blood flow; CytC, cytochrome C; DO_2, oxygen delivery; ECG, electrocardiogram; fMRI, functional magnetic resonance imaging; HRV, heart rate variability; iEEG, integrated electro encephalography; O_2ER, oxygen extraction ratio; P(v-a)CO_2, veno-arterial carbon; PbO_2, Oxygen partial pressure in brain; dioxide gradient; $ScvO_2$, central venous oxygen saturation; ST "delta', ST segment changes; StO_2 (NIRS), tissue O_2 saturation (near infra red spectroscopy); VO_2, oxygen consumption; XeCT, xenon computed tomography.

Table 3
Physiologic metrics and biomarkers reporting failure of O_2 delivery homeostasis (eg, anaerobic metabolism and aerobic supply dependency)

	Parameter	Normal Values	Developmental Variation	Suggested Threshold	References (Pediatric)	References (General)
Physiologic Metric	Global V_{O_2}	3.0–3.5 mL/O_2/kg/min	Yes	3.0 mL/O_2/kg/min, or 80%–90% of baseline	?	3,5,9,54,80,81
	$P(v-a)_{CO_2}$	—	?	—	82,83	82,84,85
Biomarkers	Lactate	<2.0 mM	No	3.0 mM/L	86	87–90
	Gastric pH (tonometry)	—	?	—	91,92	93–97
	Tissue microdialysis	—	?	—	—	98–100
	Cytochrome oxidase redox	—	?	—	—	101–106

Table 4
Physiologic metrics and biomarkers reporting loss of reserve in compensating for O_2 delivery insufficiency

	Parameter	Normal Values	Developmental Variation	Suggested Threshold	References (Pediatrics)	References (General)
Physiologic metric	Heart rate	—	Yes	120%–130% of baseline	—	4,5,54,107,108
	Blood pressure	—	Yes	70%–80% of baseline	109	4,5,54,107,108
	Respiratory rate/dyspnea	—	Yes	120%–130% of baseline	—	110,111
	Capillary refill time	—	No	—	112–114	115
	Core-peripheral temperature gradient (°)	—	Yes	—	112,116	117,118
	Sto_2 (NIRS)	—	No	—	119–121	63,64,122–130
	Dynamic Sto_2 (NIRS)	?	?	?	131,132	65,74,123,133–136
	Heart rate variability	?	Yes	?	137	138–141
	Do_2	11.0–14 mL O_2/kg/min	Yes	7.0 mL O_2/kg/min	7	3,5,9,54,80,81
	O_2ER	20%–30%	?	40%–50%	7,142	3–5,143,144
	FCD	—	?	—	145,146	147–151
Biomarkers	$ScvO_2$	65–75 (%)	No	~50–60 (%)	7,83,152	5,54,66,153
	metHb%	—	?	?	—	154

Abbreviations: DO_2, oxygen delivery; FCD, functional capillary density; metHb%, methemoglobin percentage; NIRS, near-infrared spectroscopy; O2ER, oxygen extraction ratio; $ScvO_2$, central vein oximetry.

Table 5
Physiologic metrics and biomarkers reporting vital organ-specific anemia intolerance

	Organ	Parameter	Normal Values	Developmental Variation	Suggested Threshold	References (Pediatric)	References (General)
Physiologic Metric	Heart	ST elevation	None	No	Any	—	73,155–157
		Heart rate variability	—	Yes	—	158	159,160
	Brain	Cognitive impairment	—	Yes	Deviation from baseline	—	62,110,161–164
		Cerebral NIRS	—	No	20% ↓ from baseline	165–167	127,168–175
		$PbtO_2$	—	No	—	176	177,178
		Jug. bulb $Hbo_2\%$	—	?	—	—	179
	Kidney	Various (none clearly useful)	—	?	—	—	180
	Liver	Various (none clearly useful)	—	?	—	—	181
Biomarkers	Heart	Troponin	None	No	Any	—	182
	Brain	Various (none clearly useful)	—	?	—	—	183
	Kidney	Various (none clearly useful)	—	?	—	184	180,185,186
	Liver	Various (none clearly useful)	—	?	—	—	187,188

Abbreviation: $PbtO_2$, brain tissue oxygenation.

decision making as threshold values for all metrics and biomarkers. In addition, the relative weighting (in decision making) that should be given to each metric and biomarker is context sensitive (eg, value of biomarkers may vary as a function of age, health condition, and illness trajectory).

As such, a systems-physiology approach to TDM may be summarized as follows: for any given level of anemia, a transfusion is indicated when (1) oxygen carrying capacity is thought to be rate limiting in O_2 delivery, (2) O_2 delivery fails to meet metabolic need (or failure is impending), (3) O_2 delivery failure is of sufficient magnitude to injure or threaten injury, (4) the risk and impact of this injury exceeds the risk and impact of harm anticipated from transfusion, and (5) transfusion is appropriately sequenced with other interventions (based on principles of integrative physiology, potential morbidity, likelihood to optimize O_2 delivery, and context specific to individual patient trajectories [eg, precision medicine]). In addition, once the decision to transfuse has been made, a titrated approach to administering RBCs should be used to maintain the risk of transfusion as low as reasonably achievable, while monitoring for resolution of anemia intolerance and improvement in O_2 delivery.

CALL FOR INVESTIGATION

So that the benefit of physiologic goal–directed strategies may be defined and evaluated in critically ill populations (vs [Hb] thresholds), specific physiologic goals most linked to outcome must first be identified, as well as determining appropriate thresholds for putative goals. A knowledge gap has limited progress to this end: investigators must improve the current means to assess functionality of the circulating RBC mass and its specific relationship to tissue O_2 delivery, an area of preclinical investigation that has progressed[5,74–79] and is ripe for translation.

Moreover, there is a lack of studies examining physiologic tolerance of anemia in the critically ill and specific subpopulations likely to have unique O_2 delivery/consumption relationships (hypermetabolic states, hypothermia), impaired ability to compensate for anemia (eg, respiratory disease, heart failure), or abnormal/threatened local O_2 delivery/consumption relationships (eg, brain injury, coronary insufficiency). There is also a need for studies exploring accuracy, precision, and reliability of novel approaches to quantifying and monitoring O_2 consumption and delivery (global/regional; eg, Vo_2 measurement, dynamic near-infrared spectroscopy measurements, use of novel imaging modalities, or novel markers such as nanoparticles that report either tissue O_2 levels or the abundance of specific, validated biochemical markers of perfusion sufficiency [eg, pH, lactate, reactive oxygen species, cytochrome redox state]). Investigation should also determine the relationship of these measures to clinically relevant patient outcomes, both global (eg, mortality, ventilator dependence, length of stay) and organ specific (eg, stroke, myocardial infarction, acute kidney injury). Finally, studies must evaluate the process of TDM in the setting of critical illness (eg, bayesian modeling, application of systems dynamics, and/or development of computerized decision support tools).

SUMMARY

TDM is undergoing rapid and exciting change and is on the brink of a fundamental practice change that will allow practitioners to bring details of clinical context into the difficult decision of balancing the risk of O_2 delivery failure as a result of anemia against the risk of RBC transfusion. This article considers the application of systems dynamics models to enable individualized, context-specific decision making that is based on principles of integrative physiology. Successful application of this approach will require identification of readily available clinical biomarkers for inadequate O_2 delivery as well as deployable decision support tools to offer guidance with this complex problem.

REFERENCES

1. Bateman ST, Lacroix J, Boven K, et al. Anemia, blood loss, and blood transfusions in North American children in the intensive care unit. Am J Respir Crit Care Med 2008;178(1):26–33.
2. Corwin HL, Gettinger A, Pearl RG, et al. The CRIT Study: anemia and blood transfusion in the critically ill–current clinical practice in the United States. Crit Care Med 2004;32(1):39–52.
3. Lieberman JA, Weiskopf RB, Kelley SD, et al. Critical oxygen delivery in conscious humans is less than 7.3 ml O_2 x kg^{-1} min^{-1}. Anesthesiology 2000; 92(2):407–13.
4. Madjdpour C, Spahn DR, Weiskopf RB. Anemia and perioperative red blood cell transfusion: a matter of tolerance. Crit Care Med 2006;34(5 Suppl):S102–8.
5. Weiskopf RB, Viele MK, Feiner J, et al. Human cardiovascular and metabolic response to acute, severe isovolemic anemia. JAMA 1998;279(3):217–21.
6. Ward JP. Oxygen delivery and demand. Surgery 2006;24(10):354–60.
7. Fontana JL, Welborn L, Mongan PD, et al. Oxygen consumption and cardiovascular function in children during profound intraoperative normovolemic hemodilution. Anesth Analg 1995;80(2):219–25.
8. Musallam KM, Tamim HM, Richards T, et al. Preoperative anaemia and postoperative outcomes in non-cardiac surgery: a retrospective cohort study. Lancet 2011;378(9800):1396–407.
9. Ronco JJ, Fenwick JC, Tweeddale MG, et al. Identification of the critical oxygen delivery for anaerobic metabolism in critically ill septic and nonseptic humans. JAMA 1993;270(14):1724–30.
10. Bennett-Guerrero E, Veldman TH, Doctor A, et al. Evolution of adverse changes in stored RBCs. Proc Natl Acad Sci U S A 2007;104(43):17063–8.
11. Doctor A, Spinella P. Effect of processing and storage on red blood cell function in vivo. Semin Perinatol 2012;36(4):248–59.
12. Loor G, Rajeswaran J, Li L, et al. The least of 3 evils: exposure to red blood cell transfusion, anemia, or both? J Thorac Cardiovasc Surg 2013;146(6):1480–7.e6.
13. Osawa EA, Rhodes A, Landoni G, et al. Effect of perioperative goal-directed hemodynamic resuscitation therapy on outcomes following cardiac surgery: a randomized clinical trial and systematic review. Crit Care Med 2016;44(4):724–33.
14. Spinella PC, Perkins JG, Grathwohl KW, et al. Risks associated with fresh whole blood and red blood cell transfusions in a combat support hospital. Crit Care Med 2007;35(11):2576–81.
15. Ho J, Sibbald WJ, Chin-Yee IH. Effects of storage on efficacy of red cell transfusion: when is it not safe? Crit Care Med 2003;31(12):S687–97.
16. Marik PE, Sibbald WJ. Effect of stored blood transfusion on oxygen delivery in patients with sepsis. JAMA 1993;269(23):3024–9.
17. Napolitano LM, Corwin HL. Efficacy of blood transfusion in the critically ill: does age of blood make a difference? Crit Care Med 2004;32(2):594–5.
18. Raghavan M, Marik PE. Anemia, allogenic blood transfusion, and immunomodulation in the critically ill. Chest 2005;127(1):295–307.
19. Tinmouth A, Fergusson D, Yee IC, et al. Clinical consequences of red cell storage in the critically ill. Transfusion 2006;46(11):2014–27.

20. Karam O, Tucci M, Toledano BJ, et al. Length of storage and in vitro immunomodulation induced by prestorage leukoreduced red blood cells. Transfusion 2009; 49(11):2326–34.

21. Luk CS, Gray-Statchuk LA, Cepinkas G, et al. WBC reduction reduces storage-associated RBC adhesion to human vascular endothelial cells under conditions of continuous flow in vitro. Transfusion 2003;43(2):151–6.

22. Hovav T, Yedgar S, Manny N, et al. Alteration of red cell aggregability and shape during blood storage. Transfusion 1999;39(3):277–81.

23. Yedgar S, Hovav T, Barshtein G. Red blood cell intercellular interactions in oxidative stress states. Clin Hemorheol Microcirc 1999;21(3–4):189–93.

24. Apstein CS, Dennis RC, Briggs L, et al. Effect of erythrocyte storage and oxyhemoglobin affinity changes on cardiac function. Am J Physiol 1985;248(4 Pt 2): H508–15.

25. Zallen G, Moore EE, Ciesla DJ, et al. Stored red blood cells selectively activate human neutrophils to release IL-8 and secretory PLA2. Shock 2000;13(1):29–33.

26. Opelz G, Terasaki PI. Improvement of kidney-graft survival with increased numbers of blood transfusions. N Engl J Med 1978;299(15):799–803.

27. Hill GE, Frawley WH, Griffith KE, et al. Allogeneic blood transfusion increases the risk of postoperative bacterial infection: a meta-analysis. J Trauma 2003; 54(5):908–14.

28. Silliman CC, Moore EE, Johnson JL, et al. Transfusion of the injured patient: proceed with caution. Shock 2004;21(4):291–9.

29. Kim-Shapiro DB, Lee J, Gladwin MT. Storage lesion: role of red blood cell breakdown. Transfusion 2011;51(4):844–51.

30. Xiong Z, Cavaretta J, Qu L, et al. Red blood cell microparticles show altered inflammatory chemokine binding and release ligand upon interaction with platelets. Transfusion 2011;51(3):610–21.

31. Kriebardis AG, Antonelou MH, Stamoulis KE, et al. RBC-derived vesicles during storage: ultrastructure, protein composition, oxidation, and signaling components. Transfusion 2008;48(9):1943–53.

32. Cardo LJ, Hmel P, Wilder D. Stored packed red blood cells contain a procoagulant phospholipid reducible by leukodepletion filters and washing. Transfus Apher Sci 2008;38(2):141–7.

33. Sweeney J, Kouttab N, Kurtis J. Stored red blood cell supernatant facilitates thrombin generation. Transfusion 2009;49(8):1569–79.

34. Silliman CC, Clay KL, Thurman GW, et al. Partial characterization of lipids that develop during the routine storage of blood and prime the neutrophil NADPH oxidase. J Lab Clin Med 1994;124(5):684–94.

35. Blajchman MA. Immunomodulation and blood transfusion. Am J Ther 2002;9(5): 389–95.

36. Blumberg N. Deleterious clinical effects of transfusion immunomodulation: proven beyond a reasonable doubt. Transfusion 2005;45(2 Suppl):33S–9S [discussion: 9S–40S].

37. Carson JL, Grossman BJ, Kleinman S, et al. Red blood cell transfusion: a clinical practice guideline from the AABB*. Ann Intern Med 2012;157(1):49–58.

38. Doctor A, Stamler JS. Nitric oxide transport in blood: a third gas in the respiratory cycle. Compr Physiol 2011;1(1):541–68.

39. Erzurum SC, Ghosh S, Janocha AJ, et al. Higher blood flow and circulating NO products offset high-altitude hypoxia among Tibetans. Proc Natl Acad Sci U S A 2007;104(45):17593–8.

40. Singel DJ, Stamler JS. Chemical physiology of blood flow regulation by red blood cells: role of nitric oxide and S-nitrosohemoglobin. Annu Rev Physiol 2005;67(0):99–145.
41. Gladwin MT, Kim-Shapiro DB. The functional nitrite reductase activity of the heme-globins. Blood 2008;112(7):2636–47.
42. Lacroix J, Hebert PC, Hutchison JS, et al. Transfusion strategies for patients in pediatric intensive care units. N Engl J Med 2007;356(16):1609–19.
43. Hebert PC, Wells G, Blajchman MA, et al. A multicenter, randomized, controlled clinical trial of transfusion requirements in critical care. Transfusion Requirements in Critical Care Investigators, Canadian Critical Care Trials Group. N Engl J Med 1999;340(6):409–17.
44. de Gast-Bakker DH, de Wilde RB, Hazekamp MG, et al. Safety and effects of two red blood cell transfusion strategies in pediatric cardiac surgery patients: a randomized controlled trial. Intensive Care Med 2013;39(11):2011–9.
45. Hajjar LA, Vincent JL, Galas FR, et al. Transfusion requirements after cardiac surgery: the TRACS randomized controlled trial. JAMA 2010;304(14):1559–67.
46. Jairath V, Hearnshaw S, Brunskill SJ, et al. Red cell transfusion for the management of upper gastrointestinal haemorrhage. Cochrane Database Syst Rev 2010;(9):CD006613.
47. McIntyre LA, Hebert PC. Can we safely restrict transfusion in trauma patients? Curr Opin Crit Care 2006;12(6):575–83.
48. McIntyre LA, Fergusson DA, Hutchison JS, et al. Effect of a liberal versus restrictive transfusion strategy on mortality in patients with moderate to severe head injury. Neurocrit Care 2006;5(1):4–9.
49. Villanueva C, Colomo A, Bosch A, et al. Transfusion strategies for acute upper gastrointestinal bleeding. N Engl J Med 2013;368(1):11–21.
50. Sisak K, Manolis M, Hardy BM, et al. Acute transfusion practice during trauma resuscitation: who, when, where and why? Injury 2013;44(5):581–6.
51. Lacroix J, Demaret P, Tucci M. Red blood cell transfusion: decision making in pediatric intensive care units. Semin Perinatol 2012;36(4):225–31.
52. Hebert PC, McDonald BJ, Tinmouth A. Clinical consequences of anemia and red cell transfusion in the critically ill. Crit Care Clin 2004;20(2):225–35.
53. Vincent JL. Indications for blood transfusions: too complex to base on a single number? Ann Intern Med 2012;157(1):71–2.
54. Vallet B, Adamczyk S, Barreau O, et al. Physiologic transfusion triggers. Best Pract Res Clin Anaesthesiol 2007;21(2):173–81.
55. Marshall JC. Transfusion trigger: when to transfuse? Crit Care 2004;8(Suppl 2):S31–3.
56. Adeli K, Raizman JE, Chen Y, et al. Complex biological profile of hematologic markers across pediatric, adult, and geriatric ages: establishment of robust pediatric and adult reference intervals on the basis of the Canadian Health Measures Survey. Clin Chem 2015;61:1075–86.
57. Baker SG, Kramer BS. Surrogate endpoint analysis: an exercise in extrapolation. J Natl Cancer Inst 2013;105(5):316–20.
58. Cotter DJ, Stefanik K, Zhang Y, et al. Hematocrit was not validated as a surrogate end point for survival among epoetin-treated hemodialysis patients. J Clin Epidemiol 2004;57(10):1086–95.
59. Jost MM. Surrogate end points: how well do they represent patient-relevant end points? Biomark Med 2007;1(3):437–51.
60. Prentice RL. Surrogate endpoints in clinical trials: definition and operational criteria. Stat Med 1989;8(4):431–40.

61. Prentice RL. Opportunities for enhancing efficiency and reducing cost in large scale disease prevention trials: a statistical perspective. Stat Med 1990; 9(1–2):161–70 [discussion: 70–2].

62. Spahn DR, Madjdpour C. Physiologic transfusion triggers: do we have to use (our) brain? Anesthesiology 2006;104(5):905–6.

63. van Beest PA, Vos JJ, Poterman M, et al. Tissue oxygenation as a target for goal-directed therapy in high-risk surgery: a pilot study. BMC Anesthesiol 2014;14: 122.

64. Roberson RS, Bennett-Guerrero E. Impact of red blood cell transfusion on global and regional measures of oxygenation. Mt Sinai J Med 2012;79(1):66–74.

65. Sadaka F, Aggu-Sher R, Krause K, et al. The effect of red blood cell transfusion on tissue oxygenation and microcirculation in severe septic patients. Ann Intensive Care 2011;1(1):46.

66. Sadaka F, Trottier S, Tannehill D, et al. Transfusion of red blood cells is associated with improved central venous oxygen saturation but not mortality in septic shock patients. J Clin Med Res 2014;6(6):422–8.

67. Mabry PL, Marcus SE, Clark PI, et al. Systems science: a revolution in public health policy research. Am J Public Health 2010;100(7):1161–3.

68. Stokols D, Hall KL, Taylor BK, et al. The science of team science: overview of the field and introduction to the supplement. Am J Prev Med 2008;35(2 Suppl): S77–89.

69. Thompson KM, Tebbens RJ. Eradication versus control for poliomyelitis: an economic analysis. Lancet 2007;369(9570):1363–71.

70. Tengs TO, Osgood ND, Chen LL. The cost-effectiveness of intensive national school-based anti-tobacco education: results from the tobacco policy model. Prev Med 2001;33(6):558–70.

71. Munar W, Hovmand PS, Fleming C, et al. Scaling-up impact in perinatology through systems science: bridging the collaboration and translational divides in cross-disciplinary research and public policy. Semin Perinatol 2015;39(5): 416–23.

72. Hammond RA. Complex systems modeling for obesity research. Preventing Chronic Dis 2009;6(3):A97.

73. Levy PS, Kim SJ, Eckel PK, et al. Limit to cardiac compensation during acute isovolemic hemodilution: influence of coronary stenosis. Am J Physiol 1993; 265(1 Pt 2):H340–9.

74. Creteur J, Neves AP, Vincent JL. Near-infrared spectroscopy technique to evaluate the effects of red blood cell transfusion on tissue oxygenation. Crit Care 2009;13(Suppl 5):S11.

75. Black C, Grocott MP, Singer M. Metabolic monitoring in the intensive care unit: a comparison of the Medgraphics Ultima, Deltatrac II, and Douglas bag collection methods. Br J Anaesth 2015;114(2):261–8.

76. Hare GM. Tolerance of anemia: understanding the adaptive physiological mechanisms which promote survival. Transfus Apher Sci 2014;50(1):10–2.

77. Lee J, Kim JG, Mahon SB, et al. Noninvasive optical cytochrome c oxidase redox state measurements using diffuse optical spectroscopy. J Biomed Opt 2014;19(5):055001.

78. Arakaki LS, Ciesielski WA, Thackray BD, et al. Simultaneous optical spectroscopic measurement of hemoglobin and myoglobin saturations and cytochrome aa3 oxidation in vivo. Appl Spectrosc 2010;64(9):973–9.

79. Tiba MH, Draucker GT, Barbee RW, et al. Tissue oxygenation monitoring using resonance Raman spectroscopy during hemorrhage. J Trauma Acute Care Surg 2014;76(2):402–8.
80. van Woerkens EC, Trouwborst A, van Lanschot JJ. Profound hemodilution: what is the critical level of hemodilution at which oxygen delivery-dependent oxygen consumption starts in an anesthetized human? Anesth Analg 1992;75(5): 818–21.
81. Napolitano LM, Kurek S, Luchette FA, et al. Clinical practice guideline: red blood cell transfusion in adult trauma and critical care. Crit Care Med 2009;37(12): 3124–57.
82. Lamia B, Monnet X, Teboul JL. Meaning of arterio-venous PCO_2 difference in circulatory shock. Minerva Anestesiol 2006;72(6):597–604.
83. Gergely M, Ablonczy L, Szekely EA, et al. Assessment of global tissue perfusion and oxygenation in neonates and infants after open-heart surgery. Interactive Cardiovasc Thorac Surg 2014;18(4):426–31.
84. Ho KM, Harding R, Chamberlain J. A comparison of central venous-arterial and mixed venous-arterial carbon dioxide tension gradient in circulatory failure. Anaesth Intensive Care 2007;35(5):695–701.
85. Kocsi S, Demeter G, Erces D, et al. Central venous-to-arterial CO_2-gap may increase in severe isovolemic anemia. PLoS One 2014;9(8):e105148.
86. Takahashi D, Matsui M, Shigematsu R, et al. Effect of transfusion on the venous blood lactate level in very low-birthweight infants. Pediatr Int 2009;51(3):321–5.
87. Gilbert EM, Haupt MT, Mandanas RY, et al. The effect of fluid loading, blood transfusion, and catecholamine infusion on oxygen delivery and consumption in patients with sepsis. Am Rev Respir Dis 1986;134(5):873–8.
88. Dhabangi A, Ainomugisha B, Cserti-Gazdewich C, et al. Effect of transfusion of red blood cells with longer vs shorter storage duration on elevated blood lactate levels in children with severe anemia: the TOTAL randomized clinical trial. JAMA 2015;314(23):2514–23.
89. Ohmori T, Kitamura T, Ishihara J, et al. Early predictors for massive transfusion in older adult severe trauma patients. Injury 2017;48(5):1006–12.
90. McLennan JV, Mackway-Jones KC, Horne ST, et al. Predictors of massive blood transfusion: a Delphi Study to examine the views of experts. J R Army Med Corps 2017;163(4):259–65.
91. Karaci AR, Sasmazel A, Aydemir NA, et al. Comparison of parameters for detection of splanchnic hypoxia in children undergoing cardiopulmonary bypass with pulsatile versus nonpulsatile normothermia or hypothermia during congenital heart surgeries. Artif Organs 2011;35(11):1010–7.
92. Krafte-Jacobs B, Carver J, Wilkinson JD. Comparison of gastric intramucosal pH and standard perfusional measurements in pediatric septic shock. Chest 1995;108(1):220–5.
93. Chang MC, Cheatham ML, Nelson LD, et al. Gastric tonometry supplements information provided by systemic indicators of oxygen transport. J Trauma 1994; 37(3):488–94.
94. Guzman JA, Lacoma FJ, Kruse JA. Relationship between systemic oxygen supply dependency and gastric intramucosal PCO_2 during progressive hemorrhage. J Trauma 1998;44(4):696–700.
95. McKinley BA, Butler BD. Comparison of skeletal muscle PO_2, PCO_2, and pH with gastric tonometric $P(CO_2)$ and pH in hemorrhagic shock. Crit Care Med 1999;27(9):1869–77.

96. Maynard N, Bihari D, Beale R, et al. Assessment of splanchnic oxygenation by gastric tonometry in patients with acute circulatory failure. JAMA 1993;270(10): 1203–10.

97. Ivatury RR, Simon RJ, Islam S, et al. A prospective randomized study of end points of resuscitation after major trauma: global oxygen transport indices versus organ-specific gastric mucosal pH. J Am Coll Surg 1996;183(2):145–54.

98. Bursa F, Pleva L. Anaerobic metabolism associated with traumatic hemorrhagic shock monitored by microdialysis of muscle tissue is dependent on the levels of hemoglobin and central venous oxygen saturation: a prospective, observational study. Scand J Trauma Resusc Emerg Med 2014;22:11.

99. Bursa F, Pleva L, Maca J, et al. Tissue ischemia microdialysis assessments following severe traumatic haemorrhagic shock: lactate/pyruvate ratio as a new resuscitation end point? BMC Anesthesiol 2014;14:118.

100. Ikossi DG, Knudson MM, Morabito DJ, et al. Continuous muscle tissue oxygenation in critically injured patients: a prospective observational study. J Trauma 2006;61(4):780–8 [discussion: 788–90].

101. McGown AD, Makker H, Elwell C, et al. Measurement of changes in cytochrome oxidase redox state during obstructive sleep apnea using near-infrared spectroscopy. Sleep 2003;26(6):710–6.

102. Cooper CE, Cope M, Quaresima V, et al. Measurement of cytochrome oxidase redox state by near infrared spectroscopy. Adv Exp Med Biol 1997;413:63–73.

103. Cooper CE, Springett R. Measurement of cytochrome oxidase and mitochondrial energetics by near-infrared spectroscopy. Philos Trans R Soc Lond B Biol Sci 1997;352(1354):669–76.

104. Kolyva C, Ghosh A, Tachtsidis I, et al. Cytochrome c oxidase response to changes in cerebral oxygen delivery in the adult brain shows higher brain-specificity than haemoglobin. Neuroimage 2014;85(Pt 1):234–44.

105. Tamura M. Non-invasive monitoring of the redox state of cytochrome oxidase in living tissue using near-infrared laser lights. Jpn Circ J 1993;57(8):817–24.

106. Rhee P, Langdale L, Mock C, et al. Near-infrared spectroscopy: continuous measurement of cytochrome oxidation during hemorrhagic shock. Crit Care Med 1997;25(1):166–70.

107. Feiner JR, Finlay-Morreale HE, Toy P, et al. High oxygen partial pressure decreases anemia-induced heart rate increase equivalent to transfusion. Anesthesiology 2011;115(3):492–8.

108. Spahn DR. Strategies for transfusion therapy. Best Pract Res Clin Anaesthesiol 2004;18(4):661–73.

109. Haque IU, Zaritsky AL. Analysis of the evidence for the lower limit of systolic and mean arterial pressure in children. Pediatr Crit Care Med 2007;8(2):138–44.

110. English M, Ahmed M, Ngando C, et al. Blood transfusion for severe anaemia in children in a Kenyan hospital. Lancet 2002;359(9305):494–5.

111. Akech SO, Hassall O, Pamba A, et al. Survival and haematological recovery of children with severe malaria transfused in accordance to WHO guidelines in Kilifi, Kenya. Malar J 2008;7:256.

112. Tibby SM, Hatherill M, Murdoch IA. Capillary refill and core-peripheral temperature gap as indicators of haemodynamic status in paediatric intensive care patients. Arch Dis Child 1999;80(2):163–6.

113. Fleming S, Gill P, Jones C, et al. The diagnostic value of capillary refill time for detecting serious illness in children: a systematic review and meta-analysis. PLoS One 2015;10(9):e0138155.

114. Fleming S, Gill P, Jones C, et al. Validity and reliability of measurement of capillary refill time in children: a systematic review. Arch Dis Child 2015;100(3): 239–49.

115. Schriger DL, Baraff L. Defining normal capillary refill: variation with age, sex, and temperature. Ann Emerg Med 1988;17(9):932–5.

116. Murdoch IA, Qureshi SA, Mitchell A, et al. Core-peripheral temperature gradient in children: does it reflect clinically important changes in circulatory haemodynamics? Acta Paediatr 1993;82(9):773–6.

117. Bourcier S, Pichereau C, Boelle PY, et al. Toe-to-room temperature gradient correlates with tissue perfusion and predicts outcome in selected critically ill patients with severe infections. Ann Intensive Care 2016;6(1):63.

118. Schey BM, Williams DY, Bucknall T. Skin temperature and core-peripheral temperature gradient as markers of hemodynamic status in critically ill patients: a review. Heart Lung 2010;39(1):27–40.

119. Baenziger O, Keel M, Bucher HU, et al. Oxygen extraction index measured by near infrared spectroscopy–a parameter for monitoring tissue oxygenation? Adv Exp Med Biol 2009;645:161–6.

120. Bailey SM, Hendricks-Munoz KD, Wells JT, et al. Packed red blood cell transfusion increases regional cerebral and splanchnic tissue oxygen saturation in anemic symptomatic preterm infants. Am J Perinatol 2010;27(6):445–53.

121. Chakravarti SB, Mittnacht AJ, Katz JC, et al. Multisite near-infrared spectroscopy predicts elevated blood lactate level in children after cardiac surgery. J Cardiothorac Vasc Anesth 2009;23(5):663–7.

122. Yuruk K, Bartels SA, Milstein DM, et al. Red blood cell transfusions and tissue oxygenation in anemic hematology outpatients. Transfusion 2012;52(3):641–6.

123. Duret J, Pottecher J, Bouzat P, et al. Skeletal muscle oxygenation in severe trauma patients during haemorrhagic shock resuscitation. Crit Care 2015;19:141.

124. McKinley BA, Marvin RG, Cocanour CS, et al. Tissue hemoglobin O_2 saturation during resuscitation of traumatic shock monitored using near infrared spectrometry. J Trauma 2000;48(4):637–42.

125. Torella F, Cowley R, Thorniley MS, et al. Monitoring blood loss with near infrared spectroscopy. Comp Biochem Physiol A Mol Integr Physiol 2002;132(1): 199–203.

126. Torella F, Cowley RD, Thorniley MS, et al. Regional tissue oxygenation during hemorrhage: can near infrared spectroscopy be used to monitor blood loss? Shock 2002;18(5):440–4.

127. Torella F, Haynes SL, McCollum CN. Cerebral and peripheral oxygen saturation during red cell transfusion. J Surg Res 2003;110(1):217–21.

128. Smith J, Bricker S, Putnam B. Tissue oxygen saturation predicts the need for early blood transfusion in trauma patients. Am Surg 2008;74(10):1006–11.

129. De Backer D, Ospina-Tascon G, Salgado D, et al. Monitoring the microcirculation in the critically ill patient: current methods and future approaches. Intensive Care Med 2010;36(11):1813–25.

130. Memtsoudis SG, Danninger T, Stundner O, et al. Blood transfusions may have limited effect on muscle oxygenation after total knee arthroplasty. HSS J 2015; 11(2):136–42.

131. Hassan IA, Spencer SA, Wickramasinghe YA, et al. Measurement of peripheral oxygen utilisation in neonates using near infrared spectroscopy: comparison between arterial and venous occlusion methods. Early Hum Dev 2000;57(3): 211–24.

132. Pichler G, Urlesberger B, Jirak P, et al. Forearm oxygen consumption and fore-arm blood flow in healthy children and adolescents measured by near infrared spectroscopy. J Physiol Sci 2006;56(3):191–4.

133. Girardis M, Rinaldi L, Busani S, et al. Muscle perfusion and oxygen consumption by near-infrared spectroscopy in septic-shock and non-septic-shock patients. Intensive Care Med 2003;29(7):1173–6.

134. Podbregar M, Gavric AU, Podbregar E, et al. Red blood cell transfusion and skeletal muscle tissue oxygenation in anaemic haematologic outpatients. Radiol Oncol 2016;50(4):449–55.

135. Gomez H, Torres A, Polanco P, et al. Use of non-invasive NIRS during a vascular occlusion test to assess dynamic tissue O_2 saturation response. Intensive Care Med 2008;34(9):1600–7.

136. Gomez H, Mesquida J, Simon P, et al. Characterization of tissue oxygen satura-tion and the vascular occlusion test: influence of measurement sites, probe sizes and deflation thresholds. Crit Care 2009;13(Suppl 5):S3.

137. Rajendra Acharya U, Paul Joseph K, Kannathal N, et al. Heart rate variability: a review. Med Biol Eng Comput 2006;44(12):1031–51.

138. Lauscher P, Kertscho H, Raab L, et al. Changes in heart rate variability across different degrees of acute dilutional anemia. Minerva Anestesiol 2011;77(10): 943–51.

139. Connes P, Hue O, Hardy-Dessources MD, et al. Hemorheology and heart rate variability: is there a relationship? Clin Hemorheol Microcirc 2008;38(4):257–65.

140. McCraty R, Shaffer F. Heart rate variability: new perspectives on physiological mechanisms, assessment of self-regulatory capacity, and health risk. Glob Adv Health Med 2015;4(1):46–61.

141. Fatisson J, Oswald V, Lalonde F. Influence diagram of physiological and environ-mental factors affecting heart rate variability: an extended literature overview. Heart Int 2016;11(1):e32–40.

142. Nasser B, Tageldein M, AlMesned A, et al. Effects of blood transfusion on oxy-gen extraction ratio and central venous saturation in children after cardiac sur-gery. Ann Saudi Med 2017;37(1):31–7.

143. Orlov D, O'Farrell R, McCluskey SA, et al. The clinical utility of an index of global oxygenation for guiding red blood cell transfusion in cardiac surgery. Transfu-sion 2009;49(4):682–8.

144. Yalavatti GS, DeBacker D, Vincent JL. Assessment of cardiac index in anemic patients. Chest 2000;118(3):782–7.

145. van Elteren HA, Ince C, Tibboel D, et al. Cutaneous microcirculation in preterm neonates: comparison between sidestream dark field (SDF) and incident dark field (IDF) imaging. J Clin Monit Comput 2015;29(5):543–8.

146. Genzel-Boroviczeny O, Christ F, Glas V. Blood transfusion increases functional capillary density in the skin of anemic preterm infants. Pediatr Res 2004; 56(5):751–5.

147. Aykut G, Veenstra G, Scorcella C, et al. Cytocam-IDF (incident dark field illumi-nation) imaging for bedside monitoring of the microcirculation. Intensive Care Med Exp 2015;3(1):40.

148. Frenzel T, Westphal-Varghese B, Westphal M. Role of storage time of red blood cells on microcirculation and tissue oxygenation in critically ill patients. Curr Opin Anaesthesiol 2009;22(2):275–80.

149. Sakr Y, Chierego M, Piagnerelli M, et al. Microvascular response to red blood cell transfusion in patients with severe sepsis. Crit Care Med 2007;35(7): 1639–44.

150. Tsai AG, Hofmann A, Cabrales P, et al. Perfusion vs. oxygen delivery in transfusion with "fresh" and "old" red blood cells: the experimental evidence. Transfus Apher Sci 2010;43(1):69–78.
151. Donati A, Damiani E, Luchetti M, et al. Microcirculatory effects of the transfusion of leukodepleted or non-leukodepleted red blood cells in patients with sepsis: a pilot study. Crit Care 2014;18(1):R33.
152. Kapoor PM, Dhawan I, Jain P, et al. Lactate, endothelin, and central venous oxygen saturation as predictors of mortality in patients with tetralogy of Fallot. Ann Card Anaesth 2016;19(2):269–76.
153. Vallet B, Robin E, Lebuffe G. Venous oxygen saturation as a physiologic transfusion trigger. Crit Care 2010;14(2):213.
154. Hare GM, Tsui AK, Crawford JH, et al. Is methemoglobin an inert bystander, biomarker or a mediator of oxidative stress–The example of anemia? Redox Biol 2013;1:65–9.
155. Leung JM, Weiskopf RB, Feiner J, et al. Electrocardiographic ST-segment changes during acute, severe isovolemic hemodilution in humans. Anesthesiology 2000;93(4):1004–10.
156. Spahn DR, Leone BJ, Reves JG, et al. Cardiovascular and coronary physiology of acute isovolemic hemodilution: a review of nonoxygen-carrying and oxygen-carrying solutions. Anesth Analg 1994;78(5):1000–21.
157. Jan KM, Chien S. Effect of hematocrit variations on coronary hemodynamics and oxygen utilization. Am J Physiol 1977;233(1):H106–13.
158. Yeragani VK, Berger R, Pohl R, et al. Effect of age on diurnal changes of 24-hour QT interval variability. Pediatr Cardiol 2005;26(1):39–44.
159. Ganan-Calvo AM, Fajardo-Lopez J. Universal structures of normal and pathological heart rate variability. Scientific Rep 2016;6:21749.
160. Oieru D, Moalem I, Rozen E, et al. A novel heart rate variability algorithm for the detection of myocardial ischemia: pilot data from a prospective clinical trial. Isr Med Assoc J 2015;17(3):161–5.
161. Weiskopf RB, Kramer JH, Viele M, et al. Acute severe isovolemic anemia impairs cognitive function and memory in humans. Anesthesiology 2000;92(6):1646–52.
162. Weiskopf RB, Feiner J, Hopf HW, et al. Oxygen reverses deficits of cognitive function and memory and increased heart rate induced by acute severe isovolemic anemia. Anesthesiology 2002;96(4):871–7.
163. Weiskopf RB, Toy P, Hopf HW, et al. Acute isovolemic anemia impairs central processing as determined by P300 latency. Clin Neurophysiol 2005;116(5):1028–32.
164. Weiskopf RB, Feiner J, Hopf H, et al. Fresh blood and aged stored blood are equally efficacious in immediately reversing anemia-induced brain oxygenation deficits in humans. Anesthesiology 2006;104(5):911–20.
165. van Hoften JC, Verhagen EA, Keating P, et al. Cerebral tissue oxygen saturation and extraction in preterm infants before and after blood transfusion. Arch Dis Child Fetal Neonatal Ed 2010;95(5):F352–8.
166. Smith MJ, Stiefel MF, Magge S, et al. Packed red blood cell transfusion increases local cerebral oxygenation. Crit Care Med 2005;33(5):1104–8.
167. Dhabangi A, Ainomugisha B, Cserti-Gazdewich C, et al. Cerebral oximetry in Ugandan children with severe anemia: clinical categories and response to transfusion. JAMA Pediatr 2016;170(10):995–1002.
168. Cem A, Serpil UO, Fevzi T, et al. Efficacy of near-infrared spectrometry for monitoring the cerebral effects of severe dilutional anemia. Heart Surg Forum 2014;17(3):E154–9.

169. Torella F, Haynes SL, McCollum CN. Cerebral and peripheral near-infrared spectroscopy: an alternative transfusion trigger? Vox Sang 2002;83(3):254–7.
170. Aries MJ, Coumou AD, Elting JW, et al. Near infrared spectroscopy for the detection of desaturations in vulnerable ischemic brain tissue: a pilot study at the stroke unit bedside. Stroke 2012;43(4):1134–6.
171. Moreau F, Yang R, Nambiar V, et al. Near-infrared measurements of brain oxygenation in stroke. Neurophotonics 2016;3(3):031403.
172. Shafer KM, Mann N, Hehn R, et al. Relationship between exercise parameters and noninvasive indices of right ventricular function in patients with biventricular circulation and systemic right ventricle. Congenit Heart Dis 2015;10(5):457–65.
173. Liem KD, Hopman JC, Oeseburg B, et al. The effect of blood transfusion and haemodilution on cerebral oxygenation and haemodynamics in newborn infants investigated by near infrared spectrophotometry. Eur J Pediatr 1997;156(4):305–10.
174. Torella F, McCollum CN. Regional haemoglobin oxygen saturation during surgical haemorrhage. Minerva Med 2004;95(5):461–7.
175. Nielsen HB. Systematic review of near-infrared spectroscopy determined cerebral oxygenation during non-cardiac surgery. Front Physiol 2014;5:93.
176. Figaji AA, Zwane E, Kogels M, et al. The effect of blood transfusion on brain oxygenation in children with severe traumatic brain injury. Pediatr Crit Care Med 2010;11(3):325–31.
177. Leal-Noval SR, Rincon-Ferrari MD, Marin-Niebla A, et al. Transfusion of erythrocyte concentrates produces a variable increment on cerebral oxygenation in patients with severe traumatic brain injury: a preliminary study. Intensive Care Med 2006;32(11):1733–40.
178. Leal-Noval SR, Munoz-Gomez M, Arellano-Orden V, et al. Impact of age of transfused blood on cerebral oxygenation in male patients with severe traumatic brain injury. Crit Care Med 2008;36(4):1290–6.
179. Yoshitani K, Kawaguchi M, Iwata M, et al. Comparison of changes in jugular venous bulb oxygen saturation and cerebral oxygen saturation during variations of haemoglobin concentration under propofol and sevoflurane anaesthesia. Br J Anaesth 2005;94(3):341–6.
180. Okusa MD, Jaber BL, Doran P, et al. Physiological biomarkers of acute kidney injury: a conceptual approach to improving outcomes. Contrib Nephrol 2013;182:65–81.
181. Majumdar A, Pinzani M. The holy grail of a biomarker for "liver function". Clin Liver Dis 2016;7(6):135–8.
182. Heyer L, Mebazaa A, Gayat E, et al. Cardiac troponin and skeletal muscle oxygenation in severe post-partum haemorrhage. Crit Care 2009;13(Suppl 5):S8.
183. Maestrini I, Ducroquet A, Moulin S, et al. Blood biomarkers in the early stage of cerebral ischemia. Rev Neurol (Paris) 2016;172(3):198–219.
184. Nguyen MT, Devarajan P. Biomarkers for the early detection of acute kidney injury. Pediatr Nephrol 2008;23(12):2151–7.
185. Sprenkle P, Russo P. Molecular markers for ischemia, do we have something better then creatinine and glomerular filtration rate? Arch Esp Urol 2013;66(1):99–114.
186. McCullough PA, Shaw AD, Haase M, et al. Diagnosis of acute kidney injury using functional and injury biomarkers: workgroup statements from the tenth Acute Dialysis Quality Initiative Consensus Conference. Contrib Nephrol 2013;182:13–29.

187. Kleen M, Habler O, Hutter J, et al. Effects of hemodilution on splanchnic perfusion and hepatorenal function. I. Splanchnic perfusion. Eur J Med Res 1997; 2(10):413–8.
188. Eguchi A, Wree A, Feldstein AE. Biomarkers of liver cell death. J Hepatol 2014; 60(5):1063–74.

Pathophysiology and Management of Acute Respiratory Distress Syndrome in Children

Sabrina M. Heidemann, MD[a], Alison Nair, MD[b], Yonca Bulut, MD[c], Anil Sapru, MD, MAS[b,c],*

KEYWORDS

- Acute respiratory distress syndrome • Pediatrics • Pathophysiology
- Acute lung injury • PARDS

KEY POINTS

- Acute respiratory distress syndrome (ARDS) is a clinical syndrome of noncardiogenic pulmonary edema characterized by hypoxemia, radiographic infiltrates, decreased functional residual capacity, and decreased lung compliance.
- The hallmark of pathophysiology in ARDS is the loss of the alveolar epithelial-endothelial barrier function in the setting of dysregulated inflammation and coagulation pathways complicated by concurrent loss of surfactant and impairment of lymphatic drainage.
- The mainstay of management is supportive, including lung-protective mechanical ventilation, careful attention to fluid management, treatment of underlying condition, including use of appropriate antibiotics, and general supportive care. Although several therapeutic strategies have been tested in ARDS, use of lung protective ventilation is the only universally accepted strategy to decrease mortality. Use of neuromuscular blockade and prone positioning has been shown to lead to decreased mortality among adults with severe ARDS.

INTRODUCTION

Acute respiratory distress syndrome (ARDS) is essentially a clinical syndrome of non-cardiogenic pulmonary edema and hypoxia that contributes to significant morbidity and mortality.[1,2] Initially, ARDS was described as "adult" respiratory distress syndrome to differentiate it from infant respiratory distress syndrome.[3] This name was

Disclosure Statement: The authors have nothing to disclose.
[a] Department of Pediatrics, Wayne State University, Detroit, MI 48202, USA; [b] Department of Pediatrics, University of California, San Francisco, 550 16th Street, Box 0110 San Francisco, CA 94143, USA; [c] Department of Pediatrics, David Geffen School of Medicine, University of California, Los Angeles, Los Angeles, CA, USA
* Corresponding author. 10833 Le Conte Avenue, MDCC 488, University of California, Los Angeles, Los Angeles, CA.
E-mail address: asapru@mednet.ucla.edu

Pediatr Clin N Am 64 (2017) 1017–1037
http://dx.doi.org/10.1016/j.pcl.2017.06.004
0031-3955/17/© 2017 Elsevier Inc. All rights reserved.

pediatric.theclinics.com

later modified to *acute* respiratory distress syndrome in recognition of the fact that both adults and children develop ARDS.[1,4] Lung development increases linearly with age and height until the adolescent growth spurt at 10 years in girls and 12 years in boys. Therefore, there are significant differences between adult and child ARDS pathophysiology due to remodeling, growth of the lung parenchyma, and progressive maturation of immune system.[5,6]

The traditional American-European Consensus Conference (AECC) definition proposed in 1994 classified mild ARDS as acute lung injury (ALI). ALI/ARDS was defined as acute onset of severe hypoxia (ratio of the partial pressure of arterial oxygen to the fraction of inspired oxygen or P/F ratio <300 for ALI and <200 for ARDS) with bilateral opacities on chest radiograph in the absence of clinical evidence of left ventricular failure.[7] In 2012, a panel of experts developed the Berlin definition, which replaced the AECC definition and included several significant changes, specifically, (1) ALI was eliminated and replaced with mild, moderate, and severe ARDS defined by a P/F ratio of 200–300, 100–200, or less than 100, respectively; (2) minimal ventilator settings of a positive-end expiratory pressure (PEEP) of ≥ 5 cm H_2O was required; and (3) reference to the pulmonary capillary wedge pressure was removed.[8]

The current definition of pediatric acute respiratory distress syndrome (PARDS) proposed by the Pediatric Acute Lung Injury Consensus Conference group (PALICC) followed in 2015.[9,10] PARDS is now diagnosed by the presence of hypoxia in the context of a new lung infiltrate occurring within 7 days of a known insult. Hypoxia is defined as oxygenation index (OI, determined by the mean airway pressure divided by P/F ratio) of 4 to 8 (mild), 8 to 16 (moderate), or greater than 16 (severe) for ventilated patients while on PEEP of ≥ 5 cm H_2O or the Berlin definition P/F ratio cutoffs in nonventilated patients.[10] Although there is no age limit in PARDS, the definition excludes patients with perinatal-related lung disease. It allows use of pulse oximetry oxygen saturation to calculate the S/F ratio when Pao_2 is not available. Both the use of OI (or OSI when Pao_2 is not available) to define hypoxia and the requirement for radiographic evidence of any new infiltrate are major departures from the Berlin definition used in adults.

A population-based study estimated an annual incidence of ARDS of 12.8 cases per 100,000 persons in Olmsted County in Washington. Severe sepsis (with pneumonia as the infection focus) was the most common risk factor. Reported estimates for prevalence of ARDS in single-center studies range from 1% to 10%.[11] A multinational point prevalence study of PARDS conducted by the Pediatric Acute Lung Injury and Sepsis Investigators (PALISI) is currently ongoing. The overall reported mortality from PARDS varies from 18% to 22%, but it is estimated to accompany up to 30% of all pediatric intensive care unit (ICU) deaths.[12] Although many modalities to treat PARDS have been investigated over the last decade, supportive therapies remain the mainstay of treatment.

CAUSES OF ACUTE RESPIRATORY DISTRESS SYNDROME

ARDS is associated with many different underlying clinical conditions, including pneumonia, sepsis, trauma, burns, acute pancreatitis, aspiration, toxic inhalation, transfusion, and cardiopulmonary bypass surgery[9,11–14] (**Table 1**). Although sepsis is the most common cause of ARDS for adults, the most common underlying condition for PARDS is viral respiratory infection.

PHYSIOLOGIC BASIS AND CONSEQUENCES OF NONCARDIOGENIC PULMONARY EDEMA

The lung's alveolar epithelial-capillary structure provides a large surface area for efficient gas exchange and comprises the alveolar epithelium, capillary endothelium, and

Table 1
Causes of acute respiratory distress syndrome

Direct Lung Injury (Alveolar-Epithelial)	Indirect Lung Injury (Alveolar-Capillary)
Pneumonia	Sepsis/Systemic inflammatory response syndrome
Aspiration	Major trauma
Inhalation injury	Pancreatitis
Drowning	Severe burns
Pulmonary contusion	Massive transfusion or TRALI
	Shock
	Cardiopulmonary bypass
	Head injury
	Drug overdose

basement membranes. The alveolar epithelium is coated with a thin layer of alveolar wall liquid, which is necessary for dispersion of surfactant, transfer of gases, and host defense against inhaled pathogens. Integrity of this barrier is critical for gas exchange, and separation of the aqueous and gaseous compartments (**Fig. 1**).[15,16] Disruption of the integrity of the pulmonary endothelium and alveolar epithelium leads to accumulation of protein-rich alveolar edema fluid.[1,17] Cytokines (interleukin-1 [IL-1], IL-8, tumor necrosis factor-α [TNF-α]) and lipid mediators (leukotriene B4) are attracted to alveoli and, in response to these proinflammatory mediators, neutrophils are recruited into the pulmonary interstitium and alveoli. The presence of protein, fibrinogen, and fibrin degradation products in the alveolar fluid results in surfactant degradation (**Fig. 2**).[1,2] There is decreased functional residual capacity (FRC), increased dead space, reduced respiratory system compliance, and impaired gas exchange, which leads to atelectasis and hypoxia. Loss of the epithelial barrier may also lead to sepsis in patients with bacterial pneumonia through creation of an open interface between the alveolar and circulating compartments.[1]

ALVEOLAR EPITHELIAL INJURY AND DYSFUNCTION

Alveolar epithelium is composed of 2 types of cells: flat alveolar type I cells and cuboidal alveolar type II cells, which make up 90% and 10% of the alveolar surface area, respectively. Type 1 cells are large thin cells, and they are the primary site of gas exchange, whereas type II cells are more resistant to injury and are responsible for surfactant production, ion transport, and proliferation and differentiation to type I cells after injury.[1] Type II cells are responsible for the removal of excess alveolar fluid through sodium-dependent intracellular transport.

Direct alveolar epithelial injury (infections, inhalations, aspirations, mechanical ventilation, and so forth) and indirect alveolar capillary injury (sepsis, trauma, transfusion, burns, pancreatitis, and so forth) lead to breakdown of the barrier and decrease in the ability of alveolar epithelium to remove excess alveolar fluid.[15,17,18] Decreased alveolar fluid clearance is associated with severity and worse clinical outcomes and increased mortality. Elevated plasma levels of surfactant protein D and the receptor for advance glycation end products, markers of alveolar epithelial damage, correlate with poor outcomes in patients with ARDS.[19–22]

LUNG ENDOTHELIAL INJURY

Damage to pulmonary capillary endothelium activates inflammatory and coagulation cascades.[23] There are multiple proteins along these cascades implicated in the

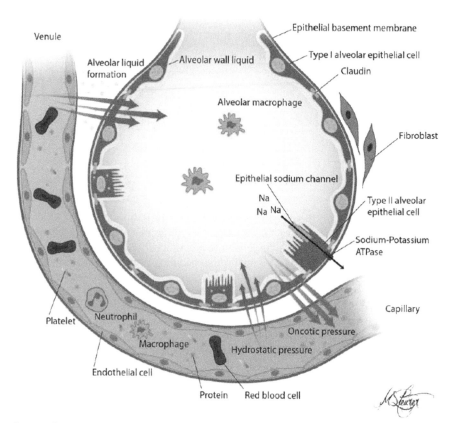

Fig. 1. Schematic of a healthy alveolus. The alveolar epithelium and capillary endothelium are intact. The characteristics of the pulmonary circulation and intact epithelial endothelial barrier allow for formation of the alveolar wall liquid (AWL) while maintaining the air-filled, fluid-free, status of the alveoli. The AWL facilitates gas exchange and is a medium for dispersal of surfactant and alveolar macrophages, which is essential for maintaining alveolar stability and host defenses. The intact sodium-dependent vectorial transport across type II alveolar epithelial cells regulates the removal of excess alveolar fluid. (*From* Sapru A, Flori H, Quasney MW, et al. Pathobiology of acute respiratory distress syndrome. Pediatr Crit Care Med 2015;16(5 Suppl 1):S6–22.)

pathogenesis of ARDS. Endothelial-specific proteins, such as von Willebrand factor and angiotensin-converting enzyme activity, correlate with ARDS mortality in children and adults.[24–26] Thrombomodulin is a transmembrane protein found on the surface of endothelial cells that facilitates the thrombin-mediated conversion of protein C to activated protein C and has roles in coagulation, fibrinolysis, and inflammation. It is highly expressed in pulmonary alveolar capillaries.[27] Elevated soluble thrombomodulin levels are associated with organ dysfunction in PARDS and with higher mortality in children with indirect lung injury.[27]

TRANSFUSIONS AND ACUTE RESPIRATORY DISTRESS SYNDROME

Over recent years, the incidence of antibody-mediated transfusion-related acute lung injury (TRALI) as a risk factor for ARDS has declined because of changes in blood

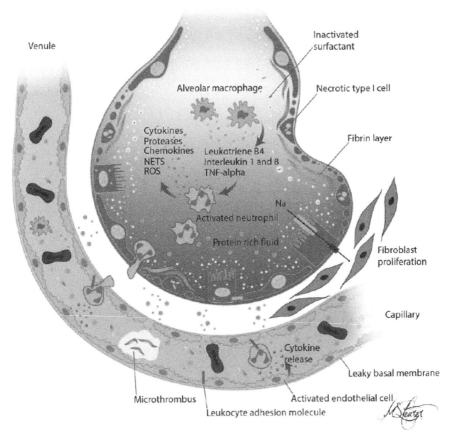

Fig. 2. Schematic of pathophysiology in ARDS. There is a loss of epithelial and endothelial barrier integrity and loss of function leading to increased permeability pulmonary edema. Solutes and large molecules such as albumin enter the alveolar space. In the presence of proinflammatory mediators and activated endothelium, leukocytes traffic into the pulmonary interstitium and alveoli. There is activation of coagulation and deposition of fibrin in capillaries and alveoli with increased concentrations of fibrinogen and fibrin-degradation products in the edema fluid. Surfactant depletion and degradation result in large increases in surface tension and loss of alveolar shape and integrity. Recovery is preceded by fibroblast proliferation. NETs, neutrophil extracellular traps; ROS, reactive oxygen species. (*From* Sapru A, Flori H, Quasney MW, et al. Pathobiology of acute respiratory distress syndrome. Pediatr Crit Care Med 2015;16(5 Suppl 1):S6–22.)

banking practice.[28] However, transfusion of red blood cells is associated with an increased risk of developing ARDS in critically ill patients with sepsis.[29] Cell-free hemoglobin (CFH) levels are increased during sepsis and ARDS because of decreased levels of haptoglobulin, hemopexin, and heme oxygenase-1 and reduced capacity to detoxify CFH.[30] Increased CFH levels may lead to injury via peroxidation of lipid membranes and increased vascular permeability.[31] In addition, massive transfusions can overwhelm the scavenging capacity of macrophages and lead to increased non-transferrin-bound iron production that can promote oxidative stress as well as increase susceptibility to infections with siderophilic bacteria.[32]

INFLAMMATORY DYSFUNCTION

Alveolar macrophages play a central role in orchestrating inflammation. When alveolar macrophages are activated, they recruit neutrophils and circulating macrophages to the alveoli. Neutrophils communicate between the vessel wall and platelets, which results in endothelial injury and releases neutrophil extracellular traps, which may also cause damage to the lung.[28,33,34]

Inflammation mediated by the innate immune system in response to infectious agents or tissue damage is triggered by the presence of pathogen-associated molecular patterns and endogenous danger (or damage) –associated molecular patterns.[33,35–37] These patterns are recognized by pattern recognition receptors such as Toll-like receptors and cytosolic nucleotide-binding oligomerization domainlike receptors, which leads to increased expression of inflammatory cytokines and chemokines, such as IL-1B, TNF-α, IL-6, and IL-8.[36,37] Several human studies have demonstrated evidence for dysregulation of inflammatory pathways in ARDS and their association with outcome.[38–40] A recent multicenter study of inflammatory pathways in PARDS identified a strong relationship between mortality and elevated plasma levels of both proinflammatory (IL-6, IL-8, IL-18, MIP-1β, TNF-α) and anti-inflammatory cytokines (IL-1RA, IL-10, and TNF-R2). These cytokines were associated with ARDS illness severity, including the P/F ratio, OI, pediatric risk of mortality score (PRISM-3), ICU morbidity, and biochemical evidence of endothelial injury, including elevated plasma angiopoietin 2 and soluble thrombomodulin. The addition of inflammatory cytokines to the OI improved risk-stratification in a heterogeneous ARDS population.[41]

SURFACTANT DYSFUNCTION

One of the hallmarks of ARDS is a reduction surfactant expression and surfactant dysfunction. Surfactant is secreted into the alveolar space by type II cells, and its main function is to lower surface tension at the air-liquid interface of the alveoli. Surfactant contains 4 major proteins: surfactant protein B and C are responsible for lowering the surface tension, whereas surfactant protein A and D are important in innate and adaptive immune responses against pathogens. Surfactant proteins A, B, and D levels are low in the bronchoalveolar lavage fluid of adults with ARDS. Loss of surfactant leads to the decreased compliance and alveolar instability observed in ARDS, and which leads to atelectasis. Furthermore, increased serum levels of these proteins in children and adults are associated with alveolar epithelial cell injury.[42–45]

COAGULATION AND FIBRINOLYSIS DYSFUNCTION

Inflammation and coagulation are critical host responses to infection and injury; however, in ARDS, there is a significant imbalance between coagulation and fibrinolysis. This process favors fibrin formation. Microthrombi and pulmonary vascular injury occur early in ARDS. Stimuli such as hypoxia, cytokines, and chemokines, and inflammatory mediators lead to activation of the endothelium.[26,46] Endothelial cells respond by shifting from their normal antithrombotic and anti-inflammatory phenotype to an "activated" state of endothelial "dysfunction,"[47] characterized by prothrombotic and proadhesive properties. Key events in this transformation are the expression of adhesion molecules, tissue factor,[48] and von Willebrand factor.[25] Furthermore, it appears that alveolar epithelium can upregulate tissue factor in response to inflammatory stimuli.[49] The procoagulant environment with ARDS is also due in part to the elevated plasminogen activator inhibitor-1 (PAI-1), and elevated PAI-1 levels are associated with increased mortality in adults and children with ARDS.[50]

Platelets can also contribute to lung injury in ARDS. Platelets can directly interact with neutrophils and monocytes and are themselves a source of proinflammatory cytokines. There is evidence that platelets can also alter the barrier function of alveolar capillaries, regulate pulmonary vascular permeability, and influence pulmonary vascular reactivity.[51]

VENTILATOR-INDUCED LUNG INJURY IN ACUTE RESPIRATORY DISTRESS SYNDROME

Current treatment regimens for ARDS include oxygen therapy and mechanical ventilation.[52] Unfortunately, side effects of these treatments include exacerbation of lung injury by barotrauma, volutrauma, and propagation of lung inflammation. These changes are clinically recognized as ventilator-induced lung injury.[53] Over the past 2 decades, except for the introduction of low-tidal volume ventilation,[54] few if any new therapeutic approaches have shown improvements in patient survival.[55,56] Recently, it has been proposed that stretch-activated ion channels, such as 2-pore-domain potassium channels, may play an important role in the development and propagation of ventilator -induced lung injury[57] by regulating inflammatory mediator secretion,[58,59] epithelial cell detachment and cytoskeletal remodeling,[60] and alveolar-capillary barrier function.[56]

RESOLUTION OF ACUTE RESPIRATORY DISTRESS SYNDROME

Although ARDS causes extensive damage to lung tissue, it can fully resolve. However, restoring the balance of proinflammatory and anti-inflammatory responses is essential to prevent lung fibrosis. Repair of the epithelium is a complex process that appears to involve epithelial cell spreading, migration, proliferation, and differentiation. Scar tissue is formed during healing to preserve alveolar integrity and prevent further alveolar edema. This fibrotic tissue is removed by matrix metalloproteinases, a family of enzymes that digest extracellular fibers.[61] Matrix metalloproteinases are upregulated during the repair process and appear to be involved in facilitating migration in the remodeling.[62] The migration and proliferation of epithelial progenitor cells are also regulated by transforming growth factor-α, fibroblast growth factor, hepatocyte growth factor, and keratinocyte growth factor. Interestingly, there is also evidence of multipotent mesenchymal stem cells that may be involved in repair of lung alveoli.[63] There is an ongoing phase 2 clinical trial to test the role of mesenchymal stem cells in ARDS in adults.

MORTALITY IN ACUTE RESPIRATORY DISTRESS SYNDROME

The overall mortality associated with PARDS is decreasing over time. The estimated mortality varies from 18% to 35%. Studies that include both invasively and noninvasively ventilated patients report 18% to 22% mortality, whereas among studies limited to invasively ventilated patients, mortality tends to be somewhat higher in the range of 26% to 35%.[14,64] Although the pooled mortality from several studies is about 30%, it is clear that children with certain comorbidities and immunodeficiency have worse outcomes.[64] Most deaths in ARDS are attributable to sepsis or multiorgan dysfunction rather than primary respiratory causes. Multiple organ system dysfunction is the single most important independent clinical risk factor for mortality in children, with only a minority of deaths attributable solely to lung failure and refractory hypoxemia.[1,64] Interestingly, a combination of OI level and history of cancer/stem cell transplant predicts mortality as well as complex models incorporating measures of overall severity of illness and severity of lung injury.[65]

MANAGEMENT OF ACUTE RESPIRATORY DISTRESS SYNDROME

Management of PARDS consists mainly of addressing gas exchange and work of breathing, and providing nutrition and general ICU supportive care, with the goal of treating the underlying cause of PARDS and minimizing iatrogenic harm. Most treatment recommendations in PARDS are based on extrapolated adult studies, small studies in pediatric populations, and the clinical expertise of bedside physicians. To promote optimization and consistency of care for children with PARDS, the PALICC published treatment recommendations in 2015.[9] Despite advances in management treatment modalities, the clinical benefits and risks of these innovations remain mixed.[9] In the following discussion, the authors review current management, citing relevant adult and pediatric studies along with the published PALICC recommendations. Because ARDS is characterized by impaired gas exchange, support of oxygenation and ventilation with supplemental oxygen, noninvasive ventilation, and invasive mechanical ventilation are the cornerstone of PARDS therapy.

HIGH-FLOW NASAL CANNULA AND NONINVASIVE VENTILATION

In adults with ARDS, some studies have demonstrated worse mortality in patients treated with these noninvasive approaches.[66–68] These poorer outcomes may be due to delay in initiation of lung-protective ventilation and tend to be more pronounced in patients with severe disease. Conversely, there may be benefit to limiting exposure of patients to invasive mechanical ventilation and its associated complications.[13,69] A recent study in adult patients with acute hypoxemic respiratory failure (defined as a P/F ratio of ≤ 300) found those randomized to receive high flow nasal cannula oxygen had more ventilator-free days at day 28 and a lower 90-day mortality than those randomized to facemask or noninvasive ventilation.[70] A prospective randomized control trial (RCT) comparing noninvasive ventilation and standard oxygen therapy in children with respiratory failure after extubation showed no difference between groups.[71] Finally, in a propensity score-matched cohort study evaluating outcomes in children admitted to the ICU, those receiving noninvasive ventilation as first-line therapy had reduced mortality, length of ventilation, and length of ICU stay.[72] Although the exact role of high-flow nasal cannula and noninvasive ventilation in PARDS remains unknown, these studies suggest that in appropriately selected patient populations these approaches may be valuable. Ongoing assessment of patients and an early change to invasive mechanical ventilation among nonresponders are key factors to successful use of noninvasive ventilation.[73]

INVASIVE MECHANICAL VENTILATION

Invasive mechanical ventilation strategies balance support of gas exchange with toxicity from volutrauma, barotrauma, and free-radical injury.[54,73] In their landmark publication on lung-protective ventilation, the ARDS Network found a decrease in mortality with lower tidal volume ventilation (6 mL/kg of predicted body weight) compared with conventional ventilation volumes at that time (12 mL/kg of predicted body weight).[54] Two subsequent meta-analyses in adult ARDS further supported that low-tidal volume ventilation reduced in-hospital mortality.[74,75] Current recommendations in adults include lung-protective ventilation with tidal volumes of less than 6 mL/kg of estimated ideal body weight, limitation of plateau pressures greater than 30 cm H_2O, and use of adequate PEEP.[54,74,75] Given the strength of the adult ARDS data, standard PARDS therapy involves lung-protective ventilation as well. PALICC recommends tidal volumes of 3 to 6 mL/kg predicted body weight for patients with poor compliance and closer to physiologic range (5–8 mL/kg predicted body weight) for patients with preserved compliance.[9] In addition, they suggest an inspiratory plateau pressure of less than 28 cm H_2O (29–32 cm H_2O in those with increased chest wall elastance).[9] Permissive hypercapnia (pH 7.15–7.30) may be used if necessary to limit further injury to the lung caused by potentially injurious ventilator pressure.[73,76] A goal-directed strategy to minimize further lung injury also includes adjusting the supplemental oxygen to maintain saturations of 92% to 97% for mild PARDS and 88% to 92% in those with PEEP of 10 cm H_2O.[73,76]

Additional invasive ventilation considerations include how best to treat hypoxia with supplemental oxygen and PEEP. The goal of applied PEEP in PARDS is to maximize alveolar recruitment, provide optimal FRC, and prevent recruitment/derecruitment cycles. When originally investigated by the ARDS Network, there was no difference in outcome between low PEEP strategies (range of 5–24 cm H_2O) and high PEEP strategies (range of 12–24 cm H_2O), so many centers favor a low PEEP strategy given the concern for barotrauma, pneumothoraces, and hemodynamic compromise that can be associated with high PEEP.[77] However, subsequent studies in adult ARDS suggest a significantly reduced mortality with a high PEEP strategy in severe ARDS.[78–80] Open lung ventilation is another emerging technique that combines low tidal-volume ventilation and setting a PEEP at least 2 cm H_2O above the lower inflection point of the patient's pressure-volume curve. Small studies suggest a reduced mortality with this strategy.[81,82] Neither high PEEP nor open lung ventilation has been evaluated in PARDS. PALICC suggests PEEP should be 10 to 15 cm H_2O with levels greater than 15 cm H_2O used in severe PARDS with careful attention to inspiratory plateau pressures.[9]

HIGH-FREQUENCY OSCILLATORY VENTILATION

Despite its widespread clinical use, studies investigating outcomes in high-frequency oscillatory ventilation (HFOV) in ARDS have not shown any benefit in lung-protective ventilation. The OSCAR trial found no difference in mortality in those randomized to HFOV compared with conventional ventilation.[83] A similar Canadian study was stopped because of futility and suggested a mortality increase in an HFOV patient.[84] Although there are no RCTs of HFOV dedicated to PARDS, 2 recent secondary analyses have shown tendency toward harm among children with PARDS managed by early HFOV.[85,86] Most recently, a propensity score matched analysis evaluating sedation in children found early (within 48 hours of intubation) initiation of HFOV to be associated with longer duration of mechanical ventilation, but no mortality difference when compared with late initiation or conventional ventilation.[86]

INHALED NITRIC OXIDE

Use of inhaled nitric oxide (iNO) in ARDS became popular when Rossaint and colleagues[87] showed that it improved oxygenation. Subsequent studies, including 3 systematic reviews with primarily adult patients, found no significant effect of iNO on mortality or number of ventilator-free days.[88–90] Furthermore, in some adults, iNO may increase renal impairment, suggesting the benefits may not outweigh the risks in certain adult populations.[90,91] Three RCTs have demonstrated an oxygenation benefit with iNO in PARDS,[92–94] but this benefit is not sustained and does not lead to improved overall outcomes. The most notable was a multicenter trial that showed iNO improved oxygenation at 12 and 24 hours, but not at 72 hours after initiation.[93] In 2014, Bronicki and colleagues[95] published an RCT that showed iNO not only improved oxygenation at 12 hours but also reduced duration of mechanical ventilation and increased extracorporeal membrane oxygenation (ECMO)-free survival. It should be noted that ECMO-free survival was not a primary endpoint, which leaves the true survival benefit of iNO still unresolved.[95] Although PALICC does not recommend routine use of iNO in PARDS, they do recommend use in severe cases or in cases complicated by pulmonary hypertension or severe right heart strain.[9]

SURFACTANT

Because there is surfactant deficiency and dysfunction in ARDS, exogenous surfactant could potentially be beneficial, particularly in early stages of lung injury.[96] However, the literature on the use of surfactant has not been conclusive. Two studies of recombinant surfactant protein in ARDS yielded improvement in oxygenation, but no effect on survival.[97,98] A post hoc analysis of this study suggested patients with severe ARDS from pneumonia or aspiration had an improvement in 28-day survival with surfactant administration[98]; however, a follow-up study in this patient population was halted for futility and demonstrated no significant benefit in mortality, oxygenation, or ventilator-free days.[99]

Several studies have shown surfactant improves lung function, oxygenation, and gas exchange.[100–102] The most notable was a multicenter RCT conducted by PALISI, which demonstrated an overall mortality benefit after early surfactant administration.[99] Of note, this was the first trial for which a post hoc analysis suggested benefit in direct lung injury. However, one of the major limitations of this trial was a greater proportion of immunocompromised patients in the control group, leading to a higher than expected mortality.[100] Another recent international, multicenter RCT on the use of lucinactant in infants with early PARDS demonstrated no significant reduction in ventilator-free days or mortality.[103] Furthermore, a 2013 study focused on PARDS secondary to direct lung injury was halted for futility, finding no significant difference in oxygenation, ventilator-free days, or 90-day mortality with surfactant administration.[104] PALICC does not recommend the routine use of surfactant in PARDS.[9]

FLUID MANAGEMENT

In addition to disrupting gas exchange, PARDS leads to fluid overload and to a proinflammatory response by the endothelium due to increasing intravascular pressure. Interstitial edema is a frequent complication.[105,106] In the FACTT trial published in 2006, an even fluid balance over the first 7 days of mechanical ventilation improved lung function, shortened duration of mechanical ventilation, and shortened duration of ICU stay.[107] There was no significant difference in 60-day mortality and no increase in nonpulmonary organ failures between conservative and liberal fluid management.[107] More recent adult ARDS literature suggests that early treatment with hemofiltration not only reduces overall lung water and improves cardiac function but also may reduce cytokine levels and systemic inflammation.[108]

Of the 4 studies to investigate fluid balance in PARDS, 3 have demonstrated an association between fluid balance and mortality. Specifically, (1) Flori and colleagues[109] demonstrated an association between cumulative fluid balance and pediatric ICU mortality; (2) Willson and colleagues[110] showed an association between cumulative fluid balance and mortality within the first week of illness; and (3) Hu and colleagues[111] found a daily fluid balance of $\leq$10 mL/kg/d was associated with lower mortality in patients with acute hypoxemic respiratory failure. Lower cumulative fluid balance was also found to increase ventilator-free days.[109,110,112] Current PALICC consensus suggests that, after initial fluid resuscitation, goal-directed fluid management should be used in order to maintain adequate intravascular volume while aiming to prevent a positive fluid balance.[9]

NUTRITION

In general, critically ill children have reduced mortality when enteral nutrition is started within 48 hours of their admission.[113] Furthermore, emerging research suggests a role for gut dysfunction in pathogenesis of ARDS.[113] The EDEN study, which attempted to address the optimal amount of enteral nutrition in ARDS, found that, compared with full enteral feeding, a strategy of initial trophic enteral feeding for up to 6 days did not improve ventilator-free days, 60-day mortality, or infectious complications, but was associated with less gastrointestinal intolerance.[114] Trials investigating omega-3 fatty acid–enriched lipid emulsion found them to be clinically safe and to modulate eicosanoid values, which may have important immunomodulatory implications.[115,116] Overall, the area of optimal nutrition is a burgeoning field within ARDS research. PALICC stresses the importance of nutrition, preferably enteral, in maintaining growth, meeting metabolic needs, and facilitating recovery.[9]

PREVENTION OF INFLAMMATION

Inflammation plays a key role in the pathophysiology of PARDS both in the lungs and systemically. Corticosteroids are used in 20% to 60% of patients with PARDS, although evaluating this use is confounded by indications including periextubation airway management, shock, and hypercytokinemia.[117–119] Despite the prevalence of corticosteroid use, a definitive role for these drugs in PARDS has not been established. In 2 adult ARDS meta-analyses, there is a suggestion of reduced mortality and increased ventilator-free days when steroids are initiated at the onset of ARDS.[120,121] In the pediatric population, data consist of small studies with wide variability in timing, duration, dose, and type of corticosteroids used.[119] In a recent RCT of low-dose methylprednisolone infusion in PARDS, there was no difference in length of mechanical ventilation, duration of ICU stay, duration of hospitalization, or mortality between intervention and control groups.[122] However, a single-center prospective observational study found corticosteroid exposure for more than 24 hours and cumulative corticosteroid dose were both independently associated with fewer ventilator-free days at 28 days and a shorter overall duration of ventilation.[117] Because of this inconsistency, the recent PALICC recommendations state that corticosteroids cannot be recommended as part of routine therapy.[9,123] That said, systemic steroids may benefit ARDS patients with certain comorbidities, including bronchopulmonary dysplasia, reactive airway disease, pneumonia in general, and pneumocystis pneumonia. Much more study of these indications is warranted.

Inflammatory pathways provide an ongoing target for novel therapies in the treatment of PARDS. Possible alternatives to systemic corticosteroids currently being investigated include the following: (1) inhaled corticosteroids, which improve dynamic lung compliance, improve oxygenation, and decrease local inflammation[124,125]; (2) angiotensin II, which induces NF-kB gene expression and blocks the renin-angiotensin axis[126]; (3) peroxisome proliferator receptor agonists, which negatively control proinflammatory gene expression[127]; and (4) hypoxia-inducible factor-1a, which inhibits the proteasome and induces anti-inflammatory effects.[128,129]

PRONE POSITIONING

Prone positioning improves oxygenation in ARDS, likely through a combination of improved lung ventilation-perfusion matching, recruitment of lower-lobe atelectasis, reduced ventilator-induced lung injury due to maintenance of open lung units, improved secretion clearance, and improved right ventricular dysfunction.[53,130] The Supine-Prone Study Group was among the first to demonstrate improved oxygenation in adult ARDS patients.[113,131] However, improvement in oxygenation in this study and several others that followed did not translate into a mortality benefit for the general ARDS population.[132–136]

In the pediatric population, an RCT investigating prone position in PARDS was halted early for futility.[137] Like previous adult studies, despite improved oxygenation this investigation demonstrated no significant benefit of prone positioning on ventilator-free days or 28-day mortality.[137] However, the mortality in the control group was unusually low at 8%, suggesting the true utility of prone positioning in PARDS may still be unknown.[137] Guerin and colleagues[138] found a 28-day and 90-day mortality benefit in patients with moderate to severe ARDS who were placed prone more than 16 hours per day. The difference between this outcome and that of previous studies is likely due to targeting children with more severe ARDS, longer time periods spent prone, and improved expertise in the prone position procedure. Lack of expertise in prone positioning, the potential for complications, and uncertainty as to which population most benefits from this therapy has led to variability in the adoption of prone positioning for PARDS.[53,132] PALICC currently recommends consideration of prone positioning in severe cases of PARDS.[9]

SEDATION AND NEUROMUSCULAR BLOCKADE

Deep sedation and neuromuscular blockade (NMB) likely benefits ARDS patients by limiting the following: (1) lung injury arising from ventilator-patient asynchrony; (2) expiratory muscle function, which can cause collapse and derecruitment; and (3) the potential release of inflammatory cytokines.[53] A multicenter RCT in adults with moderate to severe ARDS (specifically patients with a P/F ratio <150) found lower adjusted 90-day in-hospital mortality and increased ventilator-free days in patients with NMB and deep sedation compared with deep sedation alone.[139] Currently, a multicenter study is being conducted by the National Heart, Lung, and Blood Institute–funded PETAL network to assess the benefits and risks of NMB. There have been no studies investigating the effects of sedation and NMB in PARDS. PALICC recommends the use of NMB at the minimum effective dose in patients who are unable to achieve effective mechanical ventilation with sedation alone.[9] Furthermore, they recommend close monitoring, titration, and consideration of a daily NMB holiday in patients in which full chemical paralysis is used.[9]

EXTRACORPOREAL LIFE SUPPORT

Extracorporeal life support (ECLS) is likely beneficial in PARDS because it limits the volutrauma, barotrauma, and oxygen toxicity associated with mechanical ventilation.[140,141] The CESAR trial showing a survival benefit for adult patients with respiratory failure randomized to receive care in ECLS centers. ECLS is now an important therapeutic option for adult ARDS.[142]

The proper timing of initiation ECLS in respiratory failure is not defined and must balance the potential benefit of lung rest against morbidities associated with ECLS. Several observational adult ARDS studies have found that improved outcome is associated with a shorter duration of mechanical ventilation before initiation of ECLS.[143–146] Current adult ARDS recommendations suggest that patients mechanically ventilated for more than 7 days may be less likely to benefit from ECLS for their respiratory failure.[147] Zabrocki and colleagues[148] evaluated this question in the PARDS population. They found that patients mechanically ventilated for ≤ 14 days before ECLS initiation had similar survivals (56%–61%), whereas those ventilated greater than 14 days dropped their survival to 38%.[148] Nance and colleagues[149] reported a statistically significant survival decrease of 2.9% for each pre-ECLS ventilator day. Therefore, the most current ELSO guidelines for pediatrics suggest that implementing ECLS is most appropriate within the first 7 days of mechanical ventilation at high levels of support.[148]

Many other variables are important in applying ECLS in the PARDS population, including the method of support (venovenous in patients with respiratory failure and preserved cardiac function or venoarterial for patients with cardiopulmonary failure), type of cannula, location of cannulation, and approach to anticoagulation.[150,151] Although venovenous ECLS can replace lung function, this is correlated with the efficiency of ECLS, which is affected by the maximum achievable flow and the extent of recirculation. Therefore, some ventilator support might be required to augment ventilation and/or oxygenation.[150] However, in some patient populations, extubation while on ECLS is an emerging management strategy.[75,152] Finally, new data suggest that ECLS for carbon dioxide removal may be a beneficial adjuvant for patients without life-threatening hypoxia.[151] ECLS is an important and growing management strategy in PARDS. PALICC recommends consideration of ECLS in severe PARDS, where the cause is likely to be reversible or the child is suitable for consideration of lung transplantation.[153]

REFERENCES

1. Ware LB, Matthay MA. The acute respiratory distress syndrome. N Engl J Med 2000;342(18):1334–49.
2. Sapru A, Flori H, Quasney MW, et al. Pathobiology of acute respiratory distress syndrome. Pediatr Crit Care Med 2015;16(5):S6–22.
3. Ashbaugh DG, Bigelow DB, Petty TL, et al. Acute respiratory distress in adults. Lancet 1967;2(7511):319–23.
4. Katz R. Adult respiratory distress syndrome in children. Clin Chest Med 1987; 8(4):635–9.
5. Sherrill DL, Camilli A, Lebowitz MD. On the temporal relationships between lung function and somatic growth. Am Rev Respir Dis 1989;140(3):638–44.
6. Wang X, Dockery DW, Wypij D, et al. Pulmonary function between 6 and 18 years of age. Pediatr Pulmonol 1993;15(2):75–88.
7. Bernard GR, Artigas A, Brigham KL, et al. Report of the American-European consensus conference on ARDS: definitions, mechanisms, relevant outcomes and clinical trial coordination. Intensive Care Med 1994;20(3):225–32.
8. The ARDS Definition Task Force, Ranieri V, Rubenfeld G, Thompson BT, et al. Acute respiratory distress syndrome. JAMA 2012;307(23):2526–33.
9. Jouvet P, Thomas NJ, Willson DF, et al. Pediatric acute respiratory distress syndrome: consensus recommendations from the pediatric acute lung injury consensus conference. Pediatr Crit Care Med 2015;16(5):428–39.
10. Khemani RG, Smith LS, Zimmerman JJ, et al. Pediatric acute respiratory distress syndrome. Pediatr Crit Care Med 2015;16(5):S23–40.

11. Zimmerman JJ, Akhtar SR, Caldwell E, et al. Incidence and outcomes of pediatric acute lung injury. Pediatrics 2009;124(1):87–95.
12. Yehya N, Servaes S, Thomas NJ. Characterizing degree of lung injury in pediatric acute respiratory distress syndrome. Crit Care Med 2015;43(5):937–46.
13. Cheifetz IM. Year in review 2015: pediatric ARDS. Respir Care 2016;61(7): 980–5.
14. Flori H, Glidden D, Rutherford G, et al. Pediatric acute lung injury: prospective evaluation of risk factors associated with mortality. Am J Respir Crit Care Med 2005;171(9):995–991001.
15. Lai-Fook SJ. Perivascular interstitial fluid pressure measured by micropipettes in isolated dog lung. J Appl Physiol 1982;52(1):9–15.
16. Bhattacharya J, Nakahara K, Staub N. Effect of edema on pulmonary blood flow in the isolated perfused dog lung lobe. J Appl Physiol 1980;48(3):444–9.
17. Bhattacharya J, Matthay MA. Regulation and repair of the alveolar-capillary barrier in acute lung injury. Annu Rev Physiol 2013;75:593–615.
18. Bhattacharya J. Hydraulic conductivity of lung venules determined by split-drop technique. J Appl Physiol 1988;64(6):2562–7. Available at: http://www.ncbi.nlm.nih.gov/pubmed/3403440.
19. Calfee CS, Ware LB, Eisner MD, et al. Plasma receptor for advanced glycation end products and clinical outcomes in acute lung injury. Thorax 2008;63(12): 1083–9.
20. Eisner MD, Parsons P, Matthay MA, et al. Plasma surfactant protein levels and clinical outcomes in patients with acute lung injury. Thorax 2003;58(11):983–8.
21. Guo WA, Knight PR, Raghavendran K. The receptor for advanced glycation end products and acute lung injury/acute respiratory distress syndrome. Intensive Care Med 2012;38(10):1588–98.
22. Determann RM, Royakkers AA, Haitsma JJ, et al. Plasma levels of surfactant protein D and KL-6 for evaluation of lung injury in critically ill mechanically ventilated patients. BMC Pulm Med 2010;10:6.
23. Wort SJ, Evans TW. The role of the endothelium in modulating vascular control in sepsis and related conditions. Br Med Bull 1999;55(1):30–48.
24. Orfanos SE, Armaganidis A, Glynos C, et al. Pulmonary capillary endothelium-bound angiotensin-converting enzyme activity in acute lung injury. Circulation 2000;102(16):2011–8.
25. Sabharwal AK, Bajaj SP, Ameri A, et al. Tissue factor pathway inhibitor and von Willebrand factor antigen levels in adult respiratory distress syndrome and in a primate model of sepsis. Am J Respir Crit Care Med 1995;151(3 Pt 1):758–67.
26. Ware LB, Eisner MD, Thompson BT, et al. Significance of von Willebrand factor in septic and nonseptic patients with acute lung injury. Am J Respir Crit Care Med 2004;170(7):766–72.
27. Orwoll BE, Spicer AC, Zinter MS, et al. Elevated soluble thrombomodulin is associated with organ failure and mortality in children with acute respiratory distress syndrome (ARDS): a prospective observational cohort study. Crit Care 2015;19:435.
28. Toy P, Gajic O, Bacchetti P, et al. Transfusion-related acute lung injury: incidence and risk factors. Blood 2012;119(7):1757–67.
29. Janz DR, Zhao Z, Koyama T, et al. Longer storage duration of red blood cells is associated with an increased risk of acute lung injury in patients with sepsis. Ann Intensive Care 2013;3(1):33.
30. Janz DR, Ware LB. The role of red blood cells and cell-free hemoglobin in the pathogenesis of ARDS. J Intensive Care 2015;3:20.

31. Vermeulen Windsant IC, de Wit NCJ, Sertorio JTC, et al. Blood transfusions increase circulating plasma free hemoglobin levels and plasma nitric oxide consumption: a prospective observational pilot study. Crit Care 2012;16(3):R95.

32. Arezes J, Jung G, Gabayan V, et al. Hepcidin-induced hypoferremia is a critical host defense mechanism against the siderophilic bacterium Vibrio vulnificus. Cell Host Microbe 2015;17(1):47–57.

33. Aggarwal NR, King LS, D'Alessio FR. Diverse macrophage populations mediate acute lung inflammation and resolution. Am J Physiol Lung Cell Mol Physiol 2014;306(8):L709–25.

34. Caudrillier A, Kessenbrock K, Gilliss BM, et al. Platelets induce neutrophil extracellular traps in transfusion-related acute lung injury. J Clin Invest 2012;122(7):2661–71.

35. Kovach MA, Standiford TJ. Toll like receptors in diseases of the lung. Int Immunopharmacol 2011;11(10):1399–406.

36. Tolle LB, Standiford TJ. Danger-associated molecular patterns (DAMPs) in acute lung injury. J Pathol 2013;229(2):145–56.

37. Xiang M, Fan J. Pattern recognition receptor-dependent mechanisms of acute lung injury. Mol Med 2010;16(1–2):69–82.

38. Park WY, Goodman RB, Steinberg KP, et al. Cytokine balance in the lungs of patients with acute respiratory distress syndrome. Am J Respir Crit Care Med 2001;164(10 Pt 1):1896–903.

39. Parsons PE, Matthay MA, Ware LB, et al. Elevated plasma levels of soluble TNF receptors are associated with morbidity and mortality in patients with acute lung injury. Am J Physiol Lung Cell Mol Physiol 2005;288(3):L426–31.

40. Parsons PE, Eisner MD, Thompson BT, et al. Lower tidal volume ventilation and plasma cytokine markers of inflammation in patients with acute lung injury. Crit Care Med 2005;33(1):1–2.

41. Zinter MS, Orwoll BE, Spicer AC, et al. Incorporating inflammation into mortality risk in pediatric acute respiratory distress syndrome. Crit Care Med 2017. http://dx.doi.org/10.1097/CCM.0000000000002370.

42. Gregory TJ, Longmore WJ, Moxley MA, et al. Surfactant chemical composition and biophysical activity in acute respiratory distress syndrome. J Clin Invest 1991;88(6):1976–81.

43. Gunther A, Schmidt R, Feustel A, et al. Surfactant subtype conversion is related to loss of surfactant apoprotein B and surface activity in large surfactant aggregates. Experimental and clinical studies. Am J Respir Crit Care Med 1999;159(1):244–51.

44. Greene KE, Wright JR, Steinberg KP, et al. Serial changes in surfactant-associated proteins in lung and serum before and after onset of ARDS. Am J Respir Crit Care Med 1999;160(6):1843–50.

45. Cheng IW, Ware LB, Greene KE, et al. Prognostic value of surfactant proteins A and D in patients with acute lung injury. Crit Care Med 2003;31(1):20–7.

46. Flori HR, Ware LB, Milet M, et al. Early elevation of plasma von Willebrand factor antigen in pediatric acute lung injury is associated with an increased risk of death and prolonged mechanical ventilation. Pediatr Crit Care Med 2007;8(2):96–101.

47. Feletou M, Vanhoutte PM. Endothelial dysfunction: a multifaceted disorder (The Wiggers award lecture). Am J Physiol Heart Circ Physiol 2006;291(3):H985–1002.

48. Scarpati EM, Sadler JE. Regulation of endothelial cell coagulant properties. Modulation of tissue factor, plasminogen activator inhibitors, and thrombomodulin by phorbol 12-myristate 13-acetate and tumor necrosis factor. J Biol Chem 1989;264(34):20705–13.

49. Bastarache JA, Wang L, Geiser T, et al. The alveolar epithelium can initiate the extrinsic coagulation cascade through expression of tissue factor. Thorax 2007; 62(7):608–16.

50. Sapru A, Curley MAQ, Brady S, et al. Elevated PAI-1 is associated with poor clinical outcomes in pediatric patients with acute lung injury. Intensive Care Med 2010;36(1):157–63.

51. Weyrich AS, Zimmerman GA. Platelets in lung biology. Annu Rev Physiol 2013; 75:569–91.

52. Dushianthan A, Grocott MPW, Postle AD, et al. Acute respiratory distress syndrome and acute lung injury. Postgrad Med J 2011;87(1031):612–22.

53. Baron RM, Levy BD. Recent advances in understanding and treating ARDS. F1000Research 2016;5. http://dx.doi.org/10.12688/f1000research.7646.1.

54. Brower RG, Matthay MA, Morris A, et al. Ventilation with lower tidal volumes as compared with traditional tidal volumes for acute lung injury and the acute respiratory distress syndrome. N Engl J Med 2000;342(18):1301–8.

55. Needham CJ, Brindley PG. Best evidence in critical care medicine: the role of neuromuscular blocking drugs in early severe acute respiratory distress syndrome. Can J Anaesth 2012;59(1):105–8.

56. Schwingshackl A, Teng B, Makena P, et al. Deficiency of the two-pore-domain potassium channel TREK-1 promotes hyperoxia-induced lung injury. Crit Care Med 2014;42(11):e692–701.

57. Schwingshackl A, Meduri GU. Rationale for prolonged glucocorticoid use in pediatric ARDS: what the adults can teach us. Front Pediatr 2016;4:58.

58. Schwingshackl A, Teng B, Ghosh M, et al. Regulation of Monocyte Chemotactic Protein-1 secretion by the Two-Pore-Domain Potassium (K2P) channel TREK-1 in human alveolar epithelial cells. Am J Transl Res 2013;5(5):530–42.

59. Schwingshackl A, Teng B, Ghosh M, et al. Regulation of interleukin-6 secretion by the two-pore-domain potassium channel Trek-1 in alveolar epithelial cells. Am J Physiol Lung Cell Mol Physiol 2013;304(4):L276–86.

60. Roan E, Waters CM, Teng B, et al. The 2-pore domain potassium channel TREK-1 regulates stretch-induced detachment of alveolar epithelial cells. PLoS One 2014;9(2):e89429.

61. Davey A, McAuley DF, O'Kane CM. Matrix metalloproteinases in acute lung injury: mediators of injury and drivers of repair. Eur Respir J 2011;38(4):959–70.

62. Crosby LM, Waters CM. Epithelial repair mechanisms in the lung. Am J Physiol Lung Cell Mol Physiol 2010;298(6):L715–31.

63. Kajstura J, Rota M, Hall SR, et al. Evidence for human lung stem cells. N Engl J Med 2011;364(19):1795–806.

64. Flori H, Dahmer MK, Sapru A, et al. Pediatric Acute Lung Injury Consensus Conference Group. Comorbidities and assessment of severity of pediatric acute respiratory distress syndrome: proceedings from the Pediatric Acute Lung Injury Consensus Conference. Pediatr Crit Care Med 2015;16(5 Suppl 1):S41–50.

65. Spicer AC, Calfee CS, Zinter MS, et al. A simple and robust bedside model for mortality risk in pediatric patients with acute respiratory distress syndrome. Pediatr Crit Care Med 2016;17(10):1.

66. Messika J, Ben Ahmed K, Gaudry S, et al. Use of high-flow nasal cannula oxygen therapy in subjects with ARDS: a 1-year observational study. Respir Care 2015;60(2):162–9.

67. Antonelli M, Conti G, Esquinas A, et al. A multiple-center survey on the use in clinical practice of noninvasive ventilation as a first-line intervention for acute respiratory distress syndrome. Crit Care Med 2007;35(1):18–25.

68. Bellani G, Laffey JG, Pham T, et al. Noninvasive ventilation of patients with acute respiratory distress syndrome. Insights from the LUNG SAFE Study. Am J Respir Crit Care Med 2017;195(1):67–77.

69. Chiumello D, Brioni M. Severe hypoxemia: which strategy to choose. Crit Care 2016;20(1):132.

70. Frat J-P, Thille AW, Mercat A, et al. High-flow oxygen through nasal cannula in acute hypoxemic respiratory failure. N Engl J Med 2015;372(23):2185–96.

71. Fioretto JR, Ribeiro CF, Carpi MF, et al. Comparison between noninvasive mechanical ventilation and standard oxygen therapy in children up to 3 years old with respiratory failure after extubation: a pilot prospective randomized clinical study. Pediatr Crit Care Med 2015;16(2):124–30.

72. Morris JV, Ramnarayan P, Parslow RC, et al. Outcomes for children receiving noninvasive ventilation as the first-line mode of mechanical ventilation at intensive care admission: a propensity score-matched cohort study. Crit Care Med 2017. http://dx.doi.org/10.1097/CCM.0000000000002369.

73. Cheifetz IM. Pediatric acute respiratory distress syndrome. Respir Care 2011; 56(10):1589–99.

74. Putensen C, Theuerkauf N, Zinserling J, et al. Meta-analysis: ventilation strategies and outcomes of the acute respiratory distress syndrome and acute lung injury. Ann Intern Med 2009;151(8):566–76.

75. Petrucci N, De Feo C. Lung protective ventilation strategy for the acute respiratory distress syndrome. Cochrane Database Syst Rev 2013;(2):CD003844.

76. Abdelsalam M, Cheifetz IM. Goal-directed therapy for severely hypoxic patients with acute respiratory distress syndrome: permissive hypoxemia. Respir Care 2010;55(11):1483–90.

77. Brower RG, Lanken PN, MacIntyre N, et al. Higher versus lower positive end-expiratory pressures in patients with the acute respiratory distress syndrome. N Engl J Med 2004;351(4):327–36.

78. Mercat A, Richard J-CM, Vielle B, et al. Positive end-expiratory pressure setting in adults with acute lung injury and acute respiratory distress syndrome: a randomized controlled trial. JAMA 2008;299(6):646–55.

79. Briel M, Meade M, Mercat A, et al. Higher vs lower positive end-expiratory pressure in patients with acute lung injury and acute respiratory distress syndrome: systematic review and meta-analysis. JAMA 2010;303(9):865–73.

80. Santa Cruz R, Rojas JI, Nervi R, et al. High versus low positive end-expiratory pressure (PEEP) levels for mechanically ventilated adult patients with acute lung injury and acute respiratory distress syndrome. Cochrane Database Syst Rev 2013;(6):CD009098.

81. Amato MB, Barbas CS, Medeiros DM, et al. Effect of a protective-ventilation strategy on mortality in the acute respiratory distress syndrome. N Engl J Med 1998;338(6):347–54.

82. Villar J, Kacmarek RM, Perez-Mendez L, et al. A high positive end-expiratory pressure, low tidal volume ventilatory strategy improves outcome in persistent acute respiratory distress syndrome: a randomized, controlled trial. Crit Care Med 2006;34(5):1311–8.

83. Young D, Lamb SE, Shah S, et al. High-frequency oscillation for acute respiratory distress syndrome. N Engl J Med 2013;368(9):806–13.

84. Ferguson ND, Cook DJ, Guyatt GH, et al. High-frequency oscillation in early acute respiratory distress syndrome. N Engl J Med 2013;368(9):795–805.

85. Gupta P, Green JW, Tang X, et al. Comparison of high-frequency oscillatory ventilation and conventional mechanical ventilation in pediatric respiratory failure. JAMA Pediatr 2014;168(3):243–9.

86. Bateman ST, Borasino S, Asaro LA, et al. Early high-frequency oscillatory ventilation in pediatric acute respiratory failure. a propensity score analysis. Am J Respir Crit Care Med 2016;193(5):495–503.

87. Rossaint R, Falke KJ, Lopez F, et al. Inhaled nitric oxide for the adult respiratory distress syndrome. N Engl J Med 1993;328(6):399–405.

88. Adhikari NKJ, Burns KEA, Friedrich JO, et al. Effect of nitric oxide on oxygenation and mortality in acute lung injury: systematic review and meta-analysis. BMJ 2007;334(7597):779.

89. Adhikari NKJ, Dellinger RP, Lundin S, et al. Inhaled nitric oxide does not reduce mortality in patients with acute respiratory distress syndrome regardless of severity: systematic review and meta-analysis. Crit Care Med 2014;42(2): 404–12.

90. Afshari A, Brok J, Moller AM, et al. Inhaled nitric oxide for acute respiratory distress syndrome and acute lung injury in adults and children: a systematic review with meta-analysis and trial sequential analysis. Anesth Analg 2011;112(6): 1411–21.

91. Hunt JL, Bronicki RA, Anas N. Role of inhaled nitric oxide in the management of severe acute respiratory distress syndrome. Front Pediatr 2016;4:74.

92. Dobyns EL, Cornfield DN, Anas NG, et al. Multicenter randomized controlled trial of the effects of inhaled nitric oxide therapy on gas exchange in children with acute hypoxemic respiratory failure. J Pediatr 1999;134(4):406–12.

93. Day RW, Allen EM, Witte MK. A randomized, controlled study of the 1-hour and 24-hour effects of inhaled nitric oxide therapy in children with acute hypoxemic respiratory failure. Chest 1997;112(5):1324–31.

94. Ibrahim T, El-Mohamady H. Inhaled nitric oxide and prone position: how far they can improve oxygenation in pediatric patients with acute respiratory distress syndrome? J Med Sci 2007;7(3):390–5.

95. Bronicki RA, Fortenberry J, Schreiber M, et al. Multicenter randomized controlled trial of inhaled nitric oxide for pediatric acute respiratory distress syndrome. J Pediatr 2015;166(2):365–9.e1.

96. Schmidt R, Markart P, Ruppert C, et al. Time-dependent changes in pulmonary surfactant function and composition in acute respiratory distress syndrome due to pneumonia or aspiration. Respir Res 2007;8:55.

97. Spragg RG, Lewis JF, Walmrath H-D, et al. Effect of recombinant surfactant protein C-based surfactant on the acute respiratory distress syndrome. N Engl J Med 2004;351(9):884–92.

98. Taut FJH, Rippin G, Schenk P, et al. A search for subgroups of patients with ARDS who may benefit from surfactant replacement therapy: a pooled analysis of five studies with recombinant surfactant protein-C surfactant (Venticute). Chest 2008;134(4):724–32.

99. Spragg RG, Taut FJH, Lewis JF, et al. Recombinant surfactant protein C-based surfactant for patients with severe direct lung injury. Am J Respir Crit Care Med 2011;183(8):1055–61.

100. Willson DF, Thomas NJ, Markovitz BP, et al. Effect of exogenous surfactant (calfactant) in pediatric acute lung injury: a randomized controlled trial. JAMA 2005; 293(4):470–6.

101. Hermon MM, Golej J, Burda G, et al. Surfactant therapy in infants and children: three years experience in a pediatric intensive care unit. Shock 2002;17(4): 247–51.

102. Yapicioglu H, Yildizdas D, Bayram I, et al. The use of surfactant in children with acute respiratory distress syndrome: efficacy in terms of oxygenation, ventilation and mortality. Pulm Pharmacol Ther 2003;16(6):327–33.

103. Thomas NJ, Guardia CG, Moya FR, et al. A pilot, randomized, controlled clinical trial of lucinactant, a peptide-containing synthetic surfactant, in infants with acute hypoxemic respiratory failure. Pediatr Crit Care Med 2012;13(6):646–53.

104. Willson DF, Thomas NJ, Tamburro R, et al. Pediatric calfactant in acute respiratory distress syndrome trial. Pediatr Crit Care Med 2013;14(7):657–65.

105. Bein T, Grasso S, Moerer O, et al. The standard of care of patients with ARDS: ventilatory settings and rescue therapies for refractory hypoxemia. Intensive Care Med 2016;42(5):699–711.

106. Ingelse SA, Wosten-van Asperen RM, Lemson J, et al. Pediatric acute respiratory distress syndrome: fluid management in the PICU. Front Pediatr 2016;4:21.

107. Wiedemann HP, Wheeler AP, Bernard GR, et al. Comparison of two fluid-management strategies in acute lung injury. N Engl J Med 2006;354(24): 2564–75.

108. Kuzovlev A, Tishkov E, Bukaev O. Effect of continuous high-volume hemofiltration on patients with acute respiratory distress syndrome. Crit Care 2013;17: S160–1.

109. Flori HR, Church G, Liu KD, et al. Positive fluid balance is associated with higher mortality and prolonged mechanical ventilation in pediatric patients with acute lung injury. Crit Care Res Pract 2011;2011:854142.

110. Willson DF, Thomas NJ, Tamburro R, et al. The relationship of fluid administration to outcome in the pediatric calfactant in acute respiratory distress syndrome trial. Pediatr Crit Care Med 2013;14(7):666–72.

111. Hu X, Qian S, Xu F, et al. Incidence, management and mortality of acute hypoxemic respiratory failure and acute respiratory distress syndrome from a prospective study of Chinese paediatric intensive care network. Acta Paediatr 2010;99(5):715–21.

112. Valentine SL, Sapru A, Higgerson RA, et al. Fluid balance in critically ill children with acute lung injury. Crit Care Med 2012;40(10):2883–9.

113. Wilson B, Typpo K. Nutrition: a primary therapy in pediatric acute respiratory distress syndrome. Front Pediatr 2016;4:108.

114. Rice TW, Wheeler AP, Thompson BT, et al. Initial trophic vs full enteral feeding in patients with acute lung injury: the EDEN randomized trial. JAMA 2012;307(8): 795–803.

115. Sabater J, Masclans JR, Sacanell J, et al. Effects on hemodynamics and gas exchange of omega-3 fatty acid-enriched lipid emulsion in acute respiratory distress syndrome (ARDS): a prospective, randomized, double-blind, parallel group study. Lipids Health Dis 2008;7:39.

116. Sabater J, Masclans JR, Sacanell J, et al. Effects of an omega-3 fatty acid-enriched lipid emulsion on eicosanoid synthesis in acute respiratory distress syndrome (ARDS): a prospective, randomized, double-blind, parallel group study. Nutr Metab (Lond) 2011;8(1):22.

117. Yehya N, Servaes S, Thomas NJ, et al. Corticosteroid exposure in pediatric acute respiratory distress syndrome. Intensive Care Med 2015;41(9):1658–66.

118. Wong JJ-M, Loh TF, Testoni D, et al. Epidemiology of pediatric acute respiratory distress syndrome in Singapore: risk factors and predictive respiratory indices for mortality. Front Pediatr 2014;2:78.

119. Lim JKB, Lee JH, Cheifetz IM. Special considerations for the management of pediatric acute respiratory distress syndrome. Expert Rev Respir Med 2016; 10(10):1133–45.

120. Peter JV, John P, Graham PL, et al. Corticosteroids in the prevention and treatment of acute respiratory distress syndrome (ARDS) in adults: meta-analysis. BMJ 2008;336(7651):1006–9.

121. Tang BMP, Craig JC, Eslick GD, et al. Use of corticosteroids in acute lung injury and acute respiratory distress syndrome: a systematic review and meta-analysis. Crit Care Med 2009;37(5):1594–603.

122. Drago BB, Kimura D, Rovnaghi CR, et al. Double-blind, placebo-controlled pilot randomized trial of methylprednisolone infusion in pediatric acute respiratory distress syndrome. Pediatr Crit Care Med 2015;16(3):e74–81.

123. Tamburro RF, Kneyber MCJ. Pulmonary specific ancillary treatment for pediatric acute respiratory distress syndrome: proceedings from the pediatric acute lung injury consensus conference. Pediatr Crit Care Med 2015;16(5 Suppl 1):S61–72.

124. Walther S, Jansson I, Berg S, et al. Pulmonary granulocyte accumulation is reduced by nebulized corticosteroid in septic pigs. Acta Anaesthesiol Scand 1992;36(7):651–5.

125. Festic E, Ortiz-Diaz E, Lee A, et al. Prehospital use of inhaled steroids and incidence of acute lung injury among patients at risk. J Crit Care 2013;28(6): 985–91.

126. Yao S, Feng D, Wu Q, et al. Losartan attenuates ventilator-induced lung injury. J Surg Res 2008;145(1):25–32.

127. Di Paola R, Cuzzocrea S. Peroxisome proliferator-activated receptors and acute lung injury. PPAR Res 2007;2007:63745.

128. Orlicky S, Tang X, Neduva V, et al. An allosteric inhibitor of substrate recognition by the SCF(Cdc4) ubiquitin ligase. Nat Biotechnol 2010;28(7):733–7.

129. Eckle T, Brodsky K, Bonney M, et al. HIF1A reduces acute lung injury by optimizing carbohydrate metabolism in the alveolar epithelium. PLoS Biol 2013; 11(9):e1001665.

130. Soo Hoo GW. In prone ventilation, one good turn deserves another. N Engl J Med 2013;368(23):2227–8.

131. Gattinoni L, Tognoni G, Pesenti A, et al. Effect of prone positioning on the survival of patients with acute respiratory failure. N Engl J Med 2001;345(8): 568–73.

132. Mok YH, Lee JH, Rehder KJ, et al. Adjunctive treatments in pediatric acute respiratory distress syndrome. Expert Rev Respir Med 2014;8(6):703–16.

133. Gattinoni L, Vagginelli F, Carlesso E, et al. Decrease in PaCO2 with prone position is predictive of improved outcome in acute respiratory distress syndrome. Crit Care Med 2003;31(12):2727–33.

134. Guerin C, Gaillard S, Lemasson S, et al. Effects of systematic prone positioning in hypoxemic acute respiratory failure: a randomized controlled trial. JAMA 2004;292(19):2379–87.

135. Taccone P, Pesenti A, Latini R, et al. Prone positioning in patients with moderate and severe acute respiratory distress syndrome: a randomized controlled trial. JAMA 2009;302(18):1977–84.

136. Sud S, Sud M, Friedrich JO, et al. Effect of mechanical ventilation in the prone position on clinical outcomes in patients with acute hypoxemic respiratory failure: a systematic review and meta-analysis. CMAJ 2008;178(9):1153–61.
137. Curley MAQ, Hibberd PL, Fineman LD, et al. Effect of prone positioning on clinical outcomes in children with acute lung injury: a randomized controlled trial. JAMA 2005;294(2):229–37.
138. Guerin C, Reignier J, Richard J-C, et al. Prone positioning in severe acute respiratory distress syndrome. N Engl J Med 2013;368(23):2159–68.
139. Papazian L, Forel J-M, Gacouin A, et al. Neuromuscular blockers in early acute respiratory distress syndrome. N Engl J Med 2010;363(12):1107–16.
140. Bartlett RH, Gazzaniga AB, Jefferies MR, et al. Extracorporeal membrane oxygenation (ECMO) cardiopulmonary support in infancy. Trans Am Soc Artif Intern Organs 1976;22:80–93.
141. Lewandowski K. Extracorporeal membrane oxygenation for severe acute respiratory failure. Crit Care 2000;4(3):156–68.
142. Peek GJ, Mugford M, Tiruvoipati R, et al. Efficacy and economic assessment of conventional ventilatory support versus extracorporeal membrane oxygenation for severe adult respiratory failure (CESAR): a multicentre randomised controlled trial. Lancet 2009;374(9698):1351–63.
143. Pranikoff T, Hirschl RB, Steimle CN, et al. Mortality is directly related to the duration of mechanical ventilation before the initiation of extracorporeal life support for severe respiratory failure. Crit Care Med 1997;25(1):28–32.
144. Beiderlinden M, Eikermann M, Boes T, et al. Treatment of severe acute respiratory distress syndrome: role of extracorporeal gas exchange. Intensive Care Med 2006;32(10):1627–31.
145. Mols G, Loop T, Geiger K, et al. Extracorporeal membrane oxygenation: a ten-year experience. Am J Surg 2000;180(2):144–54.
146. Lewandowski K, Rossaint R, Pappert D, et al. High survival rate in 122 ARDS patients managed according to a clinical algorithm including extracorporeal membrane oxygenation. Intensive Care Med 1997;23(8):819–35.
147. Brodie D, Bacchetta M. Extracorporeal membrane oxygenation for ARDS in adults. N Engl J Med 2011;365(20):1905–14.
148. Zabrocki LA, Brogan TV, Statler KD, et al. Extracorporeal membrane oxygenation for pediatric respiratory failure: survival and predictors of mortality. Crit Care Med 2011;39(2):364–70.
149. Nance ML, Nadkarni VM, Hedrick HL, et al. Effect of preextracorporeal membrane oxygenation ventilation days and age on extracorporeal membrane oxygenation survival in critically ill children. J Pediatr Surg 2009;44(8):1606–10.
150. Fan E, Villar J, Slutsky AS. Novel approaches to minimize ventilator-induced lung injury. BMC Med 2013;11:85.
151. Morelli A, Del Sorbo L, Pesenti A, et al. Extracorporeal carbon dioxide removal (ECCO2R) in patients with acute respiratory failure. Intensive Care Med 2017; 43(4):519–30.
152. Marhong JD, Munshi L, Detsky M, et al. Mechanical ventilation during extracorporeal life support (ECLS): a systematic review. Intensive Care Med 2015;41(6): 994–1003.
153. Dalton HJ, Macrae DJ. Extracorporeal support in children with pediatric acute respiratory distress syndrome: proceedings from the pediatric acute lung injury consensus conference. Pediatr Crit Care Med 2015;16(5 Suppl 1):S111–7.

Ventilator-Associated Pneumonia in Critically Ill Children: A New Paradigm

Peter M. Mourani, MD[a],*, Marci K. Sontag, PhD[b]

KEYWORDS

- Ventilator-associated pneumonia • Mechanical ventilation • Microbiome
- Metagenomics • Pediatric intensive care

KEY POINTS

- Surveillance definitions for ventilator-associated pneumonia (VAP) are in the process of being updated. Further evaluation is needed to assure that the patients who are most amenable to targeted prevention strategies are identified.
- VAP is the most common indication for antibiotic use in the pediatric intensive care unit. Present approaches to clinical cultures and antibiotic use may actually increase risk for VAP by depleting protective commensal organisms and selecting for antibiotic resistant pathogens.
- Recent metagenomic and proteomic technologies offer the potential to better interrogate the relationships between an intubated individual's respiratory microbiota, the host's immune response, and the underlying disease process to provide important insights into the pathogenesis of VAP.
- The normal lung is colonized with diverse microbial communities. It seems likely that critical illness and its care contribute to a dysbiosis and the selection of a disease-promoting microbiome or pathobiome that increases risk for nosocomial infection, including VAP.

INTRODUCTION

Mechanically ventilated children are at high risk for nosocomial infections, including ventilator-associated pneumonia (VAP). Children who develop VAP have an increased risk of mortality[1] and morbidities such as prolonged intubation and intensive care unit (ICU) stays and the need for extensive rehabilitation.[2] VAP is the most common nosocomial infection in mechanically ventilated patients,[1] occurring in up to 32% of pediatric ICU (PICU) patients who require mechanical ventilation (MV) for more than

Disclosure: The authors have no financial relationships or conflicts of interest to report.
[a] Section of Critical Care, Department of Pediatrics, University of Colorado Denver, School of Medicine, Children's Hospital Colorado, 13121 East 17th Avenue, MS8414, Aurora, CO 80045, USA; [b] Department of Epidemiology, Colorado School of Public Health, University of Colorado Denver Anschutz Medical Campus, 13001 East 17th, B119, Aurora, CO 80045, USA
* Corresponding author.
E-mail address: Peter.Mourani@childrenscolorado.org

24 hours.[3,4] VAP is associated with a 2-fold to 3-fold increase in mortality in ventilated children,[5,6] and increases total hospitalization costs and resource utilization, increasing duration of MV by 5 to 11 days and PICU length of stay by 11 to 34 days.[3,4,6,7] The suspicion and/or the diagnosis of VAP remain the primary reason for antibiotic administration in the PICU.[8] Thus, VAP remains a significant obstacle to the management of pediatric critical illnesses and injuries.

The traditional view of the pathogenesis of pneumonia was based on the premise that the lung was sterile, and that infection occurred by the introduction of pathogens either by direct inoculation from the environment or through the blood stream. However, recent evidence has revealed that the lungs contain diverse microbial populations.[9,10] The endogenous microbiota are likely critical regulators of both pathogen behavior and host responses in the airways. Infection, therefore, occurs as a result of the combination of dysbiosis and failure of the host immune response. Because the lungs are inhabited by microbial populations (akin to the intestinal tract albeit in far lower density,[9–12]), the simple paradigm of a single pathogen gaining access to a sterile lower respiratory tract to cause infection has evolved. Pathogens are introduced to a pre-existing and often complex microbial community[9,11] that either allows, facilitates, or hinders the potential pathogen, and consequently determines whether progression to VAP occurs. Limited understanding of the microbial and host factors associated with VAP pathogenesis has precluded development of truly effective prevention and treatment strategies.[13,14]

This article briefly discusses the changing criteria by which VAP is diagnosed and the limitations of these definitions for both surveillance and clinical research attempting to identify risk factors for and the pathogenesis of VAP. It also discusses the prospects for a deeper understanding of the pathogenesis of VAP in the new era of metagenomics and proteomics, together with the recent evidence about the role of microbiome in health and disease.

SURVEILLANCE DEFINITION

In the absence of a readily available microbiologic gold standard, standardized clinical criteria for VAP were first developed in 2002 by the Centers for Disease Control (CDC) and National Nosocomial Infections Surveillance (NNIS) to allow for consistent diagnosis and reporting.[15] The CDC/NNIS definitions, which underwent some minor modifications during the subsequent decade, relied on combinations of radiographic, clinical, and laboratory evidence in the consideration of a VAP diagnosis. Because traditional culture from respiratory samples depends on the chosen medium, positive cultures from these methods were optional parts of the pediatric criteria.[16–19] When rigorously applied, CDC/NNIS VAP criteria have been shown to be associated with predictably poor outcomes.[20–22] However, application of these criteria is time-consuming and inconsistent because definitions of components of the criteria are subjective and imprecise.[23,24] Several studies demonstrate this variability. Among 64 PICUs reporting data to CDC's National Healthcare Safety Network (NHSN) between 2007 and 2012, the incidence of VAP decreased from 1.9 to 0.7 per 1000 ventilator-days.[25] However, other published prospective pediatric studies report rates as high as 7.1 per 1000 ventilator-days in the United States.[6] That different studies report markedly different VAP rates suggest that diverse populations of children have unique risk for VAP or that interpretation of the criteria by investigators is subjective. Similarly, from 2006 to 2012, adult medical ICUs reporting data to NHSN demonstrated a decline in VAP rates from 3.1 to 0.9 per 1000 ventilator-days, whereas other evaluations have concluded that VAP rates have not declined during this period with a consistent rate of approximately 10% of ventilated patients.[26] The data suggested that surveillance using previous definitions may be unreliable, and efforts to identify more objective and consistently applied VAP criteria are justified.

A comprehensive revision of the VAP criteria was undertaken by the CDC/NNIS in 2013 to develop a more objective and easily applied definition. The revision created a 3-tier definition algorithm for ventilator-associated events (VAEs). The first tier, ventilator-associated condition (VAC), defines mechanically ventilated patients following a sustained period of stability or improvement after intubation who then experience a sustained respiratory deterioration (defined by elevations in positive-end expiratory pressure [PEEP] or fractional inspired oxygen [Fio_2]). The second tier, infectious VAC (IVAC), describes patients with VAC and evidence of infection defined by changes in temperature or white blood cell count (WBC) and the clinician's decision to initiate antibiotics. The third tier defines possible and probable VAP and requires that patients with IVAC also have laboratory and/or microbiological evidence of respiratory infection (**Table 1**).[27]

These definitions were only implemented for adult patients, whereas the diagnosis of VAP in children continues to use the older criteria. Recent efforts by the CDC's Pediatric Ventilator-Associated Pneumonia Surveillance Definition Working Group, based on work by the Pediatric Ventilator-Associated Conditions Study Team,[28] have resulted in a new set of definitions patterned after the adult criteria. The main difference is that pediatric VAC determination is based on elevation of mean airway pressure as opposed to PEEP, and the threshold increase in Fio_2 is 0.25 versus 0.2 in adults.[29] The pediatric definition eliminated temperature and WBC because most patients with VAC met the derangement thresholds in these categories. Thus, instead of a category of IVAC, the pediatric criteria suggest categories of (1) pediatric VAC with antimicrobial use (pediatric AVAC), and (2) antimicrobial VAC with a positive respiratory diagnostic test (pediatric PVAP). This proposal is being pilot tested in select centers in 2017 with a goal of full implementation in 2018.

There have been few studies comparing the application of these definitions. In a single-center retrospective study of 58 children ventilated longer than 48 hours, 70 evaluations for different definitions of ventilator-associated infection were applied. Six subjects met the 2008 CDC/NHSN pediatric VAP definition, and 5 met the 2013 adult IVAC definition. Only 1 subject satisfied both definitions.[30] In another single-center prospective study conducted over a 6-month period that included 325 invasively ventilated children, application of the new 2013 adult VAE criteria resulted in 7 subjects classified with VAC, 6 with IVAC, and 3 with possible VAP. By comparison, 4 had VAP based on 2008 pediatric CDC definitions.[31] The investigators did not comment on the overlap between definitions. In an unpublished review of a cohort of 133 critically ill children ventilated for longer than 72 hours at our center (Mourani, PM and Sontag, MK), we found 12 (9%) met 2013 adult VAC criteria, of whom 5 met IVAC and 1 met possible VAP criteria. In comparison, only 5 met the newly proposed pediatric VAC criteria (no subjects satisfied the pediatric possible or probable VAP definition), whereas 27 subjects (20%) met the 2008 pediatric CDC VAP criteria. Only 5 of the 12 adult VAC criteria subjects and 3 of the 5 proposed pediatric VAC subjects met the 2008 pediatric CDC VAP criteria. In contrast, 22 of 27 subjects diagnosed by 2008 pediatric CDC VAP criteria met neither the 2013 adult nor the newly proposed CDC pediatric VAC criteria. Thus, these definitions seem to identify different cohorts of children with seemingly little overlap. All seem to be associated with worse outcomes, including increased duration of MV and length of stay. The question remains which criteria identifies the subjects who are most amenable to targeted prevention strategies.

Table 1
Comparison of recent surveillance definitions for ventilator-associated pneumonia

Criteria	Chest Radiograph Changes	Respiratory Deterioration	Temperature	White Cell Count	Antibiotic Therapy	Microbiological Evidence
2008 Pediatric Criteria	New or increasing infiltrates. consolidation, or cavitation (need to be present ≥2 radiographs for patients with pre-existing lung disease), consolidation	Combination of nonspecific worsening of gas exchange and clinical evidence of increased secretions, cough, and rales	>38.5°C or <36.5°C	≤4000 or ≥15,000 cells/mL	NA	Can be used but not required
2013 Adult Criteria[a]	NA	—	—	—	—	—
VAC	—	Increase in Fio_2 ≥0.2 or PEEP ≥3 cm H_2O	NA	NA	—	—
IVAC	—	Increase in Fio_2 ≥0.2 or PEEP ≥3 cm H_2O	>38° or <36° C	≤4000 or ≥12,000 cells/mL	New agent started and continued ≥4 d	—
Possible VAP	—	Increase in Fio_2 ≥0.2 or PEEP ≥3 cm H_2O	>38°C or <36°C	≤4000 or ≥12,000 cells/mL	New agent started and continued ≥4 d	Purulent respiratory secretions or positive respiratory specimen culture

Probable VAP	—	Increase in Fio2 ≥0.2 or PEEP ≥3 cm H2O	>38°C or <36°C	<4000 or ≥12,000 cells/mL	New agent started and continued ≥4 d	Purulent respiratory secretions and positive quantitative respiratory specimen culture or positive pleural culture, lung histopathology, legionella test, or viral test
2017 Pediatric VAP Criteria[a]	NA	NA	NA	NA	—	—
VAC	—	Increase in Fio2 ≥0.25 or MAP ≥4 cm H2O	—	—	—	—
AVAC	—	Increase in Fio2 ≥0.25 or MAP ≥4 cm H2O	—	—	New agent started and continued ≥4 d	—
VAP	—	Increase in Fio2 ≥0.25 or MAP ≥4 cm H2O	—	—	New agent started and continued ≥4 d	Same criteria as adult possible or probable VAP

Abbreviations: AVAC, antimicrobial VAC; MAP, mean airway pressure; NA, not applicable.

[a] Patient has a baseline period of stability or improvement on the ventilator, defined by 2 or more days of stable or decreasing daily minimum Fio2, PEEP (for adult), or MAP (for pediatric) values. The baseline period is defined as the 2 calendar days immediately preceding the first day of increased daily minimum Fio2, PEEP (adult), or MAP (pediatric).

RISK FACTORS FOR VENTILATOR-ASSOCIATED PNEUMONIA

The airway microbiome may play a major role in regulating both bacterial pathogen outgrowth and host immune responses.[32] As such, risk factors for developing VAP primarily affect airway colonization or the host response, including sedation or neuromuscular blockers that suppress the cough reflex, duration of MV, continuous enteral nutrition, antibiotic exposures, immunosuppression, and foreign bodies in the airway (bronchoscopy and replacement of the endotracheal tube).[3,4,6,7,33–35] Although enteral nutrition was identified as a risk factor in some of these studies, a prospective cohort study including 1245 subjects from an international group of PICUs did not find an association between the route of delivery or duration of enteral nutrition and VAP. However, they did find that the use of acid-suppression medications was associated with increase in the odds of developing VAP.[36]

The relationship between acid-suppression and VAP has been examined in multiple studies in adults. These studies have yielded inconsistent findings. In a case-control study evaluating potential risk factors for VAP in adults, stress ulcer prophylaxis was not found to be associated with risk for VAP.[37] A recent randomized controlled study of pantoprazole or placebo in ventilated adults who were suitable for enteral nutrition found no difference in the rate of VAP.[38] In contrast, a meta-analysis conducted in 2011 found that use of either proton pump inhibitor or histamine-2 receptor antagonists increases the risk of hospital-acquired pneumonias.[39] Few studies have directly examined the relationship between acid suppression and changes in the gastric microbial content, which many have hypothesized as a possible mechanism by which acid suppression alters risk for VAP. In studies of general proton pump inhibitor use, increases in gastric pH have been associated with gastric bacterial overgrowth.[40] One meta-analysis comparing histamine-2 receptor antagonists to sucralfate for ulcer prophylaxis in mechanically ventilated adults found that VAP was decreased among the subjects treated with sucralfate.[41] They also found that sucralfate use had lower rates of gastric colonization (quantitative culture of at least 1 gastric specimen had more than 100 colony-forming units/mL) compared with histamine-2 receptor antagonist use. In a study examining the gastric and oropharyngeal microbiota via traditional culture techniques in elderly subjects fed via nasogastric tubes, the investigators found remarkable similarity in the bacterial communities isolated from both sites.[42] Isolation of pathogenic bacteria was correlated with higher pH of gastric specimens, suggesting that acid suppression may lead to higher risk of pneumonia due to aspiration. Recent applications of molecular microbial identification will likely advance the pace of such investigations.

THE IMPACT OF OMICS TECHNOLOGY ON INFECTION-RELATED RESEARCH

The historical approach to diagnosis and treatment of infections relies on cultivation of the infecting organism. The 1 organism–1 disease paradigm for microbial involvement in disease has been successful for diagnosis and treatment of many acute infectious diseases. However, this paradigm may not adequately apply to all acute pneumonias, especially in the context of VAP, which may occur as a superinfection to a community-acquired bacterial or viral lower respiratory tract infection (LRTI). For critically ill children on mechanical ventilators, targeting a single microbe isolated from a tracheal aspirate or other lung specimen can be misleading because it overlooks the complex process by which that organism arrived in the lower airways and its role in disease.

Study of the microbiome, the genomic content of the microbiota, is a novel approach to expand understanding of the complexities of human environments normally colonized with microbial communities, such as the gut and the lung. Although genomics is the study of the DNA content of an organism, metagenomics applies genomic technologies and bioinformatics tools to study all the genomes recovered from a specific environmental sample. In reference to human health, this emerging powerful set of tools analyzes nucleic acids isolated from specimens collected from organ systems to provide simultaneous and sensitive quantification of the bacterial, fungal, and viral constituents of the microbiome.[43–48] One approach to identification of the microbial constituents of a sample is called shotgun sequencing. With this technique, DNA extracted from a sample is randomly sheared, and the resulting short sequences (>700 base pairs) are deciphered and then reconstructed into a consensus sequence that is aligned to known genomic databases to identify the organism from which it was extracted. Next-generation sequencing (NGS), using platforms such as the Illumina MiSeq or HiSeq (Illumina Inc, San Diego, CA), generate much shorter DNA fragments (<700 base pairs), but the limitation is offset by the significantly larger number of sequence reads generated. NGS is now the most often used technology because it has become the most economical choice. Many studies of human health have focused only on the bacterial constituents of the microbiota, acknowledging the limited contribution of viruses and fungi in many of the human compartments. For these studies, an even cheaper and more rapid sequencing alternative to NGS entails sequencing of the 16S rRNA gene of bacteria, which is highly conserved between different species but also contains hypervariable regions that presents species-specific signature sequences for identification of bacteria.

There are several bioinformatics processes that are required to decipher the large data generated by these technologies. For example, a human gut microbiome project identified 3.3 million genes assembled from more than 565 gigabases.[49] The initial sequence reads contain many redundant, low-quality, and human sequences that need to be removed in a filtering step before being inserted in to assembly programs that constructs the reads into specific genomes. Once assembled into genomes, the data are moved through informatics pipelines to determine which sequences belong to which species from the sample. Identification is performed through 2 main techniques. The first matches sequences to those that are already publicly available in sequence databases. For microbes that lack matching homologous sequences in these databases, the second method uses intrinsic characteristics of the sequences to predict the coding regions of bacterial species.

Many diseases have now been associated with changes in composition of bacterial communities in the gut.[50–52] Specifically, microbiota of limited diversity and relative absence of commensal organisms are associated with increased inflammation, barrier permeability, and disease states.[53,54] Metagenomic techniques applied to investigations of the lung have demonstrated that the lungs of healthy children and adults are rich with bacteria, contradicting the traditional theory that human lower airways are sterile.[9,10,12] These studies also demonstrate that microbial communities play an important role in human physiology.[55–58] The gut microbiota in children has been shown to have a strong influence on the development and function of the immune system and has been postulated to modulate the risk of subsequent asthma risk in infants infected with respiratory syncytial virus.[59]

In addition to molecular detection of microbial communities, metagenomics can facilitate investigations of the host response to the microbiome by providing simultaneous evaluations of both the microbial and human messenger RNA (mRNA), also known as the transcriptome. Further, comprehensive proteomic and metabolomic evaluations have the potential to add considerable depth to these investigations by not only detecting the presence of organisms but also by describing what they are doing and how they are interacting with each other and the host.[60] Proteomics refers to the study of the structure and function of proteins within cells, tissues, and organisms.

Analogous to the microbiome, the proteome refers to all expressed proteins in a specific environment, typically a cell, tissue, or organism. All organisms produce small molecules (<1200 Da), known as metabolites, that are by-products of life-sustaining biochemical process. Metabolomics is the study of these small molecules in relation to the physiology or pathophysiology of organisms. Mass spectroscopy is the usual method to identify proteins and metabolites. In this method, ions are generated from proteins or metabolites, which can be used to separate them according to their mass-to-charge ratio to create a mass spectrum. Several analytical techniques, each with their respective advantages and limitations may be used to identify specific proteins or metabolites. Application of these strategies to investigations of the intestinal tract generated the concept that dysbiosis leads to generation of disease-promoting microbiome or pathobiome,[61] increasing risk for infection, as well as promoting perturbations of the immune system and persistent organ dysfunction.[60] Combining these approaches simultaneously has been used in a study of subjects with human immunodeficiency virus and pneumonia, in which the investigators identified that the composition of the lower airway microbiome is associated with discrete local host immune responses and systemic metabolic signatures.[32] Further, these complex phenotypes were directly associated with mortality.

Translating these approaches to interrogate the relationships between an intubated individual's respiratory microbiota, the host's immune response, and the underlying disease process will likely provide important insights into the pathogenesis of VAP, help identify at-risk children early in the course of illness, and suggest new and more effective prevention and therapeutic strategies to improve outcomes and reduce resource utilization and costs.

MICROBIAL INTERACTIONS AFFECTING RISK FOR VENTILATOR-ASSOCIATED PNEUMONIA

Emerging evidence about how organisms interact with each other (including viral-bacterial interactions), environmental elements, and the host have shed light on the enormous complexity of infection pathogenesis. Microorganisms have evolved the ability to detect local environmental signals such pH, metabolites, microbial population density (quorum sensing), and host immune cells.[62–64] These sensing mechanisms allow pathogens to regulate expression of their virulence factors, masking infection until the advantage to them is greatest. Bacteria can also express structural appendages and secrete products that bind pathogen-recognition receptors on epithelial cells, which then transduce specific downstream pathways that impair local and systemic immune function.[65] Critical illness alone has been demonstrated to alter the intestinal microbiome by diminishing populations and activity of commensal bacteria.[66] Pathogen populations then proliferate as a result of unimpeded strategies to either evade detection of the host or render immune cells ineffective.[67] The impact of changes in the microbiome and bacterial virulence has not yet been routinely incorporated into the approach to infection.[68]

Numerous studies have demonstrated that viral LRTIs are frequently associated with bacterial pneumonia, including VAP and invasive bacterial infections.[69–76] The highest rates of bacterial coinfections occur in patients admitted to the ICU.[73] Pneumococcal vaccine provides protection against influenza-related hospitalization,[77] suggesting an important role for the bacterial infection in determining the severity of illness in viral LRTI. Among children admitted to the PICU with influenza during the 2009 pandemic, those with *Staphylococcus aureus* coinfection had a higher mortality risk.[78] Rhinovirus infection in chronic obstructive pulmonary disease (COPD) patients is associated with an increase in the bacterial load of *Haemophilus influenza*, suggesting that viral infection increases risk of secondary bacterial pneumonia.[79]

Historically, this complication of viral infection has been attributed to degradation of epithelial barrier function by direct cytopathologic effects of the virus. Recent work, however, has strongly implicated endogenous immune suppressive pathways that limit inflammation-mediated damage and may permit bacterial outgrowth from the microbiota into clinical infection.[80–84] Understanding the delicate balance between the immune activation required to clear infections and the immune suppression needed to reduce excessive inflammation-mediated damage is critically important for targeting new strategies to reduce VAP and its associated morbidity and mortality (**Fig. 1**).

THE MICROBIOME AND HOST IMMUNE RESPONSE

The microbiome has a critical role in immune activation and host defense against infections. The gut microbiome is crucial for priming of defenses against infection not only in the gastrointestinal tract but also in distant organs, including the lung.[83,85] Inflammasomes, receptors that regulate the activation of caspase-1 and propagate inflammatory responses to infectious organisms and molecules derived from the host, are recognized to be vital elements of host defense and innate immunity. Recent evidence suggests that systemic priming of inflammasome activation by endogenous microbes changes the set point of innate immune responses to respiratory infection, in effect priming host immune response.[83,86] This process involves activation of signaling via toll-like receptors, which then leads to production of type I interferon (INF) and the precursor molecules pro-interleukin (IL)-1β and pro-IL-18. A second insult, perhaps other products of damaged tissues, then activates caspase-1 and caspase-mediated cleavage of the pro-forms into active IL-1β and IL-18, which are released from the cell and upregulate several key cytokines and chemokines (a subfamily of cytokines that serve as chemotactic factors for different cell types). Animal models suggest that viral infections suppress immune responses and increase risk

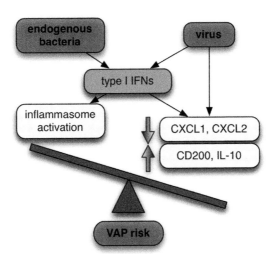

Fig. 1. Endogenous airway bacteria achieve a balance between host immune activation and suppression. Deleterious shifts in the airway ecology likely lead to VAP. Viral infection (and many other triggering factors) may initiate these shifts by suppressing host immune responses that control the bacterial populations and prevent emergence of pathogens. CXCL, of chemokine ligand; IL, interleukin; INF, interferon.

of bacterial infection. Influenza virus infections induce highly polarized type 1 T helper cell responses, producing large amounts of INF-γ and IL-10.[84] In mouse models, INF-γ contributes to postviral immune suppression by impeding alveolar macrophage function, leading to reduced bacterial clearance.[87] Influenza-mediated type I INF production also attenuates production of chemokine ligand (CXCL)-1 and CXCL2, impairing neutrophil responses and predisposing to secondary bacterial infection.[88] CD200 ligand is a membrane glycoprotein expressed on epithelial cells or other apoptotic cells that activates CD200 receptor (R) on airway macrophages, suppressing their activity. Expression of CD200 and CD200R are increased in experimental animals with viral respiratory infection, and CD200R knockout mice are less susceptible to postviral bacterial infection, suggesting that the CD200 system is a critical mediator of postviral immune suppression.[89] Commensal microbes, in particular *Staphylococcal* species, attenuate the immune-mediated lung injury and cytokine storm triggered by influenza infection by promoting the M2 immune-suppressive macrophage phenotype in airway and alveolar macrophages, leading to increased production of IL-10 and transforming growth factor (TGF)-β, and improved survival.[90] IL-10 and TGF-β have also been implicated in bacterial superinfection in other studies.[91,92] In addition to priming the immune system to prevent infection, the airway microbiota may also modulate the response to established infection. Microbial interactions with the host immune system are quite complex and may also depend on timing of exposure. For example, as these data suggest, *Staphylococcus* may prime the immune system to protect the host from influenza infection, but other studies (as previously noted) suggest that influenza and *Staphylococcal* coinfections portend a higher risk of mortality. These relationships deserve further study.

APPLICATION OF THE NEW INFECTION PARADIGM TO VENTILATOR-ASSOCIATED PNEUMONIA

Ventilator-associated tracheobronchitis can be an intermediate step between airway dysbiosis and the development of VAP,[93–95] suggesting that investigations of the changing ecology of the large airways in relation to infection are likely to augment understanding of the pathogenesis of VAP. The gold standard VAP diagnostic method of biopsy and direct culture of lung tissue is not possible for most ventilated children due to its invasive nature and risks. Yet, traditional endotracheal aspirate culture techniques are imprecise and have led to wide-spread antibiotic use, a practice which could select for drug-resistant pathogens in the airway and in other body compartments.[96–98] VAP is the most common indication for antibiotic use in the PICU, accounting for almost half of all antibiotic days.[8] Yet, rather than mitigating the adverse impact of VAP, present approaches to clinical cultures and antibiotic use may actually increase risk for VAP on an individual and unit level by depleting protective commensal organisms and selecting for antibiotic resistant pathogens. The increasing rates of antimicrobial resistance among VAP pathogens now lead many clinicians to empirically treat suspected VAP patients with a combination of broad-spectrum antibiotics, which likely perpetuates the cycle of increasing antibiotic resistance and persistent dysbiosis of the host microbiome.

To break this adverse cycle, a new paradigm is desperately needed. Moving beyond traditional culture methodologies to simultaneous employment of metagenomics, proteomics, and metabolomics will arm clinicians with critical information that has been previously unavailable. When the host organism is disturbed by disease, the profile of proteome and metabolome often changes. These changes may be in response to chronic disease that may render the host susceptible to infection or to a primary infection that may then promote organ dysfunction. Thus, simultaneous study of the proteome and metabolome along with the microbiome, may enable the discovery of biomarkers that further understanding of predisease and disease states. These data may better inform when infection is present and by what pathogens, as well as identify the risk before infection is present and point to strategies that can effectively prevent infection by restoring commensal microbial communities, strengthening the host immune response, and suppressing emergence of the detrimental pathobiome.

Early evaluations of the respiratory tract microbiota in pulmonary diseases, such as cystic fibrosis, asthma, COPD, and lung transplant,[9–11,48,99–105] reveal shifts in bacterial ecology compared with healthy patients, suggesting that the composition of the respiratory tract microbiota plays a direct role in pathophysiology of lung disease. Based on these observations, it is not unreasonable to assume that similar conclusions can be drawn for mechanically ventilated patients at risk for VAP. In fact, early application of molecular detection methods to mechanically ventilated ICU patients suggests this may be the case.[106] The authors have been evaluating changes in the airway microbiome in mechanically ventilated children. We have found that airway samples collected on intubation exhibit a relatively diverse bacterial community; however, diversity decreases in samples collected in subsequent days and the airways can rapidly become dominated by pathogenic bacteria before diagnosis of VAP (**Fig. 2**). Identification of diminishing diversity and emergence of potential pathogens

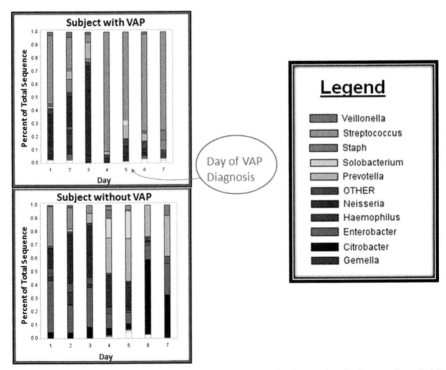

Fig. 2. Bacterial composition of tracheal aspirate samples in mechanically ventilated children as determined through 16S rRNA detection. Each bar represents a day of ventilation with relative abundance of organisms at the genus level described by the different colors. Tracheal aspirate samples are relatively diverse on intubation but may decrease over time with pathogenic bacteria dominating the community before diagnosis of VAP, Staph, Staphylococcus.

before infections occur may allow caregivers the opportunity to modulate the microbiota to increase diversity and/or limit specific pathogen outgrowth. Yet, the variability in community composition, the virulence of the pathogens involved, and the host responses belies the concept that a single approach will universally apply to all patients. Application of this new paradigm, incorporating simultaneous assessments of microbial populations and their activity, as well as the host response, may enable a personalized strategy, uniquely suited to individual patients.

SUMMARY

Despite some evidence that VAP incidence is decreasing, other data suggest that it remains a common and detrimental complication of MV support in children and is the main indication for antibiotic use in the PICU. The limitations of traditional microbial culture techniques and the lack of reliable and consistently applied diagnostic criteria have hampered the progress of understanding the pathogenesis of VAP and, thus, truly effective strategies to prevent this nosocomial infection. However, evolution of metagenomic and proteomic technologies has opened the doors to new investigations that have changed the paradigm by which infections and their impact on human health are understood. These studies have demonstrated that VAP likely results from a complex interaction of microbes, the environment, and the host immune response. Future studies evaluating the mechanisms of these interactions will improve understanding of the pathogenesis of VAP (and pneumonia, in general), enable identification of at-risk patients early in the course of MV, and suggest specific preventive and therapeutic interventions to improve outcomes in this high-risk population.

REFERENCES

1. Raymond J, Aujard Y. Nosocomial infections in pediatric patients: a European, multicenter prospective study. European Study Group. Infect Control Hosp Epidemiol 2000;21(4):260–3.
2. Foglia EE, Fraser VJ, Elward AM. Effect of nosocomial infections due to antibiotic-resistant organisms on length of stay and mortality in the pediatric intensive care unit. Infect Control Hosp Epidemiol 2007;28(3):299–306.
3. Srinivasan R, Asselin J, Gildengorin G, et al. A prospective study of ventilator-associated pneumonia in children. Pediatrics 2009;123(4):1108–15.
4. Elward AM, Warren DK, Fraser VJ. Ventilator-associated pneumonia in pediatric intensive care unit patients: risk factors and outcomes. Pediatrics 2002;109(5): 758–64.
5. Bigham MT, Amato R, Bondurrant P, et al. Ventilator-associated pneumonia in the pediatric intensive care unit: characterizing the problem and implementing a sustainable solution. J Pediatr 2009;154(4):582–7.e2.
6. Gupta S, Boville BM, Blanton R, et al. A multicentered prospective analysis of diagnosis, risk factors, and outcomes associated with pediatric ventilator-associated pneumonia. Pediatr Crit Care Med 2015;16(3):e65–73.
7. Almuneef M, Memish ZA, Balkhy HH, et al. Ventilator-associated pneumonia in a pediatric intensive care unit in Saudi Arabia: a 30-month prospective surveillance. Infect Control Hosp Epidemiol 2004;25(9):753–8.
8. Fischer JE, Ramser M, Fanconi S. Use of antibiotics in pediatric intensive care and potential savings. Intensive Care Med 2000;26(7):959–66.
9. Hilty M, Burke C, Pedro H, et al. Disordered microbial communities in asthmatic airways. PLoS One 2010;5(1):e8578.

10. Sze MA, Dimitriu PA, Hayashi S, et al. The lung tissue microbiome in chronic obstructive pulmonary disease. Am J Respir Crit Care Med 2012;185(10): 1073–80.

11. Erb-Downward JR, Thompson DL, Han MK, et al. Analysis of the lung microbiome in the "healthy" smoker and in COPD. PLoS One 2011;6(2):e16384.

12. Charlson ES, Bittinger K, Haas AR, et al. Topographical continuity of bacterial populations in the healthy human respiratory tract. Am J Respir Crit Care Med 2011;184(8):957–63.

13. Foglia E, Meier MD, Elward A. Ventilator-associated pneumonia in neonatal and pediatric intensive care unit patients. Clin Microbiol Rev 2007;20(3):409–25.

14. Venkatachalam V, Hendley JO, Willson DF. The diagnostic dilemma of ventilator-associated pneumonia in critically ill children. Pediatr Crit Care Med 2011;12(3): 286–96.

15. Centers for Disease Control and Prevention guidelines: guidelines and procedures for monitoring VAP. 2013. Available at: http://www.cdc.gov/nhsn/PDFs/pscManual/6pscVAPcurrent.pdf. Accessed September 6, 2013.

16. Gauvin F, Dassa C, Chaïbou M, et al. Ventilator-associated pneumonia in intubated children: comparison of different diagnostic methods. Pediatr Crit Care Med 2003;4(4):437–43.

17. Labenne M, Poyart C, Rambaud C, et al. Blind protected specimen brush and bronchoalveolar lavage in ventilated children. Crit Care Med 1999;27(11): 2537–43.

18. Gauvin F, Lacroix J, Guertin MC, et al. Reproducibility of blind protected bronchoalveolar lavage in mechanically ventilated children. Am J Respir Crit Care Med 2002;165(12):1618–23.

19. Zucker A, Pollack M, Katz R. Blind use of the double-lumen plugged catheter for diagnosis of respiratory tract infections in critically ill children. Crit Care Med 1984;12(10):867–70.

20. Beyersmann J, Gastmeier P, Grundmann H, et al. Use of multistate models to assess prolongation of intensive care unit stay due to nosocomial infection. Infect Control Hosp Epidemiol 2006;27(5):493–9.

21. Safdar N, Dezfulian C, Collard HR, et al. Clinical and economic consequences of ventilator-associated pneumonia: a systematic review. Crit Care Med 2005; 33(10):2184–93.

22. Suka M, Yoshida K, Uno H, et al. Incidence and outcomes of ventilator-associated pneumonia in Japanese intensive care units: the Japanese nosocomial infection surveillance system. Infect Control Hosp Epidemiol 2007;28(3): 307–13.

23. Cordero L, Ayers LW, Miller RR, et al. Surveillance of ventilator-associated pneumonia in very-low-birth-weight infants. Am J Infect Control 2002;30(1):32–9.

24. Emori TG, Edwards JR, Culver DH, et al. Accuracy of reporting nosocomial infections in intensive-care-unit patients to the National Nosocomial Infections Surveillance system: a pilot study. Infect Control Hosp Epidemiol 1998;19(5): 308–16.

25. Patrick SW, Kawai AT, Kleinman K, et al. Health care-associated infections among critically ill children in the US, 2007-2012. Pediatrics 2014;134(4): 705–12.

26. Metersky ML, Wang Y, Klompas M, et al. Trend in ventilator-associated pneumonia rates between 2005 and 2013. JAMA 2016;316(22):2427–9.

27. Magill SS, Klompas M, Balk R, et al. Developing a new, national approach to surveillance for ventilator-associated events*. Crit Care Med 2013;41(11):2467–75.

28. Cocoros NM, Kleinman K, Priebe GP, et al. Ventilator-associated events in neonates and children–a new paradigm. Crit Care Med 2016;44(1):14–22.
29. Cocoros NM, Priebe GP, Logan LK, et al. A pediatric approach to ventilator-associated events surveillance. Infect Control Hosp Epidemiol 2017;38(3):327–33.
30. Beardsley AL, Nitu ME, Cox EG, et al. An evaluation of various ventilator-associated infection criteria in a PICU. Pediatr Crit Care Med 2016;17(1):73–80.
31. Narayanan A, Dixon G, Chalkley S, et al. Ventilator-associated pneumonia in children: comparing the plethora of surveillance definitions. J Hosp Infect 2016;94(2):163–4.
32. Shenoy MK, Iwai S, Lin DL, et al. Immune response and mortality risk relate to distinct lung microbiomes in patients with HIV and pneumonia. Am J Respir Crit Care Med 2017;195(1):104–14.
33. Fayon MJ, Tucci M, Lacroix J, et al. Nosocomial pneumonia and tracheitis in a pediatric intensive care unit: a prospective study. Am J Respir Crit Care Med 1997;155(1):162–9.
34. Wright ML, Romano MJ. Ventilator-associated pneumonia in children. Semin Pediatr Infect Dis 2006;17(2):58–64.
35. Bochicchio GV, Sung J, Joshi M, et al. Persistent hyperglycemia is predictive of outcome in critically ill trauma patients. J Trauma 2005;58(5):921–4.
36. Albert BD, Zurakowski D, Bechard LJ, et al. Enteral nutrition and acid-suppressive therapy in the PICU: impact on the risk of ventilator-associated pneumonia. Pediatr Crit Care Med 2016;17(10):924–9.
37. Lewis SC, Li L, Murphy MV, et al. Risk factors for ventilator-associated events: a case-control multivariable analysis. Crit Care Med 2014;42(8):1839–48.
38. Selvanderan SP, Summers MJ, Finnis ME, et al. Pantoprazole or placebo for stress ulcer prophylaxis (POP-UP): randomized double-blind exploratory study. Crit Care Med 2016;44(10):1842–50.
39. Eom CS, Jeon CY, Lim JW, et al. Use of acid-suppressive drugs and risk of pneumonia: a systematic review and meta-analysis. CMAJ 2011;183(3):310–9.
40. Freedberg DE, Lebwohl B, Abrams JA. The impact of proton pump inhibitors on the human gastrointestinal microbiome. Clin Lab Med 2014;34(4):771–85.
41. Huang J, Cao Y, Liao C, et al. Effect of histamine-2-receptor antagonists versus sucralfate on stress ulcer prophylaxis in mechanically ventilated patients: a meta-analysis of 10 randomized controlled trials. Crit Care 2010;14(5):R194.
42. Segal R, Pogoreliuk I, Dan M, et al. Gastric microbiota in elderly patients fed via nasogastric tubes for prolonged periods. J Hosp Infect 2006;63(1):79–83.
43. Bexfield N, Kellam P. Metagenomics and the molecular identification of novel viruses. Vet J 2011;190(2):191–8.
44. Delwart EL. Viral metagenomics. Rev Med Virol 2007;17(2):115–31.
45. Haagmans BL, Andeweg AC, Osterhaus AD. The application of genomics to emerging zoonotic viral diseases. PLoS Pathog 2009;5(10):e1000557.
46. Tang P, Chiu C. Metagenomics for the discovery of novel human viruses. Future Microbiol 2010;5(2):177–89.
47. Mourani PM, Harris JK, Sontag MK, et al. Molecular identification of bacteria in tracheal aspirate fluid from mechanically ventilated preterm infants. PLoS One 2011;6(10):e25959.
48. Wootton SC, Kim DS, Kondoh Y, et al. Viral infection in acute exacerbation of idiopathic pulmonary fibrosis. Am J Respir Crit Care Med 2011;183(12):1698–702.

49. Qin J, Li R, Raes J, et al. A human gut microbial gene catalogue established by metagenomic sequencing. Nature 2010;464(7285):59–65.
50. de La Serre CB, Ellis CL, Lee J, et al. Propensity to high-fat diet-induced obesity in rats is associated with changes in the gut microbiota and gut inflammation. Am J Physiol Gastrointest Liver Physiol 2010;299(2):G440–8.
51. van Vliet MJ, Harmsen HJ, de Bont ES, et al. The role of intestinal microbiota in the development and severity of chemotherapy-induced mucositis. PLoS Pathog 2010;6(5):e1000879.
52. Yang L, Lu X, Nossa CW, et al. Inflammation and intestinal metaplasia of the distal esophagus are associated with alterations in the microbiome. Gastroenterology 2009;137(2):588–97.
53. Cani PD, Possemiers S, Van de Wiele T, et al. Changes in gut microbiota control inflammation in obese mice through a mechanism involving GLP-2-driven improvement of gut permeability. Gut 2009;58(8):1091–103.
54. Dimmitt RA, Staley EM, Chuang G, et al. Role of postnatal acquisition of the intestinal microbiome in the early development of immune function. J Pediatr Gastroenterol Nutr 2010;51(3):262–73.
55. Suerbaum S. Microbiome analysis in the esophagus. Gastroenterology 2009; 137(2):419–21.
56. Li P, Hotamisligil GS. Metabolism: host and microbes in a pickle. Nature 2010; 464(7293):1287–8.
57. Finkbeiner SR, Allred AF, Tarr PI, et al. Metagenomic analysis of human diarrhea: viral detection and discovery. PLoS Pathog 2008;4(2):e1000011.
58. Kistler A, Avila PC, Rouskin S, et al. Pan-viral screening of respiratory tract infections in adults with and without asthma reveals unexpected human coronavirus and human rhinovirus diversity. J Infect Dis 2007;196(6):817–25.
59. Lynch JP, Sikder MA, Curren BF, et al. The influence of the microbiome on early-life severe viral lower respiratory infections and asthma-food for thought? Front Immunol 2017;8:156.
60. Alverdy JC, Krezalek MA. Collapse of the microbiome, emergence of the pathobiome, and the immunopathology of sepsis. Crit Care Med 2017;45(2):337–47.
61. Gilbert JA, Quinn RA, Debelius J, et al. Microbiome-wide association studies link dynamic microbial consortia to disease. Nature 2016;535(7610):94–103.
62. Zaborina O, Lepine F, Xiao G, et al. Dynorphin activates quorum sensing quinolone signaling in *Pseudomonas aeruginosa*. PLoS Pathog 2007;3(3):e35.
63. Kohler JE, Zaborina O, Wu L, et al. Components of intestinal epithelial hypoxia activate the virulence circuitry of pseudomonas. Am J Physiol Gastrointest Liver Physiol 2005;288(5):G1048–54.
64. Patel NJ, Zaborina O, Wu L, et al. Recognition of intestinal epithelial HIF-1alpha activation by pseudomonas aeruginosa. Am J Physiol Gastrointest Liver Physiol 2007;292(1):G134–42.
65. Schreiber F, Arasteh JM, Lawley TD. Pathogen resistance mediated by IL-22 signaling at the epithelial-microbiota interface. J Mol Biol 2015;427(23):3676–82.
66. Dickson RP. The microbiome and critical illness. Lancet Respir Med 2016;4(1): 59–72.
67. Koeppen K, Hampton TH, Jarek M, et al. A novel mechanism of host-pathogen interaction through sRNA in bacterial outer membrane vesicles. PLoS Pathog 2016;12(6):e1005672.
68. Klingensmith NJ, Coopersmith CM. The gut as the motor of multiple organ dysfunction in critical illness. Crit Care Clin 2016;32(2):203–12.

69. Cherian T, Simoes EA, Steinhoff MC, et al. Bronchiolitis in tropical south India. Am J Dis Child 1990;144(9):1026–30.

70. Thorburn K, Harigopal S, Reddy V, et al. High incidence of pulmonary bacterial co-infection in children with severe respiratory syncytial virus (RSV) bronchiolitis. Thorax 2006;61(7):611–5.

71. Stockman LJ, Reed C, Kallen AJ, et al. Respiratory syncytial virus and *Staphylococcus aureus* coinfection in children hospitalized with pneumonia. Pediatr Infect Dis J 2010;29(11):1048–50.

72. Resch B, Gusenleitner W, Mueller WD. Risk of concurrent bacterial infection in preterm infants hospitalized due to respiratory syncytial virus infection. Acta Paediatr 2007;96(4):495–8.

73. Hon KL, Leung E, Tang J, et al. Premorbid factors and outcome associated with respiratory virus infections in a pediatric intensive care unit. Pediatr Pulmonol 2008;43(3):275–80.

74. Bezerra PG, Britto MC, Correia JB, et al. Viral and atypical bacterial detection in acute respiratory infection in children under five years. PLoS One 2011;6(4): e18928.

75. Madhi SA, Ludewick H, Kuwanda L, et al. Pneumococcal coinfection with human metapneumovirus. J Infect Dis 2006;193(9):1236–43.

76. Hodson A, Kasliwal M, Streetly M, et al. A parainfluenza-3 outbreak in a SCT unit: sepsis with multi-organ failure and multiple co-pathogens are associated with increased mortality. Bone Marrow Transplant 2011;46(12):1545–50.

77. Madhi SA, Klugman KP, Vaccine Trialist Group. A role for *Streptococcus pneumoniae* in virus-associated pneumonia. Nat Med 2004;10(8):811–3.

78. Randolph AG, Vaughn F, Sullivan R, et al. Critically ill children during the 2009-2010 influenza pandemic in the United States. Pediatrics 2011;128(6):e1450–8.

79. Molyneaux PL, Mallia P, Cox MJ, et al. Outgrowth of the bacterial airway microbiome after rhinovirus exacerbation of chronic obstructive pulmonary disease. Am J Respir Crit Care Med 2013;188(10):1224–31.

80. Avadhanula V, Rodriguez CA, Devincenzo JP, et al. Respiratory viruses augment the adhesion of bacterial pathogens to respiratory epithelium in a viral species-and cell type-dependent manner. J Virol 2006;80(4):1629–36.

81. McAuley JL, Hornung F, Boyd KL, et al. Expression of the 1918 influenza A virus PB1-F2 enhances the pathogenesis of viral and secondary bacterial pneumonia. Cell Host Microbe 2007;2(4):240–9.

82. Hrincius ER, Hennecke AK, Gensler L, et al. A single point mutation (Y89F) within the non-structural protein 1 of influenza A viruses limits epithelial cell tropism and virulence in mice. Am J Pathol 2012;180(6):2361–74.

83. Ichinohe T, Pang IK, Kumamoto Y, et al. Microbiota regulates immune defense against respiratory tract influenza A virus infection. Proc Natl Acad Sci U S A 2011;108(13):5354–9.

84. Braciale TJ, Sun J, Kim TS. Regulating the adaptive immune response to respiratory virus infection. Nat Rev Immunol 2012;12(4):295–305.

85. Prakash A, Sundar SV, Zhu YG, et al. Lung ischemia-reperfusion is a sterile inflammatory process influenced by commensal microbiota in mice. Shock 2015; 44(3):272–9.

86. Ganal SC, Sanos SL, Kallfass C, et al. Priming of natural killer cells by nonmucosal mononuclear phagocytes requires instructive signals from commensal microbiota. Immunity 2012;37(1):171–86.

87. Sun K, Metzger DW. Inhibition of pulmonary antibacterial defense by interferon-gamma during recovery from influenza infection. Nat Med 2008;14(5):558–64.

88. Shahangian A, Chow EK, Tian X, et al. Type I IFNs mediate development of postinfluenza bacterial pneumonia in mice. J Clin Invest 2009;119(7): 1910–20.

89. Goulding J, Godlee A, Vekaria S, et al. Lowering the threshold of lung innate immune cell activation alters susceptibility to secondary bacterial superinfection. J Infect Dis 2011;204(7):1086–94.

90. Wang J, Li F, Sun R, et al. Bacterial colonization dampens influenza-mediated acute lung injury via induction of M2 alveolar macrophages. Nat Commun 2013;4:2106.

91. van der Sluijs KF, van Elden LJ, Nijhuis M, et al. IL-10 is an important mediator of the enhanced susceptibility to pneumococcal pneumonia after influenza infection. J Immunol 2004;172(12):7603–9.

92. Neill DR, Fernandes VE, Wisby L, et al. T regulatory cells control susceptibility to invasive pneumococcal pneumonia in mice. PLoS Pathog 2012;8(4):e1002660.

93. Nseir S, Ader F, Marquette CH. Nosocomial tracheobronchitis. Curr Opin Infect Dis 2009;22(2):148–53.

94. Craven DE, Chroneou A, Zias N, et al. Ventilator-associated tracheobronchitis: the impact of targeted antibiotic therapy on patient outcomes. Chest 2009; 135(2):521–8.

95. Wheeler DS, Whitt JD, Lake M, et al. A case-control study on the impact of ventilator-associated tracheobronchitis in the PICU. Pediatr Crit Care Med 2015;16(6):565–71.

96. Willson DF, Conaway M, Kelly R, et al. The lack of specificity of tracheal aspirates in the diagnosis of pulmonary infection in intubated children. Pediatr Crit Care Med 2014;15(4):299–305.

97. Willson DF, Kirby A, Kicker JS. Respiratory secretion analyses in the evaluation of ventilator-associated pneumonia: a survey of current practice in pediatric critical care. Pediatr Crit Care Med 2014;15(8):715–9.

98. Singh N, Rogers P, Atwood CW, et al. Short-course empiric antibiotic therapy for patients with pulmonary infiltrates in the intensive care unit. A proposed solution for indiscriminate antibiotic prescription. Am J Respir Crit Care Med 2000;162(2 Pt 1):505–11.

99. Harris JK, De Groote MA, Sagel SD, et al. Molecular identification of bacteria in bronchoalveolar lavage fluid from children with cystic fibrosis. Proc Natl Acad Sci U S A 2007;104(51):20529–33.

100. Klepac-Ceraj V, Lemon KP, Martin TR, et al. Relationship between cystic fibrosis respiratory tract bacterial communities and age, genotype, antibiotics and *Pseudomonas aeruginosa*. Environ Microbiol 2010;12(5):1293–303.

101. Zemanick ET, Wagner BD, Sagel SD, et al. Reliability of quantitative real-time PCR for bacterial detection in cystic fibrosis airway specimens. PLoS One 2010;5(11):e15101.

102. Bisgaard H, Hermansen MN, Buchvald F, et al. Childhood asthma after bacterial colonization of the airway in neonates. N Engl J Med 2007;357(15): 1487–95.

103. Ege MJ, Mayer M, Normand AC, et al. Exposure to environmental microorganisms and childhood asthma. N Engl J Med 2011;364(8):701–9.

104. Charlson ES, Diamond JM, Bittinger K, et al. Lung-enriched organisms and aberrant bacterial and fungal respiratory microbiota after lung transplant. Am J Respir Crit Care Med 2012;186(6):536–45.

105. Goleva E, Jackson LP, Harris JK, et al. The effects of airway microbiome on corticosteroid responsiveness in asthma. Am J Respir Crit Care Med 2013;188(10): 1193–201.
106. Kelly BJ, Imai I, Bittinger K, et al. Composition and dynamics of the respiratory tract microbiome in intubated patients. Microbiome 2016;4:7.

Mechanical Ventilation and Decision Support in Pediatric Intensive Care

Christopher John L. Newth, MD, FRACP, FRCPC[a,*],
Robinder G. Khemani, MD, MSCI[a], Philippe A. Jouvet, MD, PhD[b],
Katherine A. Sward, RN, PhD[c]

KEYWORDS

- Mechanical ventilation • Decision support • Pediatric intensive care
- Computer-based tools • Paper-based tools

KEY POINTS

- Despite the proven effect of decision-support tools, there is no uniformity or agreement on ventilator management decisions.
- Most critical care practitioners believe they are being lung protective, but it is likely that consistent, replicable decisions are not made to minimize ventilator support across the duration of mechanical ventilation for patients with lung injury.
- Because respiratory support is required in most children in the pediatric intensive care unit and because complications may occur with its use, it is essential to develop strategies to improve patient outcome and reduce medical errors related to mechanical ventilation.

INTRODUCTION

Pediatric and neonatal critical care has been practiced formally for more than 50 years[1] and invasive mechanical ventilation is among the most common and dramatic intensive care unit (ICU) procedures, with about 30% (range 20%–60%) of patients in a pediatric ICU (PICU) supported by this technique.[2] Mechanical ventilation is a life-saving method for thousands of patients who cannot breathe on their own and is administered until patients resume independent (spontaneous) breathing. In particular, patients with acute respiratory distress syndrome (ARDS) and acute lung injury, now collectively termed pediatric ARDS (PARDS),[3] typically require days to weeks of mechanical ventilation for respiratory failure. Despite experience with mechanical ventilation, little is known about how

[a] Anesthesiology and Critical Care Medicine, University of Southern California, Children's Hospital Los Angeles, MS #12, PICU Administration, 4650 Sunset Boulevard, Los Angeles, CA 90027, USA; [b] CHU Sainte-Justine, 3175 Chemin de Côte Sainte Catherine, Montreal, Québec H3T 1C5, Canada; [c] University of Utah College of Nursing, 10 S 2000 East, Salt Lake City, UT 84112
* Corresponding author.
E-mail address: cnewth@chla.usc.edu

Pediatr Clin N Am 64 (2017) 1057–1070
http://dx.doi.org/10.1016/j.pcl.2017.06.006
0031-3955/17/© 2017 Elsevier Inc. All rights reserved.
pediatric.theclinics.com

best to ventilate patients with specific disease entities or syndromes such as PARDS. There is uncertainty about the best choice of ventilator type, mechanical ventilation mode, and the therapeutic goals of mechanical ventilation support,[4] including best practices regarding weaning from mechanical ventilation, allowing resumption of spontaneous breathing, and removing the endotracheal tube. Although the pediatric age range is wide (newborn to 18 years), normalization of important respiratory monitoring and control parameters to body weight (eg, tidal volume and compliance), allow ventilator management approaches to be consistent across the entire pediatric age spectrum.

Thirty years ago, Pollack and colleagues[5] reported that at a single US hospital, long-stay patients were 7% of the population but used 50% of the PICU care days and 48% of the technology resources. They also had a much higher mortality rate compared with short-stay patients.[5] Five years later, a prospective cohort Australian study[6] reported complications in 24% of 500 patients requiring respiratory support. Although mortality has improved markedly,[7] these overall observations about long-stay patients persist and continue to be reported in several more recent studies.[8–10] In addition, respiratory support increases the risk of complications attributable to the endotracheal tube, positive pressure ventilation, and/or sedation. A recent prospective cohort, single-center study found that nearly half of ventilated PICU patients were found to be at risk for ventilator-related volutrauma.[11] Although the basic principles of lung protective ventilation have been embraced by pediatric intensive care physicians, there is still great variability in ventilator management.[12–14] Most critical care practitioners believe they are being lung-protective, but it is likely that consistent, replicable decisions are not made to minimize ventilator support across the duration of mechanical ventilation for patients with lung injury. Because respiratory support is required in most children in PICU, and because complications may occur with its use, it is essential to develop strategies to improve patient outcome and reduce medical errors related to mechanical ventilation.

Need for Mechanical Ventilation Protocols

The observed variation in clinical practice is likely due in part to clinicians' low adherence to guidelines, and this is compounded because many facets of caring for a mechanically ventilated patient in the PICU lack high levels of evidence, or evidence is conflicting. There is good evidence, however, that clinical decision-making with a protocol decreases practice variation between clinicians,[15] standardizes patient care, and improves research and patient outcomes.[16–20] Management of mechanical ventilation is an iterative intervention encompassing many individual decisions that must be made over the course of a patient's treatment, usually by multiple practitioners. Replicable ventilator management decisions should help decrease practice variability and directly shorten the length of mechanical ventilation for children in PICUs.[14,21] Written protocols for management of respiratory support decreased ventilator days in adults when compared with usual physician orders.[22,23] Similar findings have been observed in pediatrics[24] and neonates.[25] The Pediatric Acute Lung Injury Consensus Conference (PALICC) recommendations support use of a goal-directed protocol to guide ventilator management.

Paper Versus Computer-Based Protocols

Decision-support tools, both paper and electronic, have been demonstrated to improve medical care,[26] reduce errors,[27] and improve patient outcomes.[28] However, paper-based protocols depend on caregiver availability, are often written in broad terms so they remain dependent on clinician judgment and local context for interpretation, and are, therefore, difficult to transfer from a PICU or NICU to another ICU.[15] Paper-based tools can be difficult to follow accurately, leading to low adherence rates. There was 30% compliance in a pediatric ventilator study with a paper protocol[29] compared with 94% in an adult ventilator management study with a computer-based protocol[30] and greater than 97% in a recent pediatric insulin-glucose randomized controlled trial.[31]

Computer decision-support (CDS) tools, such as computer-based protocols, were cited by the Institute of Medicine[32] as a method to reduce medical errors. Such tools aim to ensure replicable, evidence-based clinician decisions for equivalent patient states and to improve protocol compliance. The tools can generate explicit recommendations that can be carried out with little variability between clinicians[15] while remaining responsive to the patient's unique situation. The tools can assist clinicians by standardizing descriptors and procedures, by consistently performing calculations, by incorporating complex rules with patient data, and by capturing data relevant to decision-making.[33,34] Computer-based protocols can contain more extensive detail than textual guidelines or paper-based flow diagrams while protecting the user from complexity and information overload.

Pediatric Versus Adult Computer-Based Protocols

Much of the research on computer protocols in the ICU has been conducted in adult ICUs.[15,35] Research from adult ICU is commonly extrapolated for practice in the PICU, but PARDS has distinct epidemiology, outcomes, and likely pathophysiology compared with adult ARDS.[3,7] Little is known about the use of adult-derived CDS tools in pediatric medicine. An early application, an anti-infective tool,[36] seemed to be beneficial to children and allowed cost savings. A second application, a glucose-insulin protocol,[37] used a common (shared) protocol that seemed to be as applicable to children as to adults.[38] Additionally, this study demonstrated excellent protocol compliance (>97%) compared with a paper protocol and tighter adherence to the target blood glucose range. Although children are developmentally and physiologically not little adults,[39] it seems that, at least in certain domains, CDS protocols can be used with little modification for both adults and children. Nonetheless, in general, adult protocols seem likely to need modification in the granularity (detail) of the decision rules to be usable in children, and research needs to be done to investigate this issue.

Although a computer-based mechanical ventilation protocol has been developed for adult ARDS,[40] large differences between adult and pediatric critical care bring into question the practice of extrapolating adult evidence regarding ventilator management with computer protocols, to children with PARDS. In particular, pediatric clinicians may be more comfortable with smaller (more granular) changes of 0.05 in the fraction of inspired oxygen, rather than the 0.1 increments recommended in the adult ARDSNet protocol, as suggested by analysis of large datasets from both Vanderbilt Children's Hospital and Children's Hospital Los Angeles.[41] In addition, the ranges of pH (<7.15; 7.15–<7.30; 7.30–7.45; >7.45) used in the ARDSNet protocol to guide changes in ventilator rate and tidal volume may seem too broad for many pediatric intensivists, particularly those with significant postoperative cardiac surgery background in their training. There are also differences in how predicted body weight from height or length is calculated for determination of tidal volumes in lung-protective volume-controlled modes, with pediatricians needing to deal with failure to thrive, contractures, and obesity, with only the latter being of major consideration for adult practitioners. It is probable that measurement of ulna length will prove to be the best and safest predictor of height and the subsequent percentile for age used to calculate weight and thence tidal volume over the entire pediatric age range.[42,43] The adult protocol calls for recording the set volume delivered by the ventilator, whereas pediatric practice is to measure the tidal volumes directly, but this has not been standardized as either in the ventilator or at the endotracheal tube, with large differences recorded between them.[44–46] Finally, adult protocol management of ARDS is based on Assist Control volume control, a mode rarely used by pediatric intensivists who seem to prefer pressure-regulated modes.[13]

COMPUTERIZED PROTOCOLS: DEVELOPMENT AND APPLICATION

Decision-support tools vary in terms of how dynamic they are, the degree of specificity of their recommendations, and the level of integration into workflow.[15] One end of the spectrum includes general guidelines that consist of a set of broad, static recommendations.[47] At the other end of the spectrum are computerized protocols, which are CDS tools that function as a set of standardized orders, with detailed explicit instructions based on dynamic patient-specific parameters, available at the point-of-care. The latter protocol has been called an explicit computerized protocol (ECP).[48]

ECPs need to represent best-available evidence in a computable format. These typically contain validated mathematical formulae resulting from physiologic studies (eg, alveolar gas equations[49]) or rules with the formulation: if…then… (eg, if PRVC mode and pH >7.45 and tidal volume >6 mL/kg and PIP <30 cm H_2O, then decrease tidal volume by 1 mL/kg). Other formats, such as Bayesian probability computations, may also be used to represent the knowledge and associated uncertainty.[40] All potential paths that could be taken by the child during his or her PICU course need to be accounted for and should result in a specific, explicit instruction.

Simplicity in the rules and in the use of the application are essential. Data entered manually should be the exception to simplify the caregiver's work, with decision support integrated into the workflow as much as possible.[50] In the example of hemodynamic instability, data could theoretically be acquired directly from the patient's infusion pump or the electronic medical record. To get data directly, ventilator terminology must be agreed on and matched to the context of a specific computer-based decision-support tool. Standard terminologies, such as SNOMED-CT, ICD-10, and LOINC have been mandated for use in electronic health records as part of the Affordable Care Act and are used to help integrate data across different data sources. The National Library of Medicine coordinates across these terminology services but, unfortunately, pediatric-specific terms have been generally lacking. There are several ongoing national initiatives to create sharable, comparable medical data.[51] Moreover, ventilator mode descriptions and terminology are often highly variable between and within ventilator manufacturers.

Users must believe that they can count on the system to be available whenever they need it.[50] The response time must be fast, data integrity must be maintained, and data redundancy minimized. It is important that systems function at several sites for a period of time so that major problems or software bugs have been eradicated, decreasing downtime and improving acceptance. It is also essential to assess the amount of training required for users to feel comfortable with the ECP. If users become frustrated with the ECP, its performance will be suboptimal as a consequence.

The instructions should be delivered at bedside computer terminals, or even in the monitor or ventilator. ECPs are initially developed in an open-loop manner, in which a recommendation is displayed on screen and an active intervention by the clinician is required to apply this recommendation. It is important to capture specific reasons for clinician refusal to follow instructions, analyze them, and determine if iterative refinement of the rules is needed both during the initial development phase and as part of ongoing surveillance of protocol effectiveness and compliance. Capturing clinician decisions to accept or decline the recommendation, and the reason for declines, is the sine qua non to develop a robust ECP.[50]

Ultimately, after a validation phase with refinement of protocols and with clinician acceptance of safety, some or all the ECP recommendations can potentially be implemented in a closed-loop ECP, in which ventilator settings are dynamically adjusted to a patient's condition according to the ECP recommendations without caregiver intervention but still under caregiver supervision. Displaying data specific to the decision process is strongly recommended.[50] Closed-loop mechanical ventilation can be simple, with a single-output variable managed based on a single-input variable, such as in pressure support ventilation, in which flow is automatically adjusted to maintain pressure. Closed-loop ventilation can also be complex, with multiple inputs controlling multiple outputs. Some simple forms of closed-loop ventilation are quite common, whereas less is known about more complex forms.[52–55]

EXPLICIT VARIABLES AND RULES

Computerized protocols use quantifiable variables to make decisions computable. Clinicians should be able to enter data into the CDS tool but these data should be unambiguous (ie, any member of the caregiving team would enter the same data in the same circumstance). Mechanical ventilation necessitates and produces many variables that are quantifiable from devices that monitor and support the patient (SpO_2, end-tidal and transcutaneous Pco_2, blood gases, and set and measured ventilation parameters, among others). Some conditions have to be transformed by clinicians into a quantifiable variable. For example, the variable hemodynamic instability must be explicitly defined to avoid any difference in interpretation between caregivers, for example, dopamine greater than 5 μg/kg/min and/or any dose of epinephrine or norepinephrine, thus transforming this to a quantifiable variable (present or absent). In some cases, data may not exist to support decisions. Here, the team has to design observational or even clinical trials to define some thresholds or explicit rules. For example, in the development of an explicit protocol for weaning, a survey using scenarios was conducted to validate the use of tidal volume, respiratory rate, and end-tidal carbon dioxide in children.[56]

Patient Data

For illustration of the next several sections, important concepts for the development and implementation of an ECP adapted from an adult ventilator protocol for application in ventilator management for PARDS are described.

The first parameter defined is the child's lung volume. Because there is no easy way to measure this volume, a surrogate that correlates with lung volume across ages, gender, and body habitus is used. Actual body weight is not accurate enough because children may be malnourished or obese. The PALICC guidelines[3] recommend using predicted body weight. Height is a better alternative in most cases except when neuromuscular weakness or spinal deformity is present. In such circumstances, ulna length is an excellent surrogate (vide supra).[42,43]

Ventilator Input Data

Ventilator input data may include set ventilator parameters according to the ventilation mode (respiratory rate, tidal volume, PIP, positive end-expiratory pressure [PEEP], mean airway pressure, fraction of inspired oxygen [Fio_2], inspiratory/expiratory ratio) and measured ventilator parameters (spontaneous respiratory rate, expiratory tidal volume and/or air leak around the endotracheal tube, dynamic compliance, resistance). Clinicians may use various names for the modes of mechanical ventilation, particularly because different ventilator manufacturers often name same or similar modes in different ways. A recent study used an automated algorithm to reliably (Cohen's kappa of 84.5%) detect the mode of ventilation in adult patients.[57] To further complicate matters, even within a given mode of ventilation, such as volume control, many modern ventilators now allow for user-set adjustments to flow delivery (square wave vs decelerating flow), which may have important implications.

Blood Gas Data

CO_2 removal is assessed intermittently by arterial or capillary P_{CO_2} on blood gas, continuously with end-tidal CO_2 and transcutaneous P_{CO_2}, as well as indirectly by spontaneous respiratory rate and tidal volume in some assist modes when respiratory control is functioning properly. Oxygenation can be assessed intermittently by Pa_{O_2} on blood gases, and continuously by Sp_{O_2}. Blood gas analysis drives current ventilator management when ventilation is modified a few times a day. Blood gases cannot be used in an ECP in which ventilation is adjusted in real time to a patient's need. For real-time adjustment of ventilation, ECPs are currently using Sp_{O_2} and/or end-tidal CO_2 in addition to respiratory rate and tidal volume,[21] or predicting Pa_{O_2}/Fi_{O_2} ratio from Sp_{O_2}/Fi_{O_2} ratio and pH from a previous arterial to end-tidal CO_2 difference using the Henderson-Hasselbalch equation.[58,59]

Control Unit

The control unit, or inference engine,[40] is a computerized module that receives clinical information on the patient (input data) and transforms this information into orders (output data) by processing the patient data using rules or mathematical algorithms. The knowledge processed by the inference engine may be organized into several systems by which recommendations are generated from embedded rules for (1) oxygenation, (2) ventilation, (3) time between generation of recommendations, and (4) plot generation for both oxygenation and dead space, which are predictors of changing trajectory of pulmonary disease.[60–62] A further set of rules will recommend extubation when variables reach a given threshold.[21,63]

Output Data

Output data can be recommendations to the caregivers suggesting new ventilator settings, specific notes about the patient's condition such as "patient ready for separation from the ventilator," or ventilator settings being automatically adjusted by a feedback controller. During the development phase of an ECP, however, output data are usually recommendations that the caregiver then has to set (open-loop). After extensive testing, some rules or sets of rules can be switched to a closed-loop system.[64]

A simple, organized, and intuitive user interface is imperative to facilitate the understanding of the ECP decision process and for knowledge transfer at the bedside (**Fig. 1**). Ideally, the user interface should include education tools with which to train caregivers on mechanical ventilation management according to the ECP (**Fig. 2**A, B).

CLINICAL EVALUATION OF EXPLICIT COMPUTERIZED PROTOCOLS
Explicit Protocols for Respiratory Support in Adults

ECPs have been studied in adults in multicenter trials as treatment modalities for ARDS[35] and for weaning.[65] In all instances, a similar or better outcome was found when a written or electronic protocol was compared with usual care. Lellouche and colleagues[66] recently explored fully automated ventilation in cardiac patients after surgery. In a randomized, controlled trial it was found to be safe. In the seminal ARDSNet low versus high tidal volume study,[67] all participating ICUs used explicit decision-support

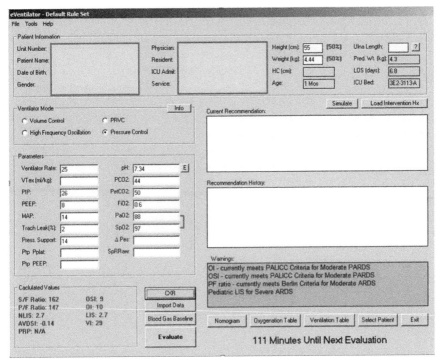

Fig. 1. The entry page for an explicit, computer-based mechanical ventilation protocol (ECP). Relevant patient data are displayed, including ideal body weight and various calculated values from the ventilator and blood gas variables either manually or automatically entered from the hospital electronic infrastructure (laboratory, monitor, and ventilator). The severity of PARDS is demonstrated, in addition to a timer displaying when the next scheduled evaluation should occur.

tools for rigorous ventilator management. Only a few units in this trial, however, used computer-based rather than paper protocols.[40]

Explicit Protocols for Respiratory Support in Pediatrics

In 2 single-center randomized clinical trials comparing a weaning ECP to usual care, Jouvet and colleagues[53,68] showed that the duration of weaning was dramatically decreased in the protocol groups when compared with the control groups.[53,68]

In children and adults, standardization of oxygenation management may involve PEEP/Fio_2 grids[69,70] that aim to maximize lung protective strategies. Such PEEP/Fio_2 scales have been used as written guidelines in several clinical trials in pediatric intensive care, including the prone positioning trial[71] and the multicenter calfactant study for direct ARDS conducted by Willson and colleagues.[72] At this time, no ECP that includes oxygenation management has been tested in pediatric clinical trials for children outside neonates, with a single exception, a single-arm, single-center pilot study of safety in 15 children.[73]

Explicit Protocol for Respiratory Support in Neonatology

Claure and Bancalari[74] developed an SpO_2-FiO_2 closed-loop system in 2001 to limit periods of hypoxemia and hyperoxemia. These investigators demonstrated that in

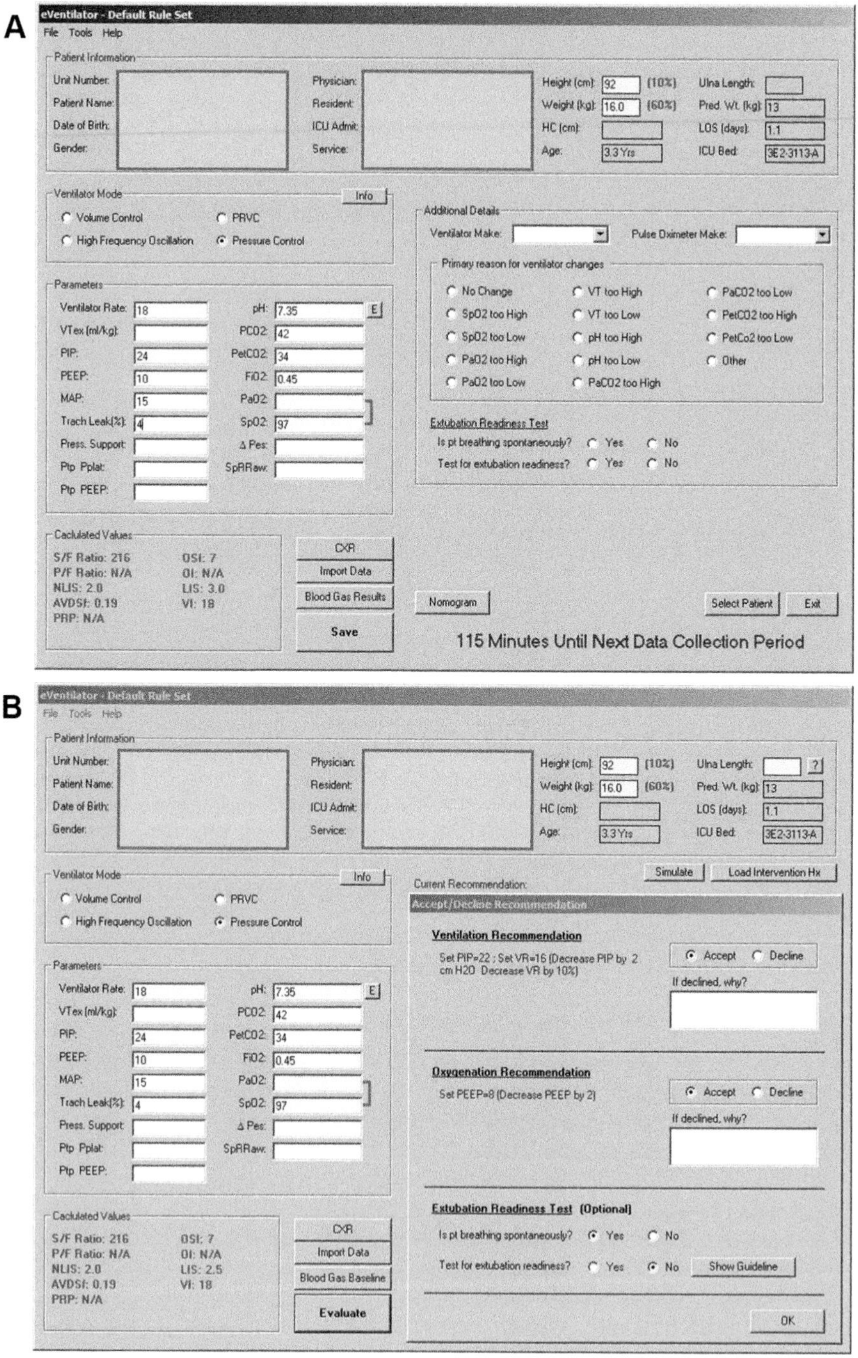

Fig. 2. (*A*) The entry page for training personnel or data collection on an explicit, computer-based mechanical ventilation protocol. The data entry sheet is essentially the same as in **Fig. 1**. However, no recommendations are offered. This approach can be used either to train personnel on the decision-support tool or for data gathering to establish a baseline of ventilator management before starting it as a full application for patient management or a study.

premature infants their explicit protocol was at least as effective as a fully dedicated nurse in maintaining SpO_2 within the target range. van Kaam and colleagues[75] performed a safety and efficacy clinical trial in 80 preterm infants with a similar computerized protocol. Periods with automatic oxygen control at 2 different target ranges were compared with periods of optimal control by a fully dedicated person. The automated control was superior in avoiding hypoxemia. These closed-loop systems could be incorporated into an ECP aimed at decreasing ventilation duration.

Challenges when Implementing an Explicit Computerized Protocol

Barriers to protocol use are many, including lack of awareness, lack of familiarity with the protocol, lack of agreement, lack of efficacy, lack of known improved outcome, and lack of ability to overcome the inertia of previous practice. There are also external barriers, including (1) protocol-related barriers (not easy to use, not convenient, cumbersome, and confusing) and (2) environment-related barriers (new resources or facilities not accessible).[76] To ensure acceptance, users must believe that they can count on the system to be available whenever they need it. The amount of downtime needed for data backup, troubleshooting, and upgrading should be minimal. The response time must be fast, data integrity must be maintained, and data redundancy minimized. It is also important to assess the amount of training necessary for users to feel comfortable with the system.

The ventilator market itself is also a barrier to the implementation of ECPs. There are numerous companies, and the competition between them results in difficulties implementing the same ECP in different ventilators. Nonetheless, for technical and regulatory issues, companies ideally should be involved in the process of implementation of ECPs on mechanical ventilation. Ventilators dedicated to pediatric and neonatal intensive care are a small market compared with the adult market. Pediatric and neonatal intensivists need to develop, test, and promote ventilation ECPs that can be adapted afterward by the different companies into the type of ventilator they sell.[52] Alternatively, standalone bedside devices or Web-based programs running on handheld electronic devices can be developed that are independent of the ventilator but can communicate with it and the monitor to get the data needed for decision support.

SUMMARY

Despite the proven effect of decision-support tools, there is no uniformity or agreement on ventilator management decisions. This results in a high variability in practice between centers and between intensivists at the same center.[12–14] Management of mechanical ventilation is an example of an iterative treatment protocol encompassing the many individual decisions that must be made over the course of a patient's treatment.[77]

◄ ───

(*B*) The recommendation-view page for on an explicit, computer-based mechanical ventilation protocol. This view displays the recommendations for oxygenation and ventilation for the ventilation and blood gas variables supplied for pressure control mode of ventilation. Various tabs provide a nomogram of acid-base status, the relevant oxygenation, and ventilation grids and plots showing the serial changes in oxygenation index, ventilation index, and SF O_2, the ratio of Oxygen saturation to Fraction of inspired oxygen; and PF O_2, the ratio of the partial pressure of Oxygen to Fraction of inspired oxygen; ratios. From a baseline arterial or capillary CO_2 to end-tidal CO_2 difference with associated pH, a new pH can be predicted from end-tidal CO_2 changes using the Henderson-Hasselbalch equation.

Decision-support tools (paper or electronic) have been shown to improve the quality of medical care,[26] reduce errors,[27] and improve patient outcomes.[28] However, paper-based tools can be difficult to follow accurately, leading to low adherence rates.

Computers can assist clinicians by standardizing descriptors and procedures, by consistently performing calculations, by incorporating complex rules with patient data, and by capturing data relevant to decision-making.[33,34,77,78] Computer-based protocols can contain extensive details while protecting the user from complexity and information overload.[33,34,78] These tools aim to ensure flexible but consistent, evidence-based clinician decisions for equivalent patient states.

REFERENCES

1. Willson DF, Dean JM, Newth C, et al. Collaborative pediatric critical care research network (CPCCRN). Pediatr Crit Care Med 2006;7:301–7.
2. Khemani RG, Markovitz BP, Curley MAQ. Characteristics of children intubated and mechanically ventilated in 16 PICUs. Chest 2009;136:765–71.
3. Pediatric Acute Lung Injury Consensus Conference Group. Pediatric acute respiratory distress syndrome: consensus recommendations from the pediatric acute lung injury consensus conference. Pediatr Crit Care Med 2015;16:428–39.
4. Randolph AG. How are children mechanically ventilated in pediatric intensive care units? Intensive Care Med 2004;30:746–7.
5. Pollack MM, Wilkinson JD, Glass NL. Long-stay pediatric intensive care unit patients: outcome and resource utilization. Pediatrics 1987;80:855–60.
6. Rivera R, Tibballs J. Complications of endotracheal intubation and mechanical ventilation in infants and children. Crit Care Med 1992;20:193–9.
7. Yehya N, Thomas NJ. Relevant outcomes in pediatric acute respiratory distress syndrome studies. Front Pediatr 2016;4:1–10.
8. Marcin JP, Slonim AD, Pollack MM, et al. Long-stay patients in the pediatric intensive care unit. Crit Care Med 2001;29:652–7.
9. Edwards JD, Houtrow AJ, Vasilevskis EE, et al. Chronic conditions among children admitted to U.S. pediatric intensive care units: their prevalence and impact on risk for mortality and prolonged length of stay. Crit Care Med 2012;40: 2196–203.
10. Traiber C, Piva JP, Fritsher CC, et al. Profile and consequences of children requiring prolonged mechanical ventilation in three Brazilian pediatric intensive care units. Pediatr Crit Care Med 2009;10:375–80.
11. Walsh BK, Smallwood CD, Rettig JS, et al. Categorization in mechanically ventilated pediatric subjects: a proposed method to improve quality. Respir Care 2016;61:1168–78.
12. Newth CJL, Sward KA, Khemani RG, et al. Variability in usual care mechanical ventilation for pediatric Acute Respiratory Distress Syndrome: Time for a decision support protocol? Pediatr Crit Care Med. 2017. In Press.
13. Santschi M, Jouvet P, Leclerc F, et al. Acute lung injury in children: therapeutic practice and feasibility of international clinical trials. Pediatr Crit Care Med 2010;11:681–9.
14. Khemani RG, Sward K, Morris A, et al. Variability in usual care mechanical ventilation for pediatric acute lung injury: the potential benefit of a lung protective computer protocol. Intensive Care Med 2011;37:1840–8.
15. Morris AH. Developing and implementing computerized protocols for standardization of clinical decisions. Ann Intern Med 2000;132:373–83.

16. Grimshaw JM, Russell IT. Effect of clinical guidelines on medical practice: a systematic review of rigorous evaluations. Lancet 1993;342:1317–22.
17. Grimm RH, Shimoni K, Harlan WR, et al. Evaluation of patient-care protocol use by various providers. N Engl J Med 1975;292:507–11.
18. Wirtschafter DD, Scalise M, Henke C, et al. Do information systems improve the quality of clinical research? Results of a randomized trial in a cooperative multi-institutional cancer group. Comput Biomed Res 1981;14:78–90.
19. Safran C, Rind DM, Davis RB, et al. Effects of a knowledge-based electronic patient record in adherence to practice guidelines. MD Comput 1996;13:55–63.
20. Garg AX, Adhikari NKJ, McDonald H, et al. Effects of computerized clinical decision support systems on practitioner performance and patient outcomes: a systematic review. JAMA 2005;293:1223–38.
21. Jouvet P, Farges C, Hatzakis G, et al. Weaning children from mechanical ventilation with a computer-driven system (closed-loop protocol): a pilot study. Pediatr Crit Care Med 2007;8:425–32.
22. Kollef MH, Shapiro SD, Silver P, et al. A randomized, controlled trial of protocol-directed versus physician-directed weaning from mechanical ventilation. Crit Care Med 1997;25:567–74.
23. Smyrnios NA, Connolly A, Wilson MM, et al. Effects of a multifaceted, multidisciplinary, hospital-wide quality improvement program on weaning from mechanical ventilation. Crit Care Med 2002;30:1224–30.
24. Schultz TR, Lin RJ, Watzman HM, et al. Weaning children from mechanical ventilation: a prospective randomized trial of protocol-directed versus physician-directed weaning. Respir Care 2001;46:772–82.
25. Hermeto F, Bottino MN, Vaillancourt K, et al. Implementation of a respiratory therapist-driven protocol for neonatal ventilation: impact on the premature population. Pediatrics 2009;123:e907–16.
26. Shortliffe EH, Cimeno JJ. Biomedical informatics: computer applications in health care and biomedicine. Third edition. New York: Springer-Verlag; 2006.
27. Slonim AD, Pollack MM. Integrating the Institute of Medicine's six quality aims into pediatric critical care: relevance and applications. Pediatr Crit Care Med 2005;6:264–9.
28. Blaser R, Schnabel M, Biber C, et al. Improving pathway compliance and clinician performance by using information technology. Int J Med Inform 2007;76:151–6.
29. Randolph AG, Wypij D, Venkataraman ST, et al. Effect of mechanical ventilator weaning protocols on respiratory outcomes in infants and children: a randomized controlled trial. JAMA 2002;288:2561–8.
30. Morris AH, Wallace CJ, Menlove RL, et al. Randomized clinical trial of pressure-controlled inverse ratio ventilation and extracorporeal CO_2 removal for adult respiratory distress syndrome. Am J Respir Crit Care Med 1994;149:295–305.
31. Agus MSD, Wypij D, Hirshberg EL, et al. Tight glycemic control in critically ill children. N Engl J Med 2017;376:729–41.
32. Kohn LT, Corrigan JM, Donaldson M. To err is human: building a safer health care system. National Academy of Sciences. Washington, DC: National Academic Press; 2000.
33. Clemmer TP. Computers in the ICU: where we started and where we are now. J Crit Care 2004;19:201–7.
34. Morris AH. Treatment algorithms and protocolized care. Curr Opin Crit Care 2003;9:236–40.

35. East TD, Heermann LK, Bradshaw RL, et al. Efficacy of computerized decision support for mechanical ventilation: results of a prospective multi-center randomized trial. Proc AMIA Symp 1999;251–5.

36. Mullett CJ, Evans RS, Christenson JC, et al. Development and impact of a computerized pediatric antiinfective decision support program. Pediatrics 2001;108:e75.

37. Morris AH, Orme JJ, Truwit JD, et al. A replicable method for blood glucose control in critically ill patients. Crit Care Med 2008;36:1787–95.

38. Thompson BT, Orme JF, Zheng H, et al. Multicenter validation of a computer-based clinical decision support tool for glucose control in adult and pediatric intensive care units. J Diabetes Sci Technol 2008;2:357–68.

39. Newth CJ. Respiratory disease and respiratory failure: implications for the young and the old. Br J Dis Chest 1986;80:209–17.

40. Sorenson D, Grissom CK, Carpenter L, et al. A frame-based representation for a bedside ventilator weaning protocol. J Biomed Inform 2008;41:461–8.

41. Khemani RG, Conti D, Alonzo TA, et al. Effect of tidal volume in children with acute hypoxemic respiratory failure. Intensive Care Med 2009;35:1428–37.

42. Gauld LM, Kappers J, Carlin JB, et al. Prediction of childhood pulmonary function using ulna length. Am J Respir Crit Care Med 2003;168:804–9.

43. Ungern-Sternberg von BS, Trachsel D, Erb TO, et al. Forced expiratory flows and volumes in intubated and paralyzed infants and children: normative data up to 5 years of age. J Appl Physiol 2009;107:105–11.

44. Kim P, Salazar A, Ross PA, et al. Comparison of tidal volumes at the endotracheal tube and at the ventilator. Pediatr Crit Care Med 2015;16:e324–31.

45. Al-Majed SI, Thompson JE, Watson KF, et al. Effect of lung compliance and endotracheal tube leakage on measurement of tidal volume. Crit Care 2004;8: R398–402.

46. Main E, Castle R, Stocks J, et al. The influence of endotracheal tube leak on the assessment of respiratory function in ventilated children. Intensive Care Med 2001;27:1788–97.

47. Roumie CL, Elasy TA, Greevy R, et al. Improving blood pressure control through provider education, provider alerts, and patient education: a cluster randomized trial. Ann Intern Med 2006;145:165–75.

48. Phansalkar S, Weir CR, Morris AH, et al. Clinicians' perceptions about use of computerized protocols: a multicenter study. Int J Med Inform 2008;77:184–93.

49. Otis AB, Fenn WO, Rahn H. Mechanics of breathing in man. J Appl Physiol 1950; 2:592–607.

50. Kawamoto K, Houlihan CA, Balas EA, et al. Improving clinical practice using clinical decision support systems: A systematic review of trials to identify features critical to success. BMJ 2005;330:765–8.

51. Sward KA, Rubin S, Jenkins TL, et al. Case study: semantic annotation of a pediatric critical care research study. Comput Inform Nurs 2016;34:101–4.

52. Rose L, Schultz MJ, Cardwell CR, et al. Automated versus non-automated weaning for reducing the duration of mechanical ventilation for critically ill adults and children: a Cochrane systematic review and meta-analysis. Crit Care 2015;19:48.

53. Jouvet PA, Payen V, Gauvin F, et al. Weaning children from mechanical ventilation with a computer-driven protocol: a pilot trial. Intensive Care Med 2013;39:919–25.

54. Burns KEA, Lellouche F, Lessard MR, et al. Automated weaning and spontaneous breathing trial systems versus non-automated weaning strategies for discontinuation time in invasively ventilated postoperative adults. Cochrane Database Syst Rev 2014;(2):CD008639.

55. Branson RD, Johannigman JA, Campbell RS, et al. Closed-loop mechanical ventilation. Respir Care 2002;47:427–51 [discussion: 451].

56. Santschi M, Gauvin F, Hatzakis G, et al. Acceptable respiratory physiologic limits for children during weaning from mechanical ventilation. Intensive Care Med 2007;33:319–25.

57. Murias G, Montanyà J, Chacón E, et al. Automatic detection of ventilatory modes during invasive mechanical ventilation. Crit Care 2016;20:938.

58. Khemani RG, Patel NR, Bart RDI, et al. Comparison of the pulse oximetric saturation/fraction of inspired oxygen ratio and the Pao(2)/fraction of inspired oxygen ratio in children. Chest 2009;135:662–8.

59. Khemani RG, Celikkaya EB, Shelton CR, et al. Algorithms to estimate PaCO2 and pH using noninvasive parameters for children with hypoxemic respiratory failure. Respir Care 2014;59:1248–57.

60. Khemani RG, Bart RD, Newth CJL. Pediatric hypoxemic respiratory failure: risk factors for mortality. Am J Respir Crit Care Med 2008;D104:3129.

61. Yehya N, Bhalla AK, Thomas NJ, et al. Alveolar dead space fraction discriminates mortality in pediatric acute respiratory distress syndrome. Pediatr Crit Care Med 2016;17:101–9.

62. Bhalla AK, Belani S, Leung D, et al. Higher dead space is associated with increased mortality in critically ill children. Crit Care Med 2015;43:2439–45.

63. Khemani RG, Hotz J, Morzov R, et al. Pediatric extubation readiness tests should not use pressure support. Intensive Care Med 2016;42(8):1214–22.

64. Wysocki M, Jouvet P, Jaber S. Closed loop mechanical ventilation. J Clin Monit Comput 2013;28:49–56.

65. Lellouche F, Mancebo J, Jolliet P, et al. A multicenter randomized trial of computer-driven protocolized weaning from mechanical ventilation. Am J Respir Crit Care Med 2006;174:894–900.

66. Lellouche F, Bouchard PA, Simard S, et al. Evaluation of fully automated ventilation: a randomized controlled study in post-cardiac surgery patients. Intensive Care Med 2013;39:463–71.

67. The Acute Respiratory Distress Syndrome Network, Brower RG, Matthay MA, Morris A, et al. Ventilation with lower tidal volumes as compared with traditional tidal volumes for acute lung injury and the acute respiratory distress syndrome. N Engl J Med 2000;342:1301–8.

68. Jouvet P, Hernert P, Wysocki M. Development and implementation of explicit computerized protocols for mechanical ventilation in children. Ann Intensive Care 2011;1:51.

69. Emeriaud G, Newth CJL, Pediatric Acute Lung Injury Consensus Conference Group. Monitoring of children with pediatric acute respiratory distress syndrome: proceedings from the pediatric acute lung injury consensus conference. Pediatr Crit Care Med 2015;16:S86–101.

70. Curley MAQ, Arnold JH, Thompson JE, et al. Clinical trial design–effect of prone positioning on clinical outcomes in infants and children with acute respiratory distress syndrome. J Crit Care 2006;21:23–32 [discussion: 32–7].

71. Curley M, Hibberd PL, Fineman LD, et al. Effect of prone positioning on clinical outcomes in children with acute lung injury - A randomized controlled trial. JAMA 2005;294:229–37.

72. Willson DF, Thomas NJ, Markovitz BP, et al. Effect of exogenous surfactant (calfactant) in pediatric acute lung injury: a randomized controlled trial. JAMA 2005;293:470–6.

73. Jouvet P, Eddington A, Payen V, et al. A pilot prospective study on closed loop controlled ventilation and oxygenation in ventilated children during the weaning phase. Crit Care 2012;16:R85.

74. Claure N, Bancalari E. Automated closed loop control of inspired oxygen concentration. Respir Care 2013;58:151–61.

75. van Kaam AH, Hummler HD, Wilinska M, et al. Automated versus manual oxygen control with different saturation targets and modes of respiratory support in preterm infants. J Pediatr 2015;167:545–50.e1-2.

76. Cabana MD, Rand CS, Powe NR, et al. Why don't physicians follow clinical practice guidelines? A framework for improvement. JAMA 1999;282:1458–65.

77. Niland JC, Rouse L, Stahl DC. An informatics blueprint for healthcare quality information systems. J Am Med Inform Assoc 2006;13:402–17.

78. Morris AH, East TD, Wallace CJ, et al. Standardization of clinical decision making for the conduct of credible clinical research in complicated medical environments. Proc AMIA Annu Fall Symp 1996;418–22.

Rationale for Adjunctive Therapies for Pediatric Sepsis Induced Multiple Organ Failure

Bradley S. Podd, MD, PhD[a], Dennis W. Simon, MD[a],
Santiago Lopez, MD[b], Andrew Nowalk, MD[b], Rajesh Aneja, MD[a],
Joseph A. Carcillo, MD[a],*

KEYWORDS

- Thrombocytopenia-associated MOF • Immune paralysis • Hyperleukocytosis
- Sequential MOF • Macrophage activation syndrome

KEY POINTS

- Adjunctive therapies are considered by clinicians for use in the management of children with sepsis inflammation pathobiology phenotypes and multiple organ failure (MOF).
- A few general themes for the management of pediatric MOF are always pertinent, including the search for and removal of sources of ongoing infection and inflammation, and support of cardiovascular and other organ functions.
- Clinicians can also use clinical criteria and confirmatory tests to identify 1 or more of 5 inflammation phenotypes that can be targeted with pathobiology-based adjunctive therapies.

INTRODUCTION

Adjunctive therapies are considered by clinicians for use in the management of children with sepsis inflammation pathobiology phenotypes and multiple organ failure (MOF). This article examines host-pathogen interaction models (or prototypes) that provide the rationale for proven, experimental, or proposed inflammation pathobiology

Funding Support: Funded in part by R01GM108616 and 5UG1HD049983 (J.A. Carcillo) from National Institute of General Medical Science and Eunice Kennedy Shriver National Institute of Child Health and Development.
[a] Department of Critical Care Medicine, Children's Hospital of Pittsburgh, University of Pittsburgh School of Medicine, 4400 Penn Avenue, Pittsburgh, PA 15214, USA; [b] Department of Pediatrics, Division of Infectious Diseases, Children's Hospital of Pittsburgh, University of Pittsburgh School of Medicine, 4400 Penn Avenue, Pittsburgh, PA 15214, USA
* Corresponding author. Children's Hospital of Pittsburgh, Suite 2000, Faculty Pavilion, 4400 Penn Avenue, Pittsburgh, PA 15214.
E-mail address: carcilloja@ccm.upmc.edu

phenotype-targeted therapies in pediatric sepsis-induced MOF. A few general themes for the management of pediatric MOF are always pertinent, including the search for and removal of sources of ongoing infection and inflammation, and support of cardiovascular and other organ functions. In addition to this general approach, clinical criteria and confirmatory tests can also be used to identify 1 or more of 5 inflammation phenotypes that can be targeted with pathobiology-based adjunctive therapies (**Table 1**).

Table 1
Five inflammation pathobiology phenotypes and putative adjunctive therapies

Phenotype	Clinical Criteria	Biomarker/Prototype	Adjunctive Therapy
Thrombocytopenia-associated MOF	Platelet level <100,000/mm³ Acute kidney injury Increased LDH level	ADAMTS13<57% Discussed prototypes = purpura fulminans/aHUS	1. Plasma exchange[9,11–15,60] removes ultralarge vWF multimers and restores ADAMTS13 activity 2. C5a antibody[16–18] inhibits activated complement (FDA approved for aHUS)
Immune paralysis–associated MOF	Persistent or secondary infections	Monocyte HLA-DR expression <30% or 8000 molecules Whole-blood ex vivo TNF response to LPS <200 pg/mL Absolute lymphocyte count <1000 mm³ Discussed prototype = H1N1/MRSA	GM-CSF[24,28,29] Immune suppressant withdrawal[27] Restores TNF response to endotoxin
Hyperleukocytosis and pulmonary hypertension–associated MOF	Age <6 mo Pulmonary HTN	WBC count >50,000 mm³ Discussed prototype = critical pertussis	Extracorporeal leukoreduction[35] removes circulating WBCs and decreases pulmonary hypertension
Sequential MOF with liver failure	Respiratory distress followed by hepatobiliary dysfunction	s-FasL level >200 pg/mL Discussed prototype = EBV lymphoproliferative disease	1. Hold immune suppressants 2. Give anti-CD20 monoclonal antibody[43,44] to remove EBV reservoir (FDA approved for PTLD)
Macrophage activation syndrome	Hepatobiliary dysfunction and disseminated intravascular coagulation	Ferritin level >500 ng/mL Discussed prototype = Viral hemorrhagic fevers	IVIG + steroids + plasma exchange[60] Anakinra[47,56] Tocilizumab[57,58] decreases macrophage inflammation

Abbreviations: aHUS, atypical hemolytic uremic syndrome; EBV, Epstein-Barr virus; FDA, US Food and Drug Administration; GM-CSF, granulocyte macrophage colony-stimulating factor; HLA-DR, human leukocyte antigen, antigen D related; HTN, hypertension; IVIG, intravenous immune globulin; LDH, lactate dehydrogenase; LPS, lipopolysaccharaide; MRSA, methicillin-resistant *Staphylococcus aureus*; PTLD, posttransplant lymphoproliferative disorder; s-FasL, soluble Fas ligand; TNF, tumor necrosis factor; vWF, von Willebrand factor; WBC, white blood cell.

Thrombocytopenia-Associated Multiple Organ Failure

Thrombocytopenia-associated MOF (TAMOF) centers on endothelial dysfunction, impairment of metalloproteinase activity of ADAMTS13, and consumptive coagulopathy that results in microvascular impairment and organ injury. This article reviews 2 host-pathogen interaction models for TAMOF: (1) *Neisseria meningitides*–induced purpura fulminans, associated with complement dysfunction, endothelial injury, production of von Willebrand factor (vWF) ultralarge multimers, and intravascular coagulation (**Fig. 1**A); and (2) atypical hemolytic uremic syndrome (aHUS) as a result of genetic polymorphisms in ADAMTS13 activity or inhibitory complement regulation (see **Fig. 1**B). In addition to microbiological source control, both types are amenable to therapeutic plasma exchange, which removes thrombogenic ultralarge vWF multimers and restores ADAMTS13 activity. aHUS is also amenable to biologic terminal complement inhibitors such as eculizumab.

There are also host genetic risk factors for the development of TAMOF, including ADAMTS13 deficiency syndrome (Upshaw-Schulman syndrome, also known as congenital thrombotic thrombocytopenic purpura), and deficiency in complement H.[1,2] Environmental risk factors include elaboration of inflammatory cytokines resulting in direct endothelial activation or injury, liver failure, and inhibitory ADAMTS13 antibodies as seen in acquired thrombotic microangiopathy.[3–5] Free hemoglobin resulting from red blood cell hemolysis in TAMOF is a driver for further endothelial and other organ injury. Other sources of pathologic free hemoglobin include any aged blood cells prone to hemolysis on transfusion, cardiopulmonary bypass, extracorporeal membrane oxygenation (ECMO), or continuous renal replacement therapy.[6–8]

There are several TAMOF-directed adjunctive therapeutic options. In a small, single-center, prospective randomized clinical study, plasma exchange therapy (1.5 volumes on day 1 followed by 1 volume on day 2 through to the end, with the end being determined by return of organ function and platelet count) was associated with removal of ultralarge vWF multimers, restoration of ADAMTS13 functional activity, and improvement in end-organ functional markers.[9,10] Meta-analyses indicate a mortality benefit with use of plasma exchange therapy in adults.[11–13] Although the data for use of plasma exchange therapy in critically adult and pediatric intensive care unit (ICU) populations for the indication of sepsis and septic shock are mixed, there is potential benefit in the TAMOF syndrome, based on biological plausibility and a track record of efficacy of its use in microangiopathies.[14,15] The decision to provide plasma exchange should be based on the clinical condition, including degree of coagulopathy and platelet count. In addition, plasma exchange should be considered in the setting of severe neurologic disease. Evidence for activation of the complement system should also prompt a consideration for plasma exchange therapy. Eculizumab, a C5 terminal complement cleavage inhibitory monoclonal antibody, can be considered in the setting of TAMOF. This therapy has been most extensively studied in the setting of aHUS associated with an ineffective inhibitory complement response, in which eculizumab has been shown to improve renal function, need for renal support, and quality of life among adult patients.[16] Eculizumab has been approved for use in pediatric aHUS.[17] Moreover, earlier administration of the antibody in an aHUS disease course is associated with improved renal recovery.[17,18]

Immunoparalysis-Associated Multiple Organ Failure

Immunoparalysis-associated MOF centers on impairment of both innate and adaptive immune function with resulting inability for the host to contain a primary or

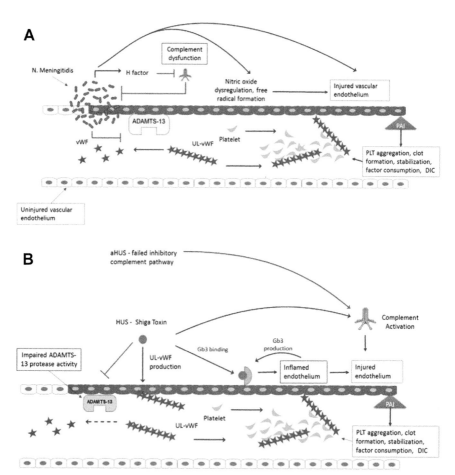

Fig. 1. TAMOF. (*A*) Purpura fulminans. *Neisseria meningitidis* can adhere to and form colonies on the vascular endothelium via pilin.[61] Meningococcal virulence factor, such as factor H binding protein, can downregulate complement response and allow bacterial proliferation.[62] Bacterial-endothelial interactions result in endothelial inflammation via nuclear factor kappa-B (NFkB) responses and can further promote endothelial infection, capillary leakage, and translocation of bacteria across the vessel.[63–65] Invasive meningococcal disease is associated with decreased activity of the metalloproteinase ADAMST13 (A disintegrin and metalloproteinase with a thrombospondin type 1 motif, member 13) and increased activity of von Willebrand factor (vWF).[66,67] Ultralarge vWF (UL vWF) multimers contribute to platelet (PLT) aggregation and intravascular thrombosis.[67,68] Endothelial inflammation contributes to platelet dysfunction via *N meningitidis*–derived NO with impaired vascular homeostasis and NO-mediated impairment of ADP-mediated platelet aggregation.[69] Inflammatory cytokines change the coagulation profile toward procoagulation with a reduction of activated protein C (APC) and antithrombin III (ATIII) and upregulation of prothrombin and the antifibrinolytic plasminogen activator inhibitor-1 (PAI-1).[70] The end result of the interaction of multiple inflammatory pathways in the organ is microthrombosis, tissue ischemia, oxidative insult, ischemia, and cell death. Plasm exchange therapy can reverse this process. (*B*) Atypical hemolytic uremic syndromes (aHUS). Sterile microangiopathies such as thrombotic thrombocytopenia purpura (TTP) are associated with inhibition of ADAMST13 activity via the presence of autoinhibitors, whereas aHUS or congenital TTP has been associated with ADAMST13 and inhibitory complement gene mutations.[71,72] On infection with Shiga toxin (ST)–producing pathogens, ST has direct effects on the vascular endothelium and

secondary infection. The host-pathogen example used here for this phenotype of MOF is H1N1 influenza A infection with impairment of monocyte function and contraction of adaptive immune populations (**Fig. 2**). In addition to antiviral and antibacterial therapy to control pathogen burden and removal (when appropriate) of pharmacologic sources of immune suppression, providing granulocyte macrophage colony-stimulating factor (GM-CSF) has been successfully used to reverse innate immune paralysis. Programmed cell death protein 1 (PD-1)/programmed cell death ligand 1 (PD-L1) blockade as well as provision of recombinant lymphocyte survival factors such as interleukin (IL)-7 are being evaluated as methods to restore adaptive immune function.

Immunoparalysis-associated MOF is associated with decreased ex vivo tumor necrosis factor (TNF) alpha response less than 200 pg/mL and decreased expression of the Major Histocompatibility Complex-II molecule human leukocyte antigen, antigen D related (HLA-DR) less than 8000 molecules or less than 30% of control level beyond 3 days of illness.[19–21] Among patients with severe sepsis, lymphopenia is an independent predictor of mortality.[22] A phenotype of prolonged lymphocyte depletion was described among spleen and other lymphoid tissue samples from pediatric and adult patients who died of sepsis-associated MOF.[19,23] Poor outcomes associated with the immunoparalysis phenotype include increased association of ventilator-associated pneumonia, reactivation of latent herpesvirus family infections, and secondary opportunistic infections, on which multiorgan failure may be superimposed.[24,25]

An examination of the clinical features associated with mortality during the 2009 to 2010 H1N1 influenza pandemic highlighted the relationship between viral immune suppression and the development of opportunistic methicillin-resistant *Staphylococcus aureus* (MRSA) infection. In a retrospective observational cohort of 838 patients less than 21 years old admitted to pediatric ICUs across the United States, overall mortality was 8.9%.[26] Leukopenia and neutropenia were associated with mortality (relative risk [RR] 1.8, 95% confidence interval [CI] 1.2–2.9; RR 2.8, 95% CI 1.5–5.5, respectively). Bacterial pneumonia (coinfection) with MRSA, but not methicillin-sensitive *S aureus*, was associated with death (RR 3.2, 95% CI 1.8–5.9). In a multivariate model, among the 251 previously healthy children enrolled in the study, only presumed MRSA infection was significantly associated with mortality (RR 8, 95% CI 3.9–20.6). Whole-blood TNF-alpha hyporesponsiveness to

---

results in increased release of ultralarge vWF multimers and to direct inhibition of ADAMST13 activity level, further promoting thrombosis formation.[72,73] ST-mediated aHUS causes a proinflammatory endothelial state by promoting leukocyte adhesion and by producing endothelial-derived cytokines such as interleukin (IL)-8, similar to the vascular pathophysiology observed in purpura fulminans. Exposure of human endothelial cells to the proinflammatory cytokines tumor necrosis factor (TNF) alpha and IL-1b increases expression of globotriaosylceramide (Gb3) on endothelial cells and results in further susceptibility to ST by a feed-forward mechanism.[74] ST causes production of complement 3a (C3a), with loss of thrombomodulin (TM), changes in cell surface adhesion molecules, and a propensity toward clot production.[2,75–77] In aHUS, mutations in the alternative complement regulatory pathway, especially mutations in the complement factor H, impair control of C3b on the cell surface by inability to recognize sialic acid and helps to explain the thrombogenic potential in these patients.[2,78] Mutations have recently been described in multiple complement regulatory genes in adult patients with aHUS, with 12% of patients having compound mutations.[79] In addition to plasma exchange therapy, the anti-C5a monoclonal antibody eculizumab is FDA approved for this process. C3a, complement 3a; DIC, disseminated intravascular coagulation; HUS, hemolytic uremic syndrome.

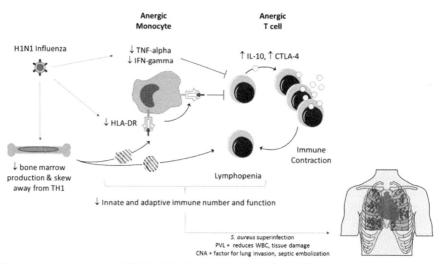

Fig. 2. Immune paralysis MOF. H1N1 influenza has adaptive and innate immune suppressive effects and is associated with the development of MRSA superinfection and death[26] in children, altered bone marrow microenvironment, and reduced leukocyte output in an animal model, with reduced human leukocyte antigen, antigen D related (HLA-DR), expression and reduction in proinflammatory TNF-a and interferon gamma (IFN-g) responses.[21,79–84] Alterations in innate immune cell function affect polarization and homeostasis of T-cell populations, because T cells interacting with anergic monocytes have increases in cytotoxic T-lymphocyte antigen 4 (CTLA-4)–mediated negative costimulation and antiinflammatory IL-10 responses.[85] Altered adaptive immune homeostasis favors contraction of immune populations and lymphopenia. Combined adaptive and innate leukopenia and decreased immune function predispose to secondary infection with methicillin-resistant *Staphylococcus aureus* (MRSA). MRSA elaboration of Panton-Valentine leukocidin (PVL) further reduces innate immune cell number and leads to cytotoxic lung and soft tissue damage.[86,87] *S aureus* collagen adhesin (CNA) is a virulence factor in invasive pulmonary disease, and may contribute to septic embolization of the pathogen.[87] Low-dose granulocyte macrophage colony-stimulating factor (GM-CSF) administration can be given to reverse immune paralysis.

endotoxin was highly and independently associated with both mortality and length of ICU stay.

The potential treatments for immune paralysis depend on the background immune status of the host. For chronically immune-suppressed patients, such as transplant recipients, withholding or reducing immune suppression is indicated in the setting of severe sepsis-associated multiple organ dysfunction syndrome (MODS).[27] Among patients with immunoparalysis-associated MOF who had a preintervention RR of death of 11 (95% CI 1.4–89), Hall and colleagues[28] showed that treatment with low-dose GM-CSF at 125 µg/meter squared per day for 7 days given over a minimum of 12 hours as an infusion prevented secondary infection, death, and restored ex vivo TNF response to LPS lipopolysaccharaide. Similarly, in a randomized double-blinded study of adults undergoing general surgical procedures with immunosuppression defined by HLA-DR expression less than 10,000 molecules on the surface of monocytes, administration of a single dose of GM-CSF, but not influenza vaccine, was associated with restored HLA-DR expression, improved white blood cell (WBC) count, and less severe delirium compared with placebo.[29] Therefore, the immune paralysis phenotype of MODS can be considered a reversible condition with appropriate modulation of the host immune response.[24]

Recent mouse model data have shown that PD-1 and PD-L1 blockade results in improved survival in a model of fungal sepsis[30] and ex vivo data have implicated PD-1 blockade as a potential therapy in patients with severe sepsis and the immune paralysis phenotype.[31] Clinical trials are currently enrolling adult patients with severe sepsis to test the role of PD-1–PD-L1 axis blockade using BMS-936559 (anti–PD-L1) in sepsis survival and organ function (https://clinicaltrials.gov/ct2/show/NCT02576457).

Critical Pertussis-Associated Multiple Organ Failure

Critical pertussis-associated MOF (**Fig. 3**) results in impairment of the innate immune response, and a poor adaptive immune response. In addition, both epithelial targeting and direct effects of pertussis toxin on leukocyte populations cause robust margination of neutrophils and lymphocytes from the tissues to the

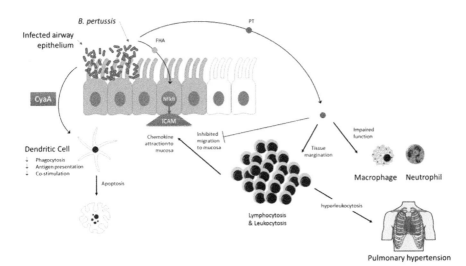

Fig. 3. Hyperleukocytosis: critical pertussis MOF. *Bordetella pertussis* infects the airway epithelium, inducing inflammation and altered mucosal immune response. Bacterial production of the virulence factor CyaA has several deleterious effects on CD11b+ dendritic cells, including decreased ability to perform phagocytosis, decreased capacity to present antigen to T cells, and decreased expression of costimulatory molecules. CyaA leads to dendritic cell apoptosis.[88] The virulence factor filamentous hemagglutinin (FHA) induces NF-kB–mediated upregulation of epithelial intercellular adhesion molecule 1 (ICAM-1) at sites of bacterial invasion.[88,92] This process, in part, results in the histopathologic findings typical of pertussis infection, including leukocyte activation and infiltration.[89] Leukocytosis and lymphocytosis and subsequent plugging of pulmonary arterioles and venules is specific to early infancy, predominantly caused by margination of cells from tissues.[89–91] Pertussis toxin (PT) decreases the ability of leukocytes to exit the blood vessel via impairment of CD62L expression and LFA-1.[91] PT has a further role in impairing macrophage and neutrophil activation and function via alterations in toll-like receptor (TLR)-4 signaling, whereas prolonged exposure of innate cells to FHA modulates NFkB responses downward.[92,93] Complement-mediated opsonization and phagocytosis and intracellular killing of *B pertussis* are impaired. Another virulence factor, ACT, leads to innate immune cell apoptosis.[93] In addition to leukocyte plugging and high blood viscosity, perturbations in NO-mediated regulation of pulmonary vascular tone contribute to pulmonary hypertension.[89–91] Infants have responded to extracorporeal leukocyte reduction therapies as well as inhaled NO and ECMO for reversal of cardiovascular collapse. ACT, Adenylate Cyclase Toxin; CD62L, L-selectin; LFA-1, lymphocyte function associated antigen 1.

circulation and the infected epithelial surfaces. The result is a unique pathophysiology of hyperleukocytosis in very young infants. The high viscosity and endothelial dysregulation with cellular plugging of pulmonary arterioles and venules results in pulmonary hypertension and cardiopulmonary collapse. The critical pertussis syndrome is associated with bacterial superinfection, and broad-spectrum antimicrobial source control should be initiated in patients with this MOF phenotype. In addition, leukoreduction therapy by therapeutic apheresis, organ support (potentially with the use of ECMO), and a trial of inhaled NO therapy are reasonable but unproven approaches to treatment.

The risk factors associated with mortality among less than 120-day-old infants include lower birth weight, younger gestational age, younger age at time of onset, higher peak WBC count, and lymphocyte count greater than 30,000 cells per microliter. In multivariate analysis, WBC count and birth weight were the only pre-ICU admission factors that were associated with death.[32] Among patients admitted to the ICU, 43% go on to require endotracheal intubation and mechanical ventilation.[33] A median WBC count greater than $27,000/mm^3$ was significantly associated with need for mechanical ventilation, the presence of pulmonary arterial hypertension, and death. Despite the brisk leukocytosis observed among infants, there is evidence that pertussis toxin has direct immune inhibitory effects on macrophage and neutrophil activation, putting the infants at risk for coinfection (see **Fig. 3**).

Therapies for critical pertussis include treatment of primary infection, prevention of secondary infection, ventilatory support, and leukoreduction to minimize the pathologic effects of hyperleukocytosis. However, limited data exist regarding whether the timing of *Bordetella pertussis*–directed antimicrobial therapy affects the important clinical outcomes of hospitalization days, need for mechanical ventilation, or death.[34] In addition to macrolide therapy, broad-spectrum antimicrobial therapy is used for critically ill patients with pertussis with severe sepsis or septic shock with special consideration for the possibility of bacterial respiratory superinfection. Rowlands and colleagues[35,36] proposed an algorithm for the use of leukoreduction therapy in critical pertussis based on WBC counts greater than $50,000/mm^3$ and presence of cardiopulmonary compromise. Additional therapies specific to pertussis pathophysiology as a toxin-driven disease include anti–pertussis toxin–enriched intravenous immune globulin (P-IVIG). Although standard intravenous immune globulin (IVIG) therapy has been shown to be ineffective in changing the severity of pertussis disease or in decreasing symptoms, preliminary trials have indicated that targeting the toxin has symptomatic benefit as well as a reduction in the degree of lymphocytosis without significant adverse events.[37,38] Further study is needed to determine the efficacy of P-IVIG or a combination of leukoreduction and antitoxin therapy in the critical pertussis cohort, specifically.

Sequential Multiple Organ Failure

Sequential MOF (SMOF) is a sequential respiratory and then hepatorenal failure syndrome that is driven by perturbation in the immune system's ability to perform activation-induced cell death (AICD) that leads to lymphoproliferation, and to perform DNA viral infection killing that leads to uncontrolled viremia (**Fig. 4**). This phenotype is most commonly found among patients with organ transplants who are maintained on T-cell immunosuppressant therapy and have Epstein-Barr virus (EBV) or other DNA viral infection. In this condition, EBV infection of B cells provides a pool for viral proliferation, resulting in posttransplant lymphoproliferative disorder (PTLD), and impairment of the normal Fas-Fas ligand (Fas-FasL)–mediated apoptotic pathways.

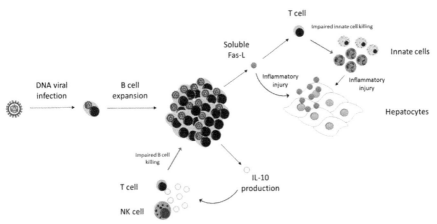

Fig. 4. Sequential MOF. The host-pathogen relationship model in sequential MOF is Epstein-Barr virus (EBV) infection of host B cells, such as occurs in transplant recipients. Virulence factors such as viral-encoded IL-10 modulate the host immune antigen-presenting, natural killer (NK) cell, and T-cell antiviral response and contribute to viral survival and lymphoproliferation.[94,95] B cells, among other cell types, have been hypothesized to be a source for soluble Fas ligand (s-FasL).[39] Membrane-bound FasL on T and NK cells interacts with Fas on target cells and results in cellular apoptosis, required to cull immune populations in AICD.[96] The production of large amounts of s-FasL by B cells may interfere with this pathway, impairing cytotoxic culling of B cells that are the cellular pool required for EBV infection. Production of s-FasL affects T cells' ability to kill innate immune cells, which leads to inflammatory injury at end organs, including hepatocytes. Furthermore, engagement of Fas on hepatocytes by anti-Fas antibody results in direct hepatic injury and s-FasL levels greater than 200 pg/mL were associated with hepatocyte destruction and mortality.[39,97–99] Immune suppressant withdrawal allows recovery of NK function and FDA-approved use of the anti-CD20 monoclonal antibody rituximab removes the reservoir of infection.

Soluble FasL interferes with the T and natural killer (NK) cells' ability to cull infected B cells, and also leads to direct hepatocyte injury through FasL-Fas interaction. Expanded innate populations further damage organs by inflammatory cytokine and direct effects. The treatment of sequential MODS includes withdrawal of immune suppression as able and B-cell reduction therapy with rituximab (anti-CD20 antibody) in addition to antiviral therapy.

The mortality has been approximately 50% once the diagnosis is made. The clinical SMOF phenotype was correlated with both high serum IL-10 concentrations and soluble Fas (s-Fas) and soluble Fas ligand (s-FasL), suggesting perturbation of Fas-FasL–mediated AICD proapoptotic pathway (see **Fig. 4**).[39,40] The at-risk host population for SMOF includes recipients of transplanted organs or tissues requiring immunosuppression, similar to the risk factor profile for PTLD. In contrast, SMOF has also been observed in viral disease without transplant in certain host genetic backgrounds, such as X-linked lymphoproliferative disease (XLP-1). Patients with XLP-1 with mutations in the SLAM-associated protein are susceptible to EBV infection because of a signal transduction defect in T cells and NK cells, rendering ineffective cytotoxic control of EBV-infected cell proliferation.[41] This process differs from X-linked inhibitor of apoptosis mutations in BIRC4 (XLP-2), in which patients are susceptible to EBV infection but present with splenomegaly and recurrent episodes of hemophagocytic syndrome, and inflammatory bowel disease.[42] In addition, mutations in this apoptotic signaling pathway have been found in approximately 75% of individuals with the autoimmune lymphoproliferative syndrome, in which immune contraction caused by AICD is impaired.

Similar to other MOF phenotypes, therapy for SMOF depends on the ascertained cause. For cases involving clinical SMOF, the magnitude of DNA viremia is important to consider. For PTLD-associated SMOF, the mainstay of therapy has been reduction of immune suppression to allow for cytotoxic T-cell and NK-cell control of the causative DNA virus. Reduction in immune suppression is balanced by risk of rejection in the setting of solid or hematopoietic organ transplant. The use of rituximab has emerged as an additional method that reduces the B-cell and, in turn, the DNA viral reservoir.[43] The therapeutic principle is that CD20 on mature B cells is engaged by the monoclonal antibody, which in turn has direct signaling effects on the B cells (apoptosis, B-cell receptor downregulation) and activation of cytotoxic response (NK cells and T cells via direct engagement and antibody-dependent cytotoxicity).[44] Based on soluble Fas levels in adult patients with diffuse large B-cell lymphomas, the measured Fas-FasL axis is related to rituximab treatment response.[45] Antiviral therapy remains critical to controlling DNA viremia and expansion of the infected pool. The observation that NK-cell cytotoxic activity is impaired in the setting of pediatric PTLD, and is associated with increased PD-1 expression, may result in new attention to monitoring NK-cell numbers and functional capacity in the host response.[46]

Severe Sepsis-Associated Macrophage Activation Syndrome

Severe sepsis-associated macrophage activation syndrome (MAS) is exemplified by the host-pathogen interaction of filoviruses (ie, Ebola virus) or other viral families associated with hemorrhagic fevers (**Fig. 5**). The hallmark of severe sepsis-associated MAS is high ferritin level, hepatobiliary dysfunction, and disseminated intravascular coagulation (DIC). In Ebola hemorrhagic fever (EHF), viral infection activates innate immune cells, impairs innate cells' ability to present antigen and costimulate T cells, and results in adaptive and NK-cell immune paralysis. The infection of vascular endothelium and macrophage production of procoagulant inflammatory mediators leads to DIC. Pathogen-associated molecular patterns and damage-associated molecular patterns (such as hemoglobin-haptoglobin complexes, and putatively ferritin) act to damage tissues and activate macrophages and also lead to direct cellular injury. The treatments for EHF specifically may include immune serum in the form of chimeric monoclonal antibodies (ie, ZMapp) to control viremia. In general terms, inflammation reduction therapy, such as steroids, IVIG, and plasma exchange, is useful in severe sepsis-associated MAS. Anticytokine therapy such as anakinra has also been shown to be beneficial as treatment of hyperinflammation in severe sepsis-associated MAS, and other cytokine blocking therapies are being evaluated.[47] The pathophysiology of hemorrhagic fever–driven MAS is based on unchecked and unabated inflammation and hemolysis-driven myeloid innate immune cell activation (see **Fig. 5**).

Viral hemorrhagic fever syndromes, such as those associated with the filoviruses (Ebola, Marburg), some flaviviruses (Dengue), and some arenaviruses (Lassa), have been reported as examples of viral disease–associated MAS. Ebola has the clinical features of MAS with associated cytopenias, DIC, ongoing capillary leak syndrome, and hepatic dysfunction.[48,49] Of note, a recent examination of 55 biomarkers in patients with EHF indicated that increases in serum thrombomodulin and serum ferritin levels were both associated with hemorrhage and mortality.[50,51] Increase of serum ferritin level has been shown to correlate with mortality among pediatric patients with MAS in multiple settings.[52,53]

Treatment of severe sepsis-associated MAS are varied but are in 2 broad categories: (1) control of source of inflammation, and (2) modulation of immune functional and

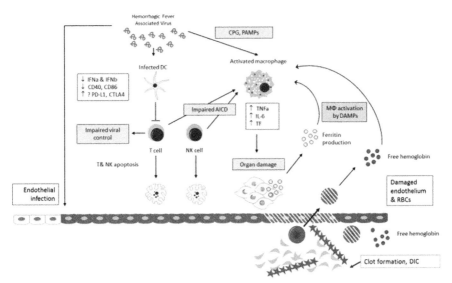

Fig. 5. Severe sepsis-associated MAS. Severe sepsis-associated MAS can be modeled after the host-pathogen interaction of the hemorrhagic fever viruses, including the filoviral family member Ebola. The unchecked inflammatory response is driven by myeloid lineage cells, including monocytes and macrophages, and functionally impaired T-cell and NK-cell responses. T cells are skewed away from robust antiviral responses and toward regulatory T-cell responses, in part because of a lack of costimulation from professional antigen-presenting cells and potentially because of negative costimulation and induction of apoptosis.[100–102] Macrophages are activated toward production of IL-6, TNF-a, and tissue factor (TF). IL-6 and TNF-a contribute to the cytokine storm phenotype, and TF promotes endothelial dysfunction and consumptive coagulopathy.[103] Danger-associated molecular pattern (DAMP) and pathogen-associated molecular pattern (PAMP) pattern recognition receptor (PRR) engagement through production of ferritin from either cellular damage or by the reticuloendothelial system, elaboration of free hemoglobin (via formation of hemoglobin-haptoglobin complexes and stimulation of CD163 receptors on monocytes and macrophages), or by TLR-9 stimulation via CpG, may provide a feed-forward mechanism by which monocytes and macrophages are further stimulated toward a proinflammatory phenotype. The proinflammatory cytokines IL-1 and TNF-alpha, which are produced at high levels by monocytes and macrophages, have been shown to have direct injurious effects on end organs and tissues (eg, heart, liver, kidney).[104,105] High ferritin levels were recently associated with mortality among patients with epidemic Ebola hemorrhagic fever.[49] Antiinflammatory therapies effective in reversing MAS have not been evaluated in patients infected with Ebola. CpG, 5'—C—phosphate—G—3' C = cytosine; p = phosphate; g = Guanine.

inflammation pathways. With regard to EHF, treatment with multiple chimeric monoclonal antibodies directed against viral components (ZMapp) was evaluated in nonhuman primates and in a clinical trial during the 2014 Sierra Leone outbreak, with inconclusive results. Although there may have been potential clinical benefit, there was an absence of statistical significance, requiring further study.[54,55] With regard to antiinflammatory and immune modulatory therapies for MAS, there are several potential approaches. One of the most studied anticytokine therapies has been IL-1 blockade with recombinant IL-1RA (anakinra), which has been associated with a 2-fold decrease in mortality in adults with severe sepsis-associated MAS.[47,56] The anti–IL-6 monoclonal antibody tocilizumab has shown efficacy in the treatment of systemic-onset juvenile idiopathic arthritis–induced MAS, and in cytokine release syndrome after chimeric antigen receptor (CAR) T-cell treatment of blood cancers.[57,58] Anti–IL-18 therapies, which may be promising for MAS, are currently under development. Unrelated to biologic therapies, a study of Turkish children with severe sepsis and features of MAS compared the hemophagocytic lymphohistiocytosis (HLH)–94 chemotherapy protocol with a regimen of plasma exchange and IVIG or methylprednisolone, and the HLH-94 protocol had an associated survival of only 50%, whereas the IVIG and steroid regimens had a survival of 100% ($P = .002$) when combined with plasma exchange therapy, supporting an anti-inflammatory approach for patients with MAS.[59,60]

SUMMARY

This article describes 5 inflammation pathobiology-driven phenotypes of pediatric sepsis-induced MOF, using specific host-pathogen interaction models to show the therapeutic opportunity for personalized precision medicine approaches that have the potential to improve outcomes in selected children. Further evaluation is necessary.

ACKNOWLEDGMENTS

The authors would like to acknowledge Dr Carol Vetterly for her ideas and expertise.

REFERENCES

1. Sadler JE, Sadler JE. Von Willebrand factor, ADAMTS13, and thrombotic thrombocytopenic purpura. Blood 2008;112(1):11–8.
2. Noris M. Complement factor H mutation in familial thrombotic thrombocytopenic purpura with ADAMTS13 deficiency and renal involvement. J Am Soc Nephrol 2005;16(5):1177–83.
3. Gando S. Microvascular thrombosis and multiple organ dysfunction syndrome. Crit Care Med 2010;38(2 Suppl):S35–42.
4. Okano E, Ko S, Kanehiro H, et al. ADAMTS13 activity decreases after hepatectomy, reflecting a postoperative liver dysfunction. Hepatogastroenterology 2010; 57(98):316–20. Available at: http://www.ncbi.nlm.nih.gov/pubmed/20583434. Accessed March 28, 2016.
5. Reuken PA, Kussmann A, Kiehntopf M, et al. Imbalance of von Willebrand factor and its cleaving protease ADAMTS 13 during systemic inflammation superimposed on advanced cirrhosis. Liver Int 2015;35(1):37–45.
6. Schaer DJ, Buehler PW, Alayash AI, et al. Hemolysis and free hemoglobin revisited: exploring hemoglobin and hemin scavengers as a novel class of therapeutic proteins. Blood 2013;121(8):1276–84.
7. Janz DR, Ware LB. The role of red blood cells and cell-free hemoglobin in the pathogenesis of ARDS. J Intensive Care 2015;3(1):1–7.
8. Gladwin MT, Kanias T, Kim-Shapiro DB. Hemolysis and cell-free hemoglobin drive an intrinsic mechanism for human disease. J Clin Invest 2012;122(4):1205–8.
9. Nguyen TC, Han YY, Kiss JE, et al. Intensive plasma exchange increases a disintegrin and metalloprotease with thrombospondin motifs-13 activity and reverses organ dysfunction in children with thrombocytopenia-associated multiple organ failure. Crit Care Med 2008;36(10):2878–87.
10. Nguyen TC, Liu A, Liu L, et al. Acquired ADAMTS-13 deficiency in pediatric patients with severe sepsis. Haematologica 2007;92(1):121–4. Available at: http://www.ncbi.nlm.nih.gov/pubmed/17229645. Accessed March 23, 2016.

11. Rimmer E, Houston BL, Kumar A, et al. The efficacy and safety of plasma exchange in patients with sepsis and septic shock: a systematic review and meta-analysis. Crit Care 2014;18(6):699.

12. Zhou F, Peng Z, Murugan R, et al. Blood purification and mortality in sepsis: a meta-analysis of randomized trials. Crit Care Med 2013;41(9):2209–20.

13. Darmon M, Azoulay E, Thiery G, et al. Time course of organ dysfunction in thrombotic microangiopathy patients receiving either plasma perfusion or plasma exchange. Crit Care Med 2006;34(8):2127–33.

14. Rock GA, Shumak KH, Buskard NA, et al. Comparison of plasma exchange with plasma infusion in the treatment of thrombotic thrombocytopenic purpura. Canadian Apheresis Study Group. N Engl J Med 1991;325(6):393–7.

15. Thejeel B, Garg AX, Clark WF, et al. Long-term outcomes of thrombotic microangiopathy treated with plasma exchange: a systematic review. Am J Hematol 2016. http://dx.doi.org/10.1002/ajh.24339.

16. Fakhouri F, Hourmant M, Campistol JM, et al. Terminal complement inhibitor eculizumab in adult patients with atypical hemolytic uremic syndrome: a single-arm, open-label trial. Am J Kidney Dis 2016;1–10. http://dx.doi.org/10.1053/j.ajkd.2015.12.034.

17. Greenbaum LA, Fila M, Ardissino G, et al. Eculizumab is a safe and effective treatment in pediatric patients with atypical hemolytic uremic syndrome. Kidney Int 2016;89(3):701–11.

18. Walle JV, Delmas Y, Ardissino G, et al. Improved renal recovery in patients with atypical hemolytic uremic syndrome following rapid initiation of eculizumab treatment. J Nephrol 2016. http://dx.doi.org/10.1007/s40620-016-0288-3.

19. Felmet KA, Hall MW, Clark RSB, et al. Prolonged lymphopenia, lymphoid depletion, and hypoprolactinemia in children with nosocomial sepsis and multiple organ failure. J Immunol 2005;174(6):3765–72.

20. Hotchkiss RS, Monneret G, Payen D. Sepsis-induced immunosuppression: from cellular dysfunctions to immunotherapy. Nat Rev Immunol 2013;13(12):862–74.

21. Hall MW, Geyer SM, Guo C-Y, et al. Innate immune function and mortality in critically ill children with influenza: a multicenter study. Crit Care Med 2013;41(1):224–36.

22. Drewry AM, Samra N, Skrupky LP, et al. Persistent lymphopenia after diagnosis of sepsis predicts mortality. Shock 2014;42(5):383–91.

23. Boomer JSJ, To K, Chang KKC, et al. Immunosuppression in patients who die of sepsis and multiple organ failure. JAMA 2011;306(23):2594–605.

24. Mathias B, Szpila BE, Moore FA, et al. A review of GM-CSF therapy in sepsis. Medicine (Baltimore) 2015;94(50):1–10.

25. Kollef KE, Schramm GE, Wills AR, et al. Predictors of 30-day mortality and hospital costs in patients with ventilator-associated pneumonia attributed to potentially antibiotic-resistant gram-negative bacteria. Chest 2008;134(2):281–7.

26. Randolph AG, Vaughn F, Sullivan R, et al. Critically ill children during the 2009-2010 influenza pandemic in the United States. Pediatrics 2011;128(6):e1450–8.

27. Mañez R, Kusne S, Linden P, et al. Temporary withdrawal of immunosuppression for life-threatening infections after liver transplantation. Transplantation 1994;57(1):149–51. Available at: http://www.pubmedcentral.nih.gov/articlerender.fcgi?artid=2977934&tool=pmcentrez&rendertype=abstract. Accessed May 19, 2016.

28. Hall MW, Knatz NL, Vetterly C, et al. Immunoparalysis and nosocomial infection in children with multiple organ dysfunction syndrome. Intensive Care Med 2011;37(3):525–32.

29. Spies C, Luetz A, Lachmann G, et al. Influence of granulocyte-macrophage colony-stimulating factor or influenza vaccination on HLA-DR, infection and delirium days in immunosuppressed surgical patients: double blind, randomised controlled trial. PLoS One 2015;10(12):e0144003.

30. Chang KC, Burnham C-A, Compton SM, et al. Blockade of the negative co-stimulatory molecules PD-1 and CTLA-4 improves survival in primary and secondary fungal sepsis. Crit Care 2013;17(3):R85.

31. Chang K, Svabek C, Vazquez-Guillamet C, et al. Targeting the programmed cell death 1: programmed cell death ligand 1 pathway reverses T cell exhaustion in patients with sepsis. Crit Care 2014;18(1):R3.

32. Winter K, Zipprich J, Harriman K, et al. Risk factors associated with infant deaths from pertussis: a case-control study. Clin Infect Dis 2015;61(7):1099–106.

33. Burr JS, Jenkins TL, Harrison R, et al. The Collaborative Pediatric Critical Care Research Network Critical Pertussis Study: collaborative research in pediatric critical care medicine. Pediatr Crit Care Med 2011;12(4):387–92.

34. Singhi S, Benkatti G. Critical pertussis. Pediatr Crit Care Med 2013;14(4):434–6.

35. Rowlands HE, Goldman AP, Harrington K, et al. Impact of rapid leukodepletion on the outcome of severe clinical pertussis in young infants. Pediatrics 2010; 126(4):e816–27.

36. Sawal M, Cohen M, Irazuzta JE, et al. Fulminant pertussis: a multi-center study with new insights into the clinico-pathological mechanisms. Pediatr Pulmonol 2009;44(10):970–80.

37. Granström M, Olinder-Nielsen AM, Holmblad P, et al. Specific immunoglobulin for treatment of whooping cough. Lancet 1991;338(8777):1230–3. Available at: http://www.ncbi.nlm.nih.gov/pubmed/1682643. Accessed October 7, 2016.

38. Bruss JB, Malley R, Halperin S, et al. Treatment of severe pertussis: a study of the safety and pharmacology of intravenous pertussis immunoglobulin. Pediatr Infect Dis J 1999;18(6):505–11. Available at: http://www.ncbi.nlm.nih.gov/pubmed/10391179. Accessed October 7, 2016.

39. Doughty L, Clark RSB, Kaplan SS, et al. sFas and sFas ligand and pediatric sepsis-induced multiple organ failure syndrome. Pediatr Res 2002;52(6):922–7.

40. Doughty L, Carcillo JA, Kaplan S, et al. The compensatory anti-inflammatory cytokine interleukin 10 response in pediatric sepsis-induced multiple organ failure. Chest 1998;113(6):1625–31.

41. Marsh RA, Madden L, Kitchen BJ, et al. XIAP deficiency: a unique primary immunodeficiency best classified as X-linked familial hemophagocytic lymphohistiocytosis and not as X-linked lymphoproliferative disease. Blood 2010; 116(7):1079–82.

42. Kelsen JR, Dawany N, Martinez A, et al. A de novo whole gene deletion of XIAP detected by exome sequencing analysis in very early onset inflammatory bowel disease: a case report. BMC Gastroenterol 2015;15:160. Available at: http://doi.org/10.1186/s12876-015-0394-z.

43. Cohen JI, Bollard CM, Khanna R, et al. Current understanding of the role of Epstein-Barr virus in lymphomagenesis and therapeutic approaches to EBV-associated lymphomas. Leuk Lymphoma 2008;49(Suppl 1):27–34. Available at: http://doi.org/10.1080/10428190802311417.

44. Weiner GJ. Rituximab: mechanism of action. Semin Hematol 2010;47(2):115–23.

45. Hara T, Tsurumi H, Goto N, et al. Serum soluble Fas level determines clinical outcome of patients with diffuse large B-cell lymphoma treated with CHOP and R-CHOP. J Cancer Res Clin Oncol 2009;135(10):1421–8.

46. Wiesmayr S, Webber SA, Macedo C, et al. Decreased NKp46 and NKG2D and elevated PD-1 are associated with altered NK-cell function in pediatric transplant patients with PTLD. Eur J Immunol 2012;42(2):541–50.
47. Shakoory B, Carcillo JA, Chatham WW, et al. Interleukin-1 receptor blockade is associated with reduced mortality in sepsis patients with features of macrophage activation syndrome: reanalysis of a prior phase III trial. Crit Care Med 2016;44(2):275–81.
48. van der Ven AJAM, Netea MG, van der Meer JWM, et al. Ebola virus disease has features of hemophagocytic lymphohistiocytosis syndrome. Front Med 2015;2:4.
49. McElroy AK, Erickson BR, Flietstra TD, et al. Ebola hemorrhagic fever: novel biomarker correlates of clinical outcome. J Infect Dis 2014;210(4):558–66.
50. Cron RQ, Behrens EM, Shakoory B, et al. Does viral hemorrhagic fever represent reactive hemophagocytic syndrome? J Rheumatol 2015;42(7):1078–80.
51. Rollin PE, Bausch DG, Sanchez A. Blood chemistry measurements and D-dimer levels associated with fatal and nonfatal outcomes in humans infected with Sudan Ebola virus. J Infect Dis 2007;196(s2):S364–71.
52. Garcia PCR, Longhi F, Branco RG, et al. Ferritin levels in children with severe sepsis and septic shock. Acta Paediatr 2007;96(12):1829–31.
53. Bennett TD, Hayward KN, Farris RWD, et al. Very high serum ferritin levels are associated with increased mortality and critical care in pediatric patients. Pediatr Crit Care Med 2011;12(6):e233–6.
54. PREVAIL II Writing Group; Multi-National PREVAIL II Study Team, Davey RT Jr, Dodd L, Proschan MA. A randomized, controlled trial of ZMapp for Ebola virus infection. N Engl J Med 2016;375(15):1448–56.
55. Qiu X, Wong G, Audet J, et al. Reversion of advanced Ebola virus disease in nonhuman primates with ZMapp. Nature 2014. http://dx.doi.org/10.1038/nature13777.
56. Rajasekaran S, Kruse K, Kovey K, et al. Therapeutic role of anakinra, an interleukin-1 receptor antagonist, in the management of secondary hemophagocytic lymphohistiocytosis/sepsis/multiple organ dysfunction/macrophage activating syndrome in critically ill children. Pediatr Crit Care Med 2014;15(5):401–8.
57. Yokota S, Imagawa T, Mori M, et al. Efficacy and safety of tocilizumab in patients with systemic-onset juvenile idiopathic arthritis: a randomised, double-blind, placebo-controlled, withdrawal phase III trial. Lancet 2008;371(9617):998–1006.
58. Teachey DT, Rheingold SR, Maude SL, et al. Cytokine release syndrome after blinatumomab treatment related to abnormal macrophage activation and ameliorated with cytokine-directed therapy. Blood 2013;121(26):5154–7.
59. Demirkol D, Yildizdas D, Bayrakci B, et al. Hyperferritinemia in the critically ill child with secondary hemophagocytic lymphohistiocytosis/sepsis/multiple organ dysfunction syndrome/macrophage activation syndrome: what is the treatment? Crit Care 2012;16(2):R52.
60. Qu L, Kiss JE, Dargo G, et al. Outcomes of previously healthy pediatric patients with fulminant sepsis-induced multisystem organ failure receiving therapeutic plasma exchange. J Clin Apher 2011;26(4):208–13.
61. Pron B, Taha MK, Rambaud C, et al. Interaction of *Neisseria meningitidis* with the components of the blood-brain barrier correlates with an increased expression of PilC. J Infect Dis 1997;176:1285–92.

62. Madico G, Welsch JA, Lewis LA, et al. The meningococcal vaccine candidate GNA1870 binds the complement regulatory protein factor H and enhances serum resistance. J Immunol 2006;177(1):501–10.

63. Miller F, Lécuyer H, Join-Lambert O, et al. *Neisseria meningitidis* colonization of the brain endothelium and cerebrospinal fluid invasion. Cell Microbiol 2013; 15(4):512–9.

64. Dixon GL, Heyderman RS, Kotovicz K, et al. Endothelial adhesion molecule expression and its inhibition by recombinant bactericidal/permeability-increasing protein are influenced by the capsulation and lipooligosaccharide structure of *Neisseria meningitidis*. Infect Immun 1999;67(11):5626–33. Available at: http://www.pubmedcentral.nih.gov/articlerender.fcgi?artid=96935&tool=pmcentrez&rendertype=abstract. Accessed March 29, 2016.

65. Dixon GLJ, Heyderman RS, van der Ley P, et al. High-level endothelial E-selectin (CD62E) cell adhesion molecule expression by a lipopolysaccharide-deficient strain of *Neisseria meningitidis* despite poor activation of NF-kappaB transcription factor. Clin Exp Immunol 2004;135(1):85–93. Available at: http://www.pubmedcentral.nih.gov/articlerender.fcgi?artid=1808929&tool=pmcentrez&rendertype=abstract. Accessed March 29, 2016.

66. Hollestelle MJ, Sprong T, Bovenschen N, et al. Von Willebrand factor activation, granzyme-B and thrombocytopenia in meningococcal disease. J Thromb Haemost 2010;8(5):1098–106.

67. Bongers TN, Emonts M, De Maat MPM, et al. Reduced ADAMTS13 in children with severe meningococcal sepsis is associated with severity and outcome. Thromb Haemost 2010;103(6):1181–7.

68. Nguyen TC, Carcillo JA. Bench-to-bedside review: thrombocytopenia-associated multiple organ failure–a newly appreciated syndrome in the critically ill. Crit Care 2006;10(6):235.

69. Kobsar A, Siauw C, Gambaryan S, et al. *Neisseria meningitidis* induces platelet inhibition and increases vascular endothelial permeability via nitric oxide regulated pathways. Thromb Haemost 2011;106(6):1127–38.

70. Pathan N, Faust SN, Levin M. Pathophysiology of meningococcal meningitis and septicaemia. Arch Dis Child 2003;88(7):601–7.

71. Feng S, Eyler SJ, Zhang Y, et al. Partial ADAMTS13 deficiency in atypical hemolytic uremic syndrome. Blood 2013;122(8):1487–94.

72. Furlan M, Robles R, Galbusera M, et al. von Willebrand factor-cleaving protease in thrombotic thrombocytopenic purpura and the hemolytic-uremic syndrome. N Engl J Med 1998;339(22):1578–84.

73. Louise CB, Obrig TG. Shiga toxin-associated hemolytic-uremic syndrome: combined cytotoxic effects of Shiga toxin, interleukin-1 beta, and tumor necrosis factor alpha on human vascular endothelial cells in vitro. Infect Immun 1991; 59(11):4173–9. Available at: http://www.pubmedcentral.nih.gov/articlerender.fcgi?artid=259013&tool=pmcentrez&rendertype=abstract.

74. Bauwens A, Betz J, Meisen I, et al. Facing glycosphingolipid-Shiga toxin interaction: dire straits for endothelial cells of the human vasculature. Cell Mol Life Sci 2013;70(3):425–57.

75. Morigi M, Galbusera M, Gastoldi S, et al. Alternative pathway activation of complement by Shiga toxin promotes exuberant C3a formation that triggers microvascular thrombosis. J Immunol 2011;187(1):172–80.

76. Müthing J, Schweppe CH, Karch H, et al. Shiga toxins, glycosphingolipid diversity, and endothelial cell injury. Thromb Haemost 2009;101(2):252–64.

77. Lehtinen MJ, Rops AL, Isenman DE, et al. Mutations of factor H impair regulation of surface-bound C3b by three mechanisms in atypical hemolytic uremic syndrome. J Biol Chem 2009;284(23):15650–8.

78. Hyvarinen S, Meri S, Jokiranta TS. Disturbed sialic acid recognition on endothelial cells and platelets in complement attack causes atypical hemolytic uremic syndrome. Blood 2016. http://dx.doi.org/10.1182/blood-2015-11-680009.

79. Maga TK, Nishimura CJ, Weaver AE, et al. Mutations in alternative pathway complement proteins in American patients with atypical hemolytic uremic syndrome. Hum Mutat 2010;31(6):1445–60.

80. Noone CM, Lewis EA, Frawely AB, et al. Novel mechanism of immunosuppression by influenza virus haemagglutinin: selective suppression of interleukin 12 p35 transcription in murine bone marrow-derived dendritic cells. J Gen Virol 2005;86(7):1885–90.

81. Ertürk M, Jennings R, Oxley KM, et al. Effect of influenza A on phagocytic cell function. Med Microbiol Immunol 1989;178(4):199–209. Available at: http://www.ncbi.nlm.nih.gov/pubmed/2747589. Accessed May 19, 2016.

82. Larson HEE, Blades R. Impairment of human polymorphonuclear leucocyte function by influenza virus. Lancet 1976;307(7954):283.

83. Hoeve MA, Nash AA, Jackson D, et al. Influenza virus A infection of human monocyte and macrophage subpopulations reveals increased susceptibility associated with cell differentiation. PLoS One 2012;7(1):e29443.

84. Lina G, Piemont Y, Godail-Gamot F, et al. Involvement of Panton-Valentine leukocidin–producing *Staphylococcus aureus* in primary skin infections and pneumonia. Clin Infect Dis 1999;29(5):1128–32.

85. Ayukawa H, Matsubara T, Kaneko M, et al. Expression of CTLA-4 (CD152) in peripheral blood T cells of children with influenza virus infection including encephalopathy in comparison with respiratory syncytial virus infection. Clin Exp Immunol 2004;137(1):151–5.

86. Löffler B, Hussain M, Grundmeier M, et al. *Staphylococcus aureus* Panton-Valentine leukocidin is a very potent cytotoxic factor for human neutrophils. PLoS Pathog 2010;6(1):e1000715.

87. Gonzalez BE, Hulten KG, Dishop MK, et al. Pulmonary manifestations in children with invasive community-acquired *Staphylococcus aureus* infection. Clin Infect Dis 2005;41(5):583–90.

88. Mattoo S, Cherry JD. Molecular pathogenesis, epidemiology, and clinical manifestations of respiratory infections due to *Bordetella pertussis* and other *Bordetella* subspecies. Clin Microbiol Rev 2005;18(2):326–82.

89. Paddock CD, Sanden GN, Cherry JD, et al. Pathology and pathogenesis of fatal *Bordetella pertussis* infection in infants. Clin Infect Dis 2008;47(3):328–38.

90. Carbonetti NH. Bordetella pertussis. Curr Opin Infect Dis 2016;29(3):287–94.

91. Carbonetti NH. Pertussis leukocytosis: mechanisms, clinical relevance and treatment. Pathog Dis 2016;74(7) [pii:ftw087].

92. Abramson T, Kedem H, Relman DA. Modulation of the NF-κB pathway by *Bordetella pertussis* filamentous hemagglutinin. PLoS One 2008;3(11):e3825.

93. de Gouw D, Diavatopoulos DA, Bootsma HJ, et al. Pertussis: a matter of immune modulation. FEMS Microbiol Rev 2011;35(3):441–74.

94. Jochum S, Moosmann A, Lang S, et al. The EBV immunoevasins vIL-10 and BNLF2a protect newly infected B cells from immune recognition and elimination. PLoS Pathog 2012;8(5):e1002704.

95. Salek-Ardakani S, Arrand JR, Mackett M. Epstein-Barr virus encoded interleukin-10 inhibits HLA-class I, ICAM-1, and B7 expression on human monocytes: implications for immune evasion by EBV. Virology 2002;304(2):342–51.

96. Waring P, Mullbacher A. Cell death induced by the Fas/Fas ligand pathway and its role in pathology. Immunol Cell Biol 1999;77(4):312–7.

97. Faouzi S, Burckhardt BE, Hanson JC, et al. Anti-Fas induces hepatic chemokines and promotes inflammation by an NF-kappa B-independent, caspase-3-dependent pathway. J Biol Chem 2001;276(52):49077–82.

98. Ogasawara J, Watanabe-Fukunaga R, Adachi M, et al. Lethal effect of the anti-Fas antibody in mice. Nature 1993;364(6440):806–9.

99. Kakinuma C, Takagaki K, Yatomi T, et al. Acute toxicity of an anti-fas antibody in mice. Toxicol Pathol 1999;27(4):412–20.

100. Bradfute SB, Braun DR, Shamblin JD, et al. Lymphocyte death in a mouse model of Ebola virus infection. J Infect Dis 2007;196(s2):S296–304.

101. Gupta M, Spiropoulou C, Rollin PE. Ebola virus infection of human PBMCs causes massive death of macrophages, CD4 and CD8 T cell sub-populations in vitro. Virology 2007;364(1):45–54.

102. Mohamadzadeh M, Chen L, Schmaljohn AL. How Ebola and Marburg viruses battle the immune system. Nat Rev Immunol 2007;7(7):556–67.

103. Geisbert TW, Hensley LE, Jahrling PB, et al. Treatment of Ebola virus infection with a recombinant inhibitor of factor VIIa/tissue factor: a study in rhesus monkeys. Lancet 2003;362(9400):1953–8.

104. Drosatos K, Lymperopoulos A, Kennel PJ, et al. Pathophysiology of sepsis-related cardiac dysfunction: driven by inflammation, energy mismanagement, or both? Curr Heart Fail Rep 2015;12(2):130–40.

105. Mizuhara H, O'Neill E, Seki N, et al. T cell activation-associated hepatic injury: mediation by tumor necrosis factors and protection by interleukin 6. J Exp Med 1994;179(5):1529–37. Available at: http://www.ncbi.nlm.nih.gov/pubmed/8163936. Accessed February 14, 2017.

Immunoparalysis in Pediatric Critical Care

Mark W. Hall, MD[a],*, Kristin C. Greathouse, MS, CPNP-AC[b], Rajan K. Thakkar, MD[c], Eric A. Sribnick, MD, PhD[d], Jennifer A. Muszynski, MD[a]

KEYWORDS

- Immunoparalysis • Pediatric • Critical care • Immune • Sepsis • Trauma
- Cardiopulmonary bypass

KEY POINTS

- The proinflammatory surge that accompanies the onset of pediatric critical illness often occurs concurrently with a compensatory anti-inflammatory response.
- When severe and persistent, this anti-inflammatory response has been termed immunoparalysis and is associated with increased risks for nosocomial infection and mortality across a wide variety of pediatric intensive care unit (PICU) diagnoses.
- Immunoparalysis is quantifiable by tests that measure monocyte human leukocyte antigen (HLA)-DR expression, ex vivo stimulated cytokine production capacities, and cell counts.
- Promising therapies exist that have the potential to reverse immunoparalysis and improve outcomes in the PICU.
- Standardized immune monitoring regimens are needed to guide clinical management and inform enrollment into clinical trials aimed at restoring immune function in the PICU.

INTRODUCTION

Although the diagnoses that result in pediatric critical illness can vary (eg, sepsis, trauma, cardiopulmonary bypass [CPB]), the initial insult is often proinflammatory in nature.

It has long been understood that the degree of hyperinflammation associated with these diagnoses predicts adverse outcomes, with greater inflammation being linked to organ failure and mortality.[1–3] Mounting evidence suggests, however, that a

Disclosure Statement: No relevant disclosures.
[a] Department of Pediatrics, Division of Critical Care Medicine, Nationwide Children's Hospital, 700 Children's Drive, Columbus, OH 43205, USA; [b] The Heart Center, Nationwide Children's Hospital, 700 Children's Drive, Columbus, OH 43205, USA; [c] Department of Pediatric Surgery, Nationwide Children's Hospital, 700 Children's Drive, Columbus, OH 43205, USA; [d] Department of Neurosurgery, Nationwide Children's Hospital, 700 Children's Drive, Columbus, OH 43205, USA
* Corresponding author.
E-mail address: mark.hall@nationwidechildrens.org

compensatory anti-inflammatory response syndrome (CARS) often occurs concurrently with the systemic inflammatory response syndrome (SIRS) (**Fig. 1**). This anti-inflammatory response, when severe and persistent, has been termed immunoparalysis and it represents a form of acquired immune deficiency that is itself associated with adverse outcomes in the pediatric intensive care unit (PICU). Immunoparalysis can affect multiple arms of the immune system and is often occult, with no physical examination or routine clinical laboratory evidence of its presence. Specialized testing, however, can identify patients with critical illness-induced immune suppression and a growing body of evidence suggests that immunoparalysis is reversible with the potential for beneficial effects on clinical outcomes.

To place the concept of immunoparalysis in context, this article begins with an overview of the immune system. Following this, the laboratory characteristics of immunoparalysis are reviewed along with detailed discussions of its clinical implications across multiple forms of pediatric critical illness. The treatment of immunoparalysis through immunostimulatory strategies is also reviewed. The overall goal is to highlight the need for immunologic balance in children with critical illness and to identify immunoparalysis as an important contributor to clinical outcomes in the PICU.

THE IMMUNOLOGY OF INFLAMMATION
The Innate Immune System

In general terms, the immune system can be divided into the innate and the adaptive arms (**Box 1**). The innate immune system is the body's first cellular line of defense. It includes cell types such as monocytes, macrophages, polymorphonuclear cells, natural killer (NK) cells, and dendritic cells. Innate immune cells are key drivers of the initial acute immune response. Their diverse roles include recognition and phagocytosis of pathogens, presentation of antigens to adaptive immune cells, and secretion of mediators that modulate the overall immune response. A characteristic feature of innate immune cells is their ability to consistently respond to pathogens regardless of prior

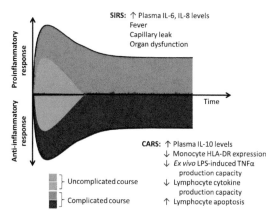

Fig. 1. The dynamic nature of the immune response to critical illness. Severe and persistent inflammation is associated with the classic symptoms of SIRS with fever, capillary leak, and organ dysfunction. CARS can occur concurrently with systemic inflammation. This can also be pathogenic when severe and prolonged, with associated increases in risk of nosocomial infection and death. More modest and transient deviations from immunologic homeostasis are typically associated with uncomplicated recovery. Both SIRS and CARS can be quantified through specific laboratory testing. HLA, human leukocyte antigen; IL, interleukin; LPS, lipopolysaccharide; TNF, tumor necrosis factor.

Box 1
Elements of the innate and adaptive immune systems

Innate	Adaptive
Cellular Elements	Cellular Elements
Phagocytosis	Antibody production
Monocytes/Macrophages	B cells/Plasma cells
Polymorphonuclear leukocytes	Cytotoxic killing
Dendritic cells	CD8+ T cells
Antigen presentation	Cytokine/chemokine production
Monocytes/Macrophages	CD4+ T cells
Dendritic cells	T_H^1 cells (proinflammatory)
Cytotoxic killing	T_H^2 cells (anti-inflammatory)
Natural killer cells	T_{reg} cells (anti-inflammatory)
Polymorphonuclear leukocytes	
Cytokine/chemokine production	
All of the above	
Noncellular Elements	Noncellular Elements
Cytokines	Immunoglobulins
Cheniokines	Cytokines
Complement	Cheniokines

exposure history. This is accomplished through the presence of constitutively expressed receptors on their plasma membranes. These receptors recognize broad classes of pathogen-associated molecular patterns. For example, bacterial lipopolysaccharide (LPS) is recognized by monocytes through its interaction with the toll-like receptor-4 on the monocyte's cell surface. A monocyte that encounters LPS should respond vigorously regardless of whether it has been exposed to LPS in the past.

Once stimulated, monocytes engulf and destroy microbes that are then processed into antigenic peptides. These are presented on the surfaces of innate immune cells on class II major histocompatibility complex (MHC) molecules such as human leukocyte antigen (HLA)-DR. Antigens presented in this way, along with costimulatory input from the innate immune cells, activate the adaptive arm of the immune response. Innate immune cells also secrete cytokines and chemokines that modulate the inflammatory response by recruiting and activating other immune effector cells and activating noncellular aspects of the immune response, such as the complement and coagulation cascades. Local production of proinflammatory cytokines, such as tumor necrosis factor (TNF)-α, results in activation of nearby immune cells and alters the vascular endothelium to promote cellular migration into the periphery. It is when these effects become systemic that the clinical signs and symptoms of hyperinflammation (fever, hemodynamic instability, and capillary leak) become evident.

The Adaptive Immune System

T and B lymphocytes are adaptive immune cells. In contrast to innate immunity, the adaptive immune system produces responses that are highly antigen-specific. Adaptive immune responses typically require antigen presentation by innate immune cells. The initial lymphocyte response to a pathogen takes more time and is of smaller magnitude than the initial innate response. Repeated exposure to an antigen, however, provokes a more rapid and powerful adaptive immune response due to the presence of antigen-specific T and B cell clones that can be maintained for decades.

On stimulation, B cells mature into plasma cells that produce antibodies that opsonize invaders, thus marking them for clearance by lymphoid organs and phagocytes. Activated T cells regulate the immune response through the production of cytokines (CD4+) and via cytotoxic killing (CD8+). Naïve CD4+ T cells can differentiate into 1 of several T cell subtypes, depending on the cytokine milieu in which they are activated. Although a detailed review of T-cell biology is beyond the scope of this article, several major classes of CD4+ T cells merit general discussion. These include the T-helper (T_H)-1, T_H2, and regulatory T cells (T_{reg}). In the presence of proinflammatory cytokines, naïve T cells will differentiate into T_H1 cells. These cells, in turn, produce proinflammatory cytokines such as interferon (INF)-γ and serve to perpetuate the inflammatory response. T_H2 cells, by contrast, arise when naïve T cells are activated in an anti-inflammatory environment. In addition to promoting host immunity against extracellular parasites (eg, helminths) and stimulating immunoglobulin E release by B cells, T_H2 cells produce anti-inflammatory cytokines, including interleukin (IL)-10 with a resultant inhibitory effect on the inflammatory response. T_{reg} are even more potently anti-inflammatory, down-regulating proinflammatory responses through elaboration of IL-10 and transforming growth factor (TGF)-β along with direct inhibition of leukocytes through cell-to-cell contact. These cells can be identified through their cell surface marker expression pattern ($CD4^+CD25^+CD127^{lo}$) and through their expression of transcription factor FOXP3.

Cytokines and Chemokines

Cytokines and chemokines are proteins that leukocytes and other cell types produce that modulate the local environment and/or recruit other immune cells to the area to combat infection (**Table 1**). Some cytokines (eg, TNFα, INF-γ, and IL-1β) have proinflammatory effects, whereas anti-inflammatory cytokines (eg, IL-10 and TGFβ) deactivate effector cells and inhibit the proinflammatory response. Chemokines, such as IL-8, are chemoattractants that result in cellular migration into an inflamed area. Some cytokines are pleiotropic, with both proinflammatory and anti-inflammatory effects. For example, IL-6 is known to stimulate the hepatic acute phase response while it also induces an adrenal glucocorticoid response.[4,5] Restoring balance between proinflammatory and anti-inflammatory forces, while maintaining the ability of immune cells to survey for and fight new infection and participate in tissue healing, is the goal of immunomodulatory therapy in the PICU.

LABORATORY CHARACTERISTICS OF IMMUNOPARALYSIS

The innate and adaptive arms of the immune system can both be affected in the setting of immunoparalysis. The 2 measures of reduced innate immune function that have been most consistently associated with adverse PICU outcomes are monocyte HLA-DR expression and whole blood ex vivo LPS-induced cytokine production capacity. As previously noted, monocytes activate the adaptive immune response through the presentation of antigens on cell-surface class II MHC molecules, of which there are several subtypes. HLA-DR is the antigen-presenting molecule that has been best characterized in critical illness, and its expression on circulating monocytes can be quantified by flow cytometry. It has been clearly shown that monocytes, which normally express HLA-DR very strongly, internalize their HLA-DR molecules in the setting of immunoparalysis.[6] Early work in critically ill adults suggested that if less than 30% of subjects' circulating monocytes stained strongly for HLA-DR then their risk of

Table 1
Selected cytokines and their effects

	Cytokine	Primary Producers	Actions
Proinflammatory	IL-1β	Monocytes or macrophages	Fever, vasodilation, activation of T cells, monocytes, or macrophages
	TNFα	Monocytes or macrophages, T cells (T$_H$1), NK cells	Fever, vasodilation, apoptosis, activation of T cells, monocytes, or macrophages
	IL-18	Macrophages	Activation of T cells and monocytes
	IL-12	Macrophages, DCs	Activation of NK cells
	IL-17	T cells (T$_H$ 17)	Induction of proinflammatory cytokines
	INF-γ	T cells (T$_H$1), NK cells	Activation of monocytes or macrophages
	GM-CSF	T cells, macrophages	Increases production and promotes growth and activation of monocytes, macrophages, PMNs, and DCs
Mixed effects	IL6	Monocytes, macrophages, vascular endothelium	Promotes acute phase response (pro), activates adrenal axis (anti)
Anti-inflammatory	IL-10	Monocytes or macrophages, T cells (T$_H$2, Treg)	Inhibits monocyte or macrophage activation
	TGFβ	Monocytes, T cells (T$_H$2, Treg)	Inhibits monocyte or macrophage proliferation and activation
	IL-13	T cells (T$_H$2)	Inhibits monocyte or macrophage cytokine production
	IL-1ra	Hepatocytes, monocytes or macrophages, PMNs	Inhibits IL-1 action by blocking the IL-1 receptor

Abbreviations: DC, dendritic cell; GM-CSF, granulocyte macrophage colony-stimulating factor; INF, interferon; IL, interleukin; PMN, polymorphonucleocyte; ra, receptor antagonist; TNF, tumor necrosis factor.

nosocomial infection and/or death was significantly higher than those with higher HLA-DR expression.[7–10] This has also been demonstrated in children with multiple organ dysfunction syndrome (MODS).[11] More recently, assays have been developed that can determine the number of HLA-DR molecules per monocyte, also using flow cytometry.[12] This method, through the use of standard beads, has the potential to avoid variability between antibody lots and cytometers, leading to more generalizable results. A threshold of fewer than 8000 HLA-DR molecules per cell has been used to define immunoparalysis, with fewer than 5000 HLA-DR molecules per cell signifying severe immunoparalysis.[13] Although few studies have used this method to evaluate pediatric innate immune function, 1 small study showed that failure to increase monocyte HLA-DR expression by at least 1000 molecules per cell over the first week of pediatric septic shock was associated with mortality.[14]

The other commonly used method for quantification of innate immune function in pediatric critical illness is through measurement of the capacity of whole blood to produce the proinflammatory cytokine TNFα when stimulated ex vivo. This type of measurement does not reflect circulating TNFα levels in the plasma but rather reflects the ability of a patient's blood to make TNFα when it is needed. Although a normal patient's whole blood will produce large amounts of TNFα when incubated with LPS, a sample from an immunoparalyzed patient's will not. In this way TNFα production capacity, when measured using highly standardized stimulation reagents and protocols, can serve as a readout of innate immune responsiveness, with a low value representing immune suppression. The largest body of evidence in critically ill children associating low innate immune function with adverse outcomes, spanning multiple diagnostic groups, uses this method of immune function testing.[11,15–18]

The adaptive immune system can fail in the context of immunoparalysis as well. Apoptosis of lymphocytes within lymphoid organs such as the spleen is common in the setting of immunoparalysis.[19–21] Similarly, persistent systemic lymphopenia with an absolute lymphocyte count less than 1000 cells/mm^3 has been associated with nosocomial infection and death in the setting of pediatric MODS.[20] In addition to low cell numbers, lymphocyte responsiveness can also be reduced in the intensive care unit (ICU). Reduction in the ability of lymphocytes to produce INF-γ when incubated ex vivo with the lymphocyte stimulants phytohemagglutinin (PHA) or anti-CD3–anti-CD28 antibody has been associated with infections, complications, and death in the setting of pediatric and adult sepsis.[21,22] These findings are in agreement with messenger RNA (mRNA) studies that suggest that early suppression of lymphocyte signaling pathways are associated with pediatric sepsis mortality.[23] Finally, expression of coinhibitory molecules such as programmed death (PD)-1 on lymphocytes, and its ligands PD-L1 and PD-L2 on antigen-presenting cells, is known to be upregulated in critically ill adults, with higher expression levels predicting adverse outcomes.[21,24]

CLINICAL IMPLICATIONS OF IMMUNOPARALYSIS
Trauma

Trauma surgeons were among the first clinicians to study the innate immune response in the setting of critical illness. In 1986, Polk and colleagues[25] undertook a systematic evaluation of adults with severe trauma to assess immunologic factors associated with the development of secondary infection and late mortality. The results of their analyses indicated that persistently impaired monocyte antigen-presenting capacity was associated with the development of nosocomial sepsis. The ability of HLA-DR expression to predict outcome in traumatized adults was strengthened by the work of Cheadle and colleagues[26] in 1989 in a study of serial monocyte HLA-DR measurements in 60 trauma victims beginning the first 24 hours after injury. In their cohort, the depth and persistence of reduction in HLA-DR expression was predictive of the development of secondary infection. Ex vivo TNFα production has also been correlated with outcome in clinical trauma studies. Majetschak and colleagues[27] in 1999 performed ex vivo LPS-induced stimulation of whole blood samples from 46 adult blunt trauma victims. They documented a profound reduction in subjects' TNFα production capacity compared with healthy controls. The degree of reduction in the TNFα response was associated with the severity of injury and this reduction was detectable in samples obtained within 90 minutes after trauma. Subjects requiring surgery to treat their injuries experienced a further impairment in their TNFα response. In 2014, Muszynski and colleagues[18] reported similar findings in a 76-subject cohort of critically injured children, with early reduction in ex vivo LPS-induced TNFα production capacity (<48 hours from injury) being associated with nosocomial infection risk. Children who went on to develop nosocomial infection also had lower TNF responses over the first week following injury compared with children who recovered without infection.

Central nervous system damage represents a particularly immunosuppressive form of injury. Injury to the brain and/or spinal cord can promote immune cell deactivation through direct neural effects mediated by the vagus nerve, through the hypothalamo-adrenal axis, and through elaboration of immunomodulatory mediators that cross the damaged blood-brain barrier into the systemic circulation.[28] It is not clear if these mechanisms are similar between pediatric and adult brain-injured patients, but in the Muszynski cohort, severe traumatic brain injury was associated with severe impairment of innate immune function and dramatically increased risk for nosocomial infection.[18]

Sepsis

Critical illness–induced immune suppression has also been well described in the setting of adult and pediatric sepsis. In the mid-1990s Volk and colleagues[7] studied monocyte HLA-DR expression in 247 septic adults. In their cohort, an HLA-DR expression level less than 30% for 5 days or more was associated with a 12% survival rate. This was in contrast to a survival rate of 88% in subjects whose reduction in monocyte HLA-DR expression was transient or less severe. Monneret and colleagues[9] in 2006 reported monocyte HLA-DR expression data from 93 adult subjects with septic shock and showed that those who survived had recovery of HLA-DR expression by day 3 or 4, whereas those who eventually died failed to recover HLA-DR expression. Multivariate logistic regression analysis showed that a monocyte HLA-DR expression less than 30% on day 3 or 4 was associated with mortality after adjusting for confounders, including initial severity of illness and presence of comorbidities. Hall and colleagues[11] found similar results in children with MODS, in that those who demonstrated monocyte HLA-DR expression less than 30% for more than 3 days had significantly increased risks for the development of nosocomial infection and death. It is notable that immunoparalysis was highly prevalent in this population, representing approximately a third of subjects.

As in the setting of trauma, impairment of the ex vivo LPS-induced TNFα response has also been shown to occur following the onset of septic disease and is also associated with adverse outcomes. Ploder and colleagues[29] described a series of adult subjects with sepsis in whom the degree of depression of the ex vivo TNFα response on the day of sepsis onset was more predictive of death than was the level of monocyte HLA-DR expression. In a cohort of 28 children with MODS (25 of whom had septic shock as the inciting event), Hall and colleagues[30] showed that nonsurvivors demonstrated lower ex vivo LPS-induced TNFα production over the first 2 weeks of MODS compared with survivors.

Innate immune function has been evaluated in single center and multicenter cohorts of children with critical illness due to viral infection. In 2013, Hall and colleagues[31] reported results from a 15-center, 55-subject study of critical influenza that spanned the recent H1N1 pandemic. Nonsurvivors had high levels of both proinflammatory and anti-inflammatory mediators in their serum but had marked reduction in their TNFα response in samples obtained within 72 hours of ICU admission compared with survivors and healthy controls. Severe innate immune suppression remained associated with mortality risk after adjusting for initial severity of illness, secondary infection, and comorbidities. Interestingly, the risk of severe reduction in TNFα response was greatest in children presenting with influenza plus Staphylococcus aureus secondary infection. Mella and colleagues[17] similarly showed, in a cohort of infants hospitalized with respiratory syncytial virus infection, that reduction in the ex vivo LPS-induced TNFα response was associated with higher severity of illness and longer lengths of PICU stay.

As previously noted, lymphocyte suppression has also been associated with adverse sepsis outcomes. Hotchkiss and colleagues[19,21] have repeatedly shown that lymphocyte apoptosis and impairment of lymphocyte cytokine production capacity are characteristic of sepsis deaths in adults. Muszynski and colleagues[22] demonstrated, in children with septic shock, that infectious complications were associated with lower lymphocyte counts and reduced ability of lymphocytes to respond to ex vivo stimulation with PHA. This reduction was not limited to proinflammatory cytokines such as INF-γ but extended to anti-inflammatory cytokines as well, implying global down-regulation of cytokine responses. These data were consistent with transcriptome profiling done by Wong and colleagues[23] that suggested that early down-regulation of lymphocyte signaling pathways predicts mortality and organ failure duration in pediatric sepsis. In addition, data from septic adults suggest that T_{reg} cells may be resistant to the apoptotic surge seen in sepsis, resulting in a T_{reg}-predominant state that may perpetuate immunoparalysis.[32–34] This T_{reg}-predominance has not been seen in pediatric sepsis to date.[22]

Cardiopulmonary Bypass

The inflammatory stimuli of leukocyte exposure to CBP circuitry and ischemia-reperfusion injury frequently result in systemic inflammation following pediatric open heart surgery. CARS, however, can also be prevalent in this population. Allen and colleagues[35] studied 82 infants and children undergoing CPB for repair of congenital heart defects and documented reduced monocyte HLA-DR expression in all subjects post-CPB compared with pre-CPB levels. Prolonged reduction of HLA-DR expression was associated with the development of SIRS and sepsis after surgery. These results were supported by the same group in a 2006 follow-up study in which 36 children undergoing CPB were evaluated.[16] Immune function was monitored serially by ex vivo LPS stimulation assays and IL-10 measurements. Higher levels of plasma IL-10 were associated with the greatest risk of developing more severe innate immune dysfunction. Patients with more profoundly reduced ex vivo TNFα responses as early as day 2 following CPB had a greater likelihood of experiencing postoperative complications, including nosocomial sepsis. More recently, Cornell and colleagues[15] demonstrated an association between reduced TNFα response on postoperative day 1 and subsequent development of sepsis in a 92 subject cohort of children undergoing CPB. Intriguingly, an epigenetic modification in the IL-10 promotor region that is predicted to enhance IL-10 production seemed to be triggered by CPB in some children.

REVERSIBILITY OF IMMUNOPARALYSIS

Evidence suggests that host immune function can be restored in the setting of immunoparalysis through several therapeutic approaches. Hershman and colleagues[36] reported in 1989 that monocytes collected from immunoparalyzed adult trauma victims upregulated their HLA-DR expression on ex vivo culture with INF-γ. In a similar cohort, Flohe and colleagues[37] showed restoration of the TNFα response in monocytes that were cultured ex vivo with the cytokine granulocyte macrophage colony-stimulating factor (GM-CSF). More recently, Lendemans and colleagues[38] showed that ex vivo treatment with INF-γ or GM-CSF (but not granulocyte colony-stimulating factor) resulted in improvement in both monocyte HLA-DR expression and whole blood LPS-induced cytokine production in blood samples from injured subjects.

Reversal of immunoparalysis in vivo seems to be possible as well. In 1997, Kox and colleagues[39] demonstrated restoration of monocyte HLA-DR expression and ex vivo

TNFα response in 9 of 10 adult septic subjects with immunoparalysis on treatment with subcutaneous INF-γ. In 2002, Nakos and colleagues[40] conducted a small randomized placebo-controlled trial of inhaled INF-γ in 21 trauma subjects with reduced HLA-DR expression on alveolar macrophages obtained by bronchoalveolar lavage (BAL). Although there was no difference in mortality between groups, the INF-γ-treated subjects showed increased HLA-DR expression on alveolar macrophages, decreased IL-10 levels in subsequent BAL fluid, and a reduced rate of ventilator-associated pneumonia compared with the placebo group.

Recombinant human GM-CSF has also been used to treat ICU patients with immunoparalysis. This drug is particularly favorable for this purpose because it has been approved by the Food and Drug Administration (FDA) since 1991 for reconstitution of bone marrow after chemotherapy. The side effect profile is low and it is known to increase granulocyte and monocyte numbers, as well as improve the function of existing cells of those lineages. In 2003, Nierhaus and colleagues[41] reported a case series in which 9 septic adults with immunoparalysis received GM-CSF by subcutaneous injection daily for 3 days. All subjects experienced increases in both monocyte HLA-DR expression and ex vivo LPS-induced TNFα production within 24 hours of initiation of GM-CSF treatment. A small randomized, controlled trial (RCT) in septic adults showed improvement in monocyte HLA-DR expression and faster resolution of infection with GM-CSF compared with placebo.[42] In 2001, Bilgin and colleagues[43] reported the results of an RCT of GM-CSF therapy versus placebo for neutropenic neonates with sepsis. Neonates receiving GM-CSF demonstrated significant improvement in mortality rate (10%) compared with those in the placebo group (30%). These RCTs, however, did not use a priori measurement of the innate immune response. It is likely, therefore, that some subjects assigned to receive GM-CSF did not have severe reductions in innate immune function, thereby diluting the treatment effect.

Two small clinical trials, 1 in adults and 1 in children, have been completed using innate immune function monitoring to screen subjects for immunoparalysis before drug treatment. Meisel and colleagues[13] reported data from 38 subjects who had immunoparalysis as evidenced by monocyte HLA-DR expression fewer than 8000 molecules per cell for 2 days. Subjects were randomized to receive GM-CSF or placebo for 8 days. Subjects in GM-CSF group showed higher HLA-DR expression and TNFα production capacity over time compared with the placebo group, with lower illness severity over time and lower resource utilization. A smaller, 14-subject RCT has been performed in children with MODS, comparing GM-CSF treatment to standard care in subjects found to have severe reduction in TNFα response.[11] In this study, GM-CSF therapy was associated with normalization of the TNFα response and dramatic reduction in risk of nosocomial infection. Importantly, in none of these studies was GM-CSF therapy associated with worsening of systemic inflammation. In fact, plasma levels of proinflammatory markers, such as IL-6 and IL-8, were the same or lower after treatment with GM-CSF.

There are several ongoing studies of GM-CSF for the restoration of innate immune function in critical illness. These include a French RCT in septic adults with immunoparalysis, targeting reduction in nosocomial infection risk (NCT02361528) and a smaller British RCT in septic adults, targeting improvement in neutrophil function (NCT01653665). The only such trial in pediatrics is the GM-CSF for Immunomodulation Following Trauma (GIFT) study that is currently being performed by the Collaborative Pediatric Critical Care Research Network (NCT01495637). In this multicenter study, critically injured children undergo immune function testing in the first few days following injury using a highly standardized and centralized approach. Immune testing kits are produced and quality controlled at the Immune Surveillance Laboratory (ISL) at The

Research Institute at Nationwide Children's Hospital and are then shipped to study sites. LPS stimulation and HLA-DR staining are done at each site, and the resulting supernatants and flow cytometry tubes are sent back to the ISL for TNFα and monocyte HLA-DR quantitation. Only children who are shown to have significant reduction in their TNFα production capacity go on to get GM-CSF. This open-label, dose-finding study is designed to determine the lowest immunostimulatory, tolerable dose of GM-CSF that will restore the TNFα response and monocyte HLA-DR expression above thresholds thought to be protective against nosocomial infection.

Less work has been done to investigate stimulation of the adaptive arm of the immune system in critical illness. Experimental evidence suggests, however, that blockade of the PD-1 pathway may confer a survival advantage in animal models of sepsis.[44,45] Recombinant human IL-7 has been shown to have similar effects in animal models.[46] Because blocking antibodies against coinhibitory molecules (checkpoint inhibitors) such as PD-1 have been tested in the adult oncology population, investigators are beginning to evaluate them as therapies for critical illness–induced immune suppression. A multicenter clinical trial of anti-PD-L1 is currently ongoing in adult septic patients with lymphopenia (NCT02576457).

IATROGENIC IMMUNOSUPPRESSION

Many patients in the PICU receive systemic immunosuppressive therapies for the management of malignancy, autoimmune disease, or transplantation. At present, most transplant specialists follow drug levels and monitor end-organ function to titrate immunosuppressive therapy (eg, tacrolimus, cyclosporine). Although these agents are classically thought of as T-cell inhibitors, they also exert a polarizing effect, skewing both innate and adaptive immune systems toward a T_H2-like phenotype. Similarly, glucocorticoids promote lymphocyte apoptosis and impair proinflammatory signaling. The tapering or withholding of these medications in the context of life-threatening infection is thought to be essential. Reinke and Volk[47] described a cohort of 45 adult kidney transplant recipients who developed nosocomial sepsis in the setting of immunoparalysis. Subjects who underwent rapid tapering of their calcineurin inhibition experienced a 90% survival rate (30/33) with 98% graft survival. In contrast, subjects who did not undergo tapering had an 8% survival rate (1/12) with the sole survivor experiencing graft loss. Pediatric data on this subject are limited, but Hoffman and colleagues[48] described a series of 13 pediatric lung transplant recipients who underwent monocyte HLA-DR monitoring weekly following transplantation. Those who developed pneumonia had lower monocyte HLA-DR expression over the 4-week study period than those who remained infection-free. Monocyte HLA-DR expression measurement and quantification of the ex vivo stimulated cytokine responses both seem to have the potential to provide insight into the degree of functional immunosuppression following transplantation and are deserving of future study.

Perhaps less obvious is that most of the medications and therapies that are used in the PICU are, in some way, immunomodulatory (**Table 2**). Catecholamines, sedatives, analgesics, insulin, and diuretics can all directly or indirectly affect leukocyte function with the bulk of their effects being immunosuppressive. The net effect of these drugs' immunologic influences in a given patient is poorly understood. Another example of unintended immunomodulation can be found in the transfusion literature. Transfusion-related immunomodulation has historically been associated with the proinflammatory effects of mediators in stored blood products, but we now know that stored blood products can be immunosuppressive.[49] These examples highlight the need for prospective immune function screening in critically ill patients to develop

Table 2
Potential sources of unintended immunomodulation in the pediatric intensive care unit

Drug or Therapy	Immune Effect	Potential Mechanisms
Antibiotics	↑	Release of bacterial components on cell death
		Direct enhancement of intracellular killing
	↓	Bone marrow suppression (β lactams)
		Decreased proinflammatory cytokine production (macrolides)
Benzodiazepines	↓	Upregulation of cortisol axis
Catecholamines	↑	Stimulation of α adrenergic receptors
	↓	Stimulation of β adrenergic receptors
Dexmedetomidine	↓	CNS-mediated and peripherally mediated reduction in cytokine production
Furosemide	↓	Decreased proinflammatory cytokine production
Insulin	↓	Indirect reduction in hyperglycemia-induced proinflammatory cytokine production
Opiates	↓	Induction of leukocyte apoptosis, upregulation of TGFβ and down-regulation of INF-γ
RBC transfusion	↑	Immune activation through cytokines and other mediators in stored blood products
	↓	Inhibition of host proinflammatory cytokine production capacity

Abbreviations: CNS, central nervous system; Downward arrow, anti-inflammatory; RBC, red blood cell; upward arrow, proinflammatory.

immunophenotype-specific management strategies designed to promote immuno-logic balance.

SUMMARY AND FUTURE DIRECTIONS

Although anti-inflammatory strategies were once thought to be promising in the setting of critical illness, the repeated failure of studies designed to reduce the in-flammatory response in the ICU called this into question. The immunologic response to critical illness is now known to be highly dynamic and often includes a phase in which systemic inflammation and functional immunosuppression coexist. Immune monitoring strategies now exist that can identify critical illness–induced im-mune suppression, or immunoparalysis. These include quantification of monocyte HLA-DR expression, whole blood ex vivo stimulation testing, and measurement of lymphocyte counts and coinhibitor molecule expression (eg, PD-1). Although these tests are not yet FDA-approved for the clinical laboratory, they can be used in the research setting for the design and execution of immune monitoring and modulation trials. By prospectively identifying patients with immunoparalysis, studies can be enriched with subjects most likely to benefit from immunostimulatory strategies. Among the highest research priorities in the field is the development of a better un-derstanding of the specific disease, treatment, and host factors that promote immu-noparalysis in the ICU. It similarly remains unknown if immunostimulatory strategies should target the innate or adaptive immune system or both. The approach of real-time, multicenter, highly standardized immunophenotype-driven clinical trials has great potential to answer these questions and improve the outcomes and lives of critically ill children.

REFERENCES

1. Kellum JA, Kong L, Fink MP, et al. Understanding the inflammatory cytokine response in pneumonia and sepsis: results of the Genetic and Inflammatory Markers of Sepsis (GenIMS) Study. Arch Intern Med 2007;167(15):1655–63.
2. Ozturk H, Yagmur Y, Ozturk H. The prognostic importance of serum IL-1beta, IL-6, IL-8 and TNF-alpha levels compared to trauma scoring systems for early mortality in children with blunt trauma. Pediatr Surg Int 2008;24(2):235–9.
3. Wong HR, Salisbury S, Xiao Q, et al. The pediatric sepsis biomarker risk model. Crit Care 2012;16(5):R174.
4. Steensberg A, Fischer CP, Keller C, et al. IL-6 enhances plasma IL-1ra, IL-10, and cortisol in humans. Am J Physiol Endocrinol Metab 2003;285(2):E433–7.
5. Diehl S, Rincon M. The two faces of IL-6 on Th1/Th2 differentiation. Mol Immunol 2002;39(9):531–6.
6. Fumeaux T, Pugin J. Role of interleukin-10 in the intracellular sequestration of human leukocyte antigen-DR in monocytes during septic shock. Am J Respir Crit Care Med 2002;166(11):1475–82.
7. Volk HD, Reinke P, Krausch D, et al. Monocyte deactivation–rationale for a new therapeutic strategy in sepsis. Intensive Care Med 1996;22(Suppl 4):S474–81.
8. Livingston DH, Appel SH, Wellhausen SR, et al. Depressed interferon gamma production and monocyte HLA-DR expression after severe injury. Arch Surg 1988;123(11):1309–12.
9. Monneret G, Lepape A, Voirin N, et al. Persisting low monocyte human leukocyte antigen-DR expression predicts mortality in septic shock. Intensive Care Med 2006;32(8):1175–83.
10. Ho YP, Sheen IS, Chiu CT, et al. A strong association between down-regulation of HLA-DR expression and the late mortality in patients with severe acute pancreatitis. Am J Gastroenterol 2006;101(5):1117–24.
11. Hall MW, Knatz NL, Vetterly C, et al. Immunoparalysis and nosocomial infection in children with multiple organ dysfunction syndrome. Intensive Care Med 2011; 37(3):525–32.
12. Docke WD, Hoflich C, Davis KA, et al. Monitoring temporary immunodepression by flow cytometric measurement of monocytic HLA-DR expression: a multicenter standardized study. Clin Chem 2005;51(12):2341–7.
13. Meisel C, Schefold JC, Pschowski R, et al. Granulocyte-macrophage colony-stimulating factor to reverse sepsis-associated immunosuppression: a double-blind, randomized, placebo-controlled multicenter trial. Am J Respir Crit Care Med 2009;180(7):640–8.
14. Manzoli TF, Troster EJ, Ferranti JF, et al. Prolonged suppression of monocytic human leukocyte antigen-DR expression correlates with mortality in pediatric septic patients in a pediatric tertiary Intensive Care Unit. J Crit Care 2016;33:84–9.
15. Cornell TT, Sun L, Hall MW, et al. Clinical implications and molecular mechanisms of immunoparalysis after cardiopulmonary bypass. J Thorac Cardiovasc Surg 2012;143(5):1160–6.e1.
16. Allen ML, Hoschtitzky JA, Peters MJ, et al. Interleukin-10 and its role in clinical immunoparalysis following pediatric cardiac surgery. Crit Care Med 2006; 34(10):2658–65.
17. Mella C, Suarez-Arrabal MC, Lopez S, et al. Innate immune dysfunction is associated with enhanced disease severity in infants with severe respiratory syncytial virus bronchiolitis. J Infect Dis 2013;207(4):564–73.

18. Muszynski JA, Nofziger R, Greathouse K, et al. Innate immune function predicts the development of nosocomial infection in critically injured children. Shock 2014; 42(4):313–21.

19. Hotchkiss RS, Tinsley KW, Swanson PE, et al. Sepsis-induced apoptosis causes progressive profound depletion of B and CD4+ T lymphocytes in humans. J Immunol 2001;166(11):6952–63.

20. Felmet KA, Hall MW, Clark RS, et al. Prolonged lymphopenia, lymphoid depletion, and hypoprolactinemia in children with nosocomial sepsis and multiple organ failure. J Immunol 2005;174(6):3765–72.

21. Boomer JS, To K, Chang KC, et al. Immunosuppression in patients who die of sepsis and multiple organ failure. JAMA 2011;306(23):2594–605.

22. Muszynski JA, Nofziger R, Greathouse K, et al. Early adaptive immune suppression in children with septic shock: a prospective observational study. Crit Care 2014;18(4):R145.

23. Wong HR, Cvijanovich NZ, Anas N, et al. Developing a clinically feasible personalized medicine approach to pediatric septic shock. Am J Respir Crit Care Med 2015;191(3):309–15.

24. Guignant C, Lepape A, Huang X, et al. Programmed death-1 levels correlate with increased mortality, nosocomial infection and immune dysfunctions in septic shock patients. Crit Care 2011;15(2):R99.

25. Polk HC Jr, Wellhausen SR, Regan M. A systematic study of host defense processes in badly injured patients. Ann Surg 1986;204(3):282–97.

26. Cheadle WG, Wilson M, Hershman MJ, et al. Comparison of trauma assessment scores and their use in prediction of infection and death. Ann Surg 1989;209(5): 541–5 [discussion: 545–6].

27. Majetschak M, Flach R, Kreuzfelder E, et al. The extent of traumatic damage determines a graded depression of the endotoxin responsiveness of peripheral blood mononuclear cells from patients with blunt injuries. Crit Care Med 1999; 27(2):313–8.

28. Meisel C, Schwab JM, Prass K, et al. Central nervous system injury-induced immune deficiency syndrome. Nat Rev Neurosci 2005;6(10):775–86.

29. Ploder M, Pelinka L, Schmuckenschlager C, et al. Lipopolysaccharide-induced tumor necrosis factor alpha production and not monocyte human leukocyte antigen-DR expression is correlated with survival in septic trauma patients. Shock 2006;25(2):129–34.

30. Hall MW, Gavrilin MA, Knatz NL, et al. Monocyte mRNA phenotype and adverse outcomes from pediatric multiple organ dysfunction syndrome. Pediatr Res 2007; 62(5):597–603.

31. Hall MW, Geyer SM, Guo CY, et al. Innate immune function and mortality in critically ill children with influenza: a multicenter study. Crit Care Med 2013;41(1):224–36.

32. Monneret G, Debard AL, Venet F, et al. Marked elevation of human circulating CD4+CD25+ regulatory T cells in sepsis-induced immunoparalysis. Crit Care Med 2003;31(7):2068–71.

33. Venet F, Chung CS, Kherouf H, et al. Increased circulating regulatory T cells (CD4(+)CD25 (+)CD127 (-)) contribute to lymphocyte anergy in septic shock patients. Intensive Care Med 2009;35(4):678–86.

34. Venet F, Pachot A, Debard AL, et al. Increased percentage of CD4+CD25+ regulatory T cells during septic shock is due to the decrease of CD4+CD25- lymphocytes. Crit Care Med 2004;32(11):2329–31.

35. Allen ML, Peters MJ, Goldman A, et al. Early postoperative monocyte deactivation predicts systemic inflammation and prolonged stay in pediatric cardiac intensive care. Crit Care Med 2002;30(5):1140–5.

36. Hershman MJ, Appel SH, Wellhausen SR, et al. Interferon-gamma treatment increases HLA-DR expression on monocytes in severely injured patients. Clin Exp Immunol 1989;77(1):67–70.

37. Flohe S, Borgermann J, Dominguez FE, et al. Influence of granulocyte-macrophage colony-stimulating factor (GM-CSF) on whole blood endotoxin responsiveness following trauma, cardiopulmonary bypass, and severe sepsis. Shock 1999;12(1):17–24.

38. Lendemans S, Kreuzfelder E, Waydhas C, et al. Differential immunostimulating effect of granulocyte-macrophage colony-stimulating factor (GM-CSF), granulocyte colony-stimulating factor (G-CSF) and interferon gamma (IFNgamma) after severe trauma. Inflamm Res 2007;56(1):38–44.

39. Kox WJ, Bone RC, Krausch D, et al. Interferon gamma-1b in the treatment of compensatory anti-inflammatory response syndrome. A new approach: proof of principle. Arch Intern Med 1997;157(4):389–93.

40. Nakos G, Malamou-Mitsi VD, Lachana A, et al. Immunoparalysis in patients with severe trauma and the effect of inhaled interferon-gamma. Crit Care Med 2002; 30(7):1488–94.

41. Nierhaus A, Montag B, Timmler N, et al. Reversal of immunoparalysis by recombinant human granulocyte-macrophage colony-stimulating factor in patients with severe sepsis. Intensive Care Med 2003;29(4):646–51.

42. Rosenbloom AJ, Linden PK, Dorrance A, et al. Effect of granulocyte-monocyte colony-stimulating factor therapy on leukocyte function and clearance of serious infection in nonneutropenic patients. Chest 2005;127(6):2139–50.

43. Bilgin K, Yaramis A, Haspolat K, et al. A randomized trial of granulocyte-macrophage colony-stimulating factor in neonates with sepsis and neutropenia. Pediatrics 2001;107(1):36–41.

44. Chang KC, Burnham CA, Compton SM, et al. Blockade of the negative co-stimulatory molecules PD-1 and CTLA-4 improves survival in primary and secondary fungal sepsis. Crit Care 2013;17(3):R85.

45. Brahmamdam P, Inoue S, Unsinger J, et al. Delayed administration of anti-PD-1 antibody reverses immune dysfunction and improves survival during sepsis. J Leukoc Biol 2010;88(2):233–40.

46. Shindo Y, Unsinger J, Burnham CA, et al. Interleukin-7 and anti-programmed cell death 1 antibody have differing effects to reverse sepsis-induced immunosuppression. Shock 2015;43(4):334–43.

47. Reinke P, Volk HD. Diagnostic and predictive value of an immune monitoring program for complications after kidney transplantation. Urol Int 1992;49(2):69–75.

48. Hoffman JA, Weinberg KI, Azen CG, et al. Human leukocyte antigen-DR expression on peripheral blood monocytes and the risk of pneumonia in pediatric lung transplant recipients. Transpl Infect Dis 2004;6(4):147–55.

49. Muszynski JA, Spinella PC, Cholette JM, et al. Transfusion-related immunomodulation: review of the literature and implications for pediatric critical illness. Transfusion 2017;57(1):195–206.

Sedation Analgesia and Neuromuscular Blockade in Pediatric Critical Care

Overview and Current Landscape

Athena F. Zuppa, MD, MSCE[a],*, Martha A.Q. Curley, RN, PhD[b]

KEYWORDS

• Sedation • Critical illness • Benzodiazepine • Opiate

KEY POINTS

• Sedation is a mainstay of therapy for critically ill children. Drugs of many classes are available to sedate children cared for in the PICU, and are used in various combinations to achieve the desired effect.

• Although necessary in the care of the critically ill child, sedative drugs are associated with adverse effects, such as disruption of circadian rhythm, altered sleep, delirium, potential neurotoxicity, and immunosuppression.

• Optimal approaches to the sedation of the critically ill child should include identification of sedation targets and sedation interruptions, allowing for a more individualized approach to sedation.

• Further research is needed to better understand the relationship between critical illness and sedation pharmacokinetics and pharmacodynamics, the impact of sedation on immune function, and the genetic implications on drug disposition and response.

In 2006 the consensus guidelines on sedation and analgesia in critically ill children was published, providing guidance for sedative use in the pediatric intensive care unit (PICU).[1] This guidance included statements supporting the assessment of sedation level using validated sedation scales, specifying that the "desired level of sedation should be identified for each patient and should be regularly reassessed" and "doses

Disclosure Statement: A.F. Zuppa serves as a paid adviser for Pfizer, which manufactures dexmedetomidine.
[a] Department of Pediatric Anesthesia and Critical Care Medicine, The Children's Hospital of Philadelphia, Center for Clinical Pharmacology, Colket Translational Research, Room 4008, 3614 Civic Center Boulevard, Philadelphia, PA 19104-4318, USA; [b] Anesthesia and Critical Care Medicine, School of Nursing, University of Pennsylvania, Claire M. Fagin Hall, 418 Curie Boulevard - #425, Philadelphia, PA 19104-4217, USA
* Corresponding author. 26 High Point Drive, Medford, NJ 08055.
E-mail address: zuppa@email.chop.edu

of sedative agents should be titrated to produce the desired level of sedation." In addition, the concepts of tolerance and withdrawal were detailed, with the recommendation for medication tapering after 7 days of therapy. These overarching concepts to sedation in the PICU still hold true a decade later. However, recent changes in knowledge about potentially deleterious effects of sedative medications in combination with addition of newer medications, such as dexmedetomidine, suggest that previous guidance in 2006 may not apply today.

In 2016, the Pediatric Cardiac Intensive Care Society 2014 consensus statement "Pharmacotherapies in Cardiac Critical Care: Sedation, Analgesia and Muscle Relaxant" was published.[2] Analgesic guidance for morphine, fentanyl, remifentanil, ketamine, and methadone was provided. In addition, guidance on the benzodiazepines midazolam, lorazepam, and diazepam was also given. Dexmedetomidine was highlighted in this statement, with an in-depth review of its pharmacokinetics and dynamics, and its potential as an antiarrhythmic especially in this setting. In conclusion, it was stated that sedation should be tailored to the individual needs of the patient.

This article provides an overview of the various drug classes that are used in the sedation of the critically ill child, and details regarding select drugs within each class. Analgesics, or medications that provide relief from pain, are also included because these agents are often included as sedation adjuncts regardless of whether there is an indication to treat pain. Afterward, an overview of concepts and issues surrounding sedation in the PICU is discussed, providing the reader with the current state of knowledge and areas that require additional scientific inquiry.

BENZODIAZEPINES

Benzodiazepines are often used to provide sedation and amnesia, and exert their anxiolytic, amnestic, anticonvulsant, and muscle-relaxing effects through interaction at specific binding sites on neuronal γ-aminobutyric acid (GABA) receptors.[3] Chronic administration of benzodiazepines can lead to decreased receptor activity and drug tolerance. Tolerance is a common finding in intensive care unit (ICU) patients receiving benzodiazepines or other sedative agents for periods longer than 24 hours, although most commonly seen clinically after 3 to 7 days. Withdrawal syndromes have been reported with cessation of midazolam and other benzodiazepine infusions. Risk factors for acute withdrawal include high infusion rates, prolonged duration, and abrupt cessation. For these reasons, gradual tapering of sedative infusions is suggested to reduce the chance of withdrawal reactions.

Midazolam undergoes extensive metabolism by the cytochrome P-450 (CYP) 3A (CYP3A) subfamily to a major (1-OH-midazolam) and a minor hydroxylated metabolite (4-OH-midazolam), both of which are subsequently metabolized to their respective glucuronide metabolites by uridine diphosphate-glucuronosyltransferases and renally cleared. The major metabolite 1-OH-glucorinide also seems to have sedative properties when concentrations are high, as has been observed in adult patients with renal failure.[4] The elimination half-life is prolonged and clearance reduced in adolescents as compared with younger children.[5] The elimination half-life of midazolam is 2 hours in young, healthy adults but increases rapidly in the elderly and following major surgery.[6] CYP3A activity reaches adult levels between 3 and 12 months of postnatal age.[7] Developmental differences in CYP3A activity may therefore alter the pharmacokinetics of midazolam in PICU patients of different ages.[4] In addition, polymorphisms in CYP3A impact midazolam disposition and response, but unfortunately are not currently accounted for in dosing decisions at the bedside.[4,8,9] The most dramatic changes in the pharmacokinetics of midazolam in the critically ill may result from altered hepatic metabolism. Accumulation occurs in critically ill patients at the peak of their illness with low or absent concentrations of 1-hydroxy midazolam, suggesting the failure of liver metabolism.[10] Several drugs, including cimetidine, erythromycin, propofol, and diltiazem, have been reported to delay midazolam metabolism and therefore increase its duration of effect. The accumulation of the active metabolite also may be important in some ICU patients. Midazolam, as do other benzodiazepines, causes dose-related respiratory depression and in large doses can cause vasodilation and hypotension.[6] As with many highly lipid soluble drugs, after continuous infusion for extended time periods drug accumulates in peripheral tissues and in the bloodstream rather than being metabolized. When the infusion is discontinued, peripheral tissue stores release midazolam back into the plasma, and the duration of clinical effect can be prolonged. Obese patients with larger volumes of distribution and elderly patients with decreased hepatic and renal function may be even more prone to prolonged sedation.[11]

Various in vitro, animal, and limited human adult studies suggest a profound inhibitory effect of inflammation and disease on CYP3A-mediated drug metabolism. Studies showing this relationship in critically ill patients are few. A recent study of 83 critically ill children (median age, 5.1 months) examining midazolam plasma concentrations, cytokines, C-reactive protein, and organ dysfunction scores (PRISM II, PIM2, PELOD), and number of failing organs using a population pharmacokinetic model showed that C-reactive protein and organ failure were significantly associated with midazolam clearance ($P<.01$). In simulations, a C-reactive protein of 300 mg/L was associated with a 65% lower clearance compared with 10 mg/L and three failing organs were associated with a 35% lower clearance compared with one failing organ. The authors concluded that inflammation and organ failure strongly reduce midazolam clearance in critically ill children, and as such, critically ill patients receiving CYP3A substrate drugs may be at risk of increased drug levels and associated toxicity.[12]

Diazepam is highly lipid-soluble, highly protein-bound, and distributes quickly into the brain. Diazepam administration results in antegrade but not retrograde amnesia. It reduces the cerebral metabolic rate for oxygen consumption and thus decreases cerebral blood flow in a dose-dependent manner. As do other benzodiazepines, diazepam raises the seizure threshold.[6] Diazepam is metabolized by hepatic microsomal enzymes (CYP2C19) to active compounds, such as desmethyldiazepam and oxazepam. Desmethyldiazepam has a long elimination half-life of 100 to 200 hours and is eliminated by the kidneys. Oxezepam has an elimination half-life of 10 hours. The elimination half-life of diazepam averages 72 hours; varies widely; and is increased in the elderly, neonates, and patients with liver disease. Metabolism also is affected by genetics, gender, endocrine status, nutritional status, smoking, and concurrent drug therapy.[6] Diazepam alone has minimal cardiovascular depressant effects, although systemic vascular resistance is reduced slightly, producing a small decline in arterial blood pressure. Respiratory drive is likewise minimally decreased by diazepam.[6]

Lorazepam is the least lipid-soluble of the three benzodiazepines and traverses the blood-brain barrier most slowly, resulting in delayed onset and prolonged duration of effect.[6] Lorazepam is metabolized to inactive products by hepatic glucuronidation. The pharmacokinetics of lorazepam does not change significantly in the elderly or critically ill populations. The elimination half-life ranges from 10 to 20 hours but is prolonged by liver and end-stage kidney disease.[6] Because lorazepam is insoluble in water, it is manufactured with polyethylene glycol. This drug vehicle may be associated with lactic acidosis, hyperosmolar coma, and a reversible nephrotoxicity after high doses or prolonged infusions.[6]

BARBITURATES

Barbiturates are weak acids that are absorbed and rapidly distributed to all tissues and fluids with high concentrations in the brain, liver, and kidneys. Lipid solubility of the barbiturates is the dominant factor in their distribution within the body. The more lipid-soluble the barbiturate, the more rapidly it penetrates all tissues of the body. Pentobarbital has a potent effect on GABA-sensitive chloride channels, and is a potent central nervous system depressant. Following intravenous administration, the onset of action is almost immediate. Pentobarbital enters the brain more rapidly than phenobarbital or diazepam, and is a potent antiepileptic drug. High-dose pentobarbital infusions have been advocated as an effective adjunct in controlling persistent intracranial hypertension after severe head trauma in patients refractory to conventional therapy. Pentobarbital has also been recommended as a sedative agent for diagnostic imaging studies.[13,14]

OPIOIDS

Opioids are endogenous or exogenous substances that bind to opiate receptors found in the central nervous system and peripheral tissue. Opioids lead to a dose-dependent, centrally mediated respiratory depression, mediated by the mu2 receptors in the medulla. Opioids have little hemodynamic effect on patients with euvolemia whose blood pressure is not sustained by the sympathetic nervous system. Opiate side effects include nausea, vomiting, decreased gastrointestinal motility, urinary retention, and pruritus.[11] Morphine is a potent mu-receptor agonist with additional kappa-receptor activity.[15] Morphine's onset of action is slow (5–10 minutes) because of low lipid solubility. The duration of action is dose dependent but is approximately 4 hours after a single dose.[11] Metabolism primarily occurs through the liver by glucuronide conjugation, and excretion occurs through the kidney. Morphine's predominate metabolite, morphine 6-glucuronide, is an active analgesic and may accumulate in patients with renal failure. This active metabolite is several times more potent than morphine itself.[15] The pharmacologic effects of morphine-like agents include analgesia, respiratory depression, gastrointestinal effects (nausea and vomiting), orthostatic hypotension, sedation, and altered mentation.[15] Morphine administration may cause histamine release and therefore may not be an ideal drug choice in the treatments of bronchoconstriction.

Hydromorphone is a morphine-like agonist and a semisynthetic opioid analgesic with roughly three- to four-fold greater potency than morphine. Hydromorphone, like morphine, provides analgesic effects within 15 to 30 minutes of administration. Its metabolism primarily occurs by the liver to hydromorphone-3-glucuronide. Although it has been recommended as an alternative to morphine for patients in renal failure, hydromorphone's metabolite may accumulate in renal failure, resulting in neuroexcitability and cognitive impairment.[15]

Meperidine is primarily a mu-receptor agonist and has approximately one-tenth the potency of morphine. Analgesic effects of meperidine are detectable within 5 minutes of intravenous administration and 10 minutes after intramuscular or subcutaneous administration. Meperidine is useful for drug-induced rigors and pain. such as those that accompany administration of amphotericin B. It is metabolized through the liver to an active metabolite, normeperidine.[15] Normeperidine accumulates in renal failure and produces neurotoxicity, which may result in tremors, myoclonic jerks, and seizures. Case reports of seizures with meperidine have been noted with administration by patient-controlled analgesia pumps.[16] Risk for seizures also is reported in patients with renal insufficiency, with sickle-cell anemia, and in those receiving high-dose meperidine, and should be used with caution in critically ill children.[15]

Fentanyl is a synthetic opioid commonly used in anesthesia and in the ICU for pain management and sedation. Fentanyl is 50 to 100 times as potent as morphine, and provides a quick onset of action and short duration (approximately 0.5–1 hour). Fentanyl is more lipid soluble than morphine and has a more rapid onset of action because of quicker penetration of the central nervous system. Fentanyl may be administered by the intravenous, intramuscular, epidural, transdermal, intranasal, and intrathecal routes.[15,17] Long-term continuous infusions of fentanyl may result in a prolonged elimination half-life and duration of action as a result of drug accumulation in peripheral tissues. Unlike morphine, fentanyl is not associated with histamine release and may be preferred in patients susceptible to the cardiovascular effects of morphine. Rapid administration has been associated with chest wall rigidity.[17]

KETAMINE

Ketamine is a racemic mixture consisting of two optical enantiomers, R(−) and S(+). Administration produces a dose-dependent central nervous system depression that leads to a dissociative state, characterized by profound analgesia and amnesia but not necessarily loss of consciousness. Ketamine is a bronchodilator and causes minimal respiratory depression. However, increased oral secretions can occur with its use. It is used clinically for such indications as induction of anesthesia in patients in hemodynamic shock or active asthmatic disease; intramuscular sedation of uncooperative patients; supplementation of incomplete regional or local anesthesia; sedation in the intensive care setting; and for analgesia for short, painful procedures, such as dressing changes in burn patients. Common side effects include emergence delirium and severe hallucinations. These effects are reduced with concomitant administration of a benzodiazepine, such as midazolam. Although ketamine administration is generally associated with increases in heart rate, cardiac output, and blood pressure, hypotension from direct myocardial depression can occur.[11] As such, it should be used in caution in patients with suspected sympathomimetic depletion. A recent review of the use of ketamine in the care of patients with traumatic brain injury (TBI) reported evidence to support that ketamine does not increase intracranial pressure in patients with severe TBI that are sedated and ventilated, and in fact may lower it in selected cases. Is role in the management of these patients continues to expand in the clinical setting.[18]

PROPOFOL

Propofol is an alkylphenol intravenous anesthetic. Propofol is highly lipid soluble and rapidly crosses the blood-brain barrier. Onset of sedation is rapid (1–5 minutes). The duration of action is dose dependent but is usually short (2–8 minutes) because of rapid redistribution to peripheral tissues. Propofol is a hypnotic agent that provides a suppression of awareness from mild depression of responsiveness to obtundation. It is a potent anxiolytic and a potent amnestic agent, but does not possess analgesic properties.[11] Apnea often occurs after a loading dose, and administration can cause significant decreases in blood pressure, especially in hypovolemic patients. This is mainly a result of preload reduction from dilation of venous capacitance vessels. A lesser effect is mild myocardial depression. Because it is delivered in a lipid carrier, hypertriglyceridemia is a possible side effect of propofol.[11] Recently the propofol binding site on $\beta 3$ subunits of GABAA receptor-complexes was described.[19] Previous research in preclinical models suggests additional mechanism for propofol's effects including glutamate modulation and cannabinoid activity.[20] Propofol may rarely cause a potentially fatal condition known as propofol infusion syndrome, characterized by refractory bradycardia plus at least one of the following: metabolic acidosis, rhabdomyolysis, hyperlipidemia, or hepatomegaly.[21] Lactic acidosis has been associated with its use in the pediatric population.[22] Reports of dysrhythmia, heart failure, metabolic acidosis, hyperkalemia, and rhabdomyolysis have been described in adults treated with high doses of propofol (>80 µg/kg/min).[23] Sebastiani and colleagues[24] used a controlled cortical impact mouse model to investigate the effects of propofol on injury and recovery from TBI. Previously, the same group found that propofol administration following the same TBI model increased mortality, worsened neurobehavioral outcomes, and reduced hippocampal neurogenesis.[25] The more recent study shows that even a single bolus dose of propofol administered 24 hours after controlled cortical impact results in increased lesion volume, increased apoptotic neuronal cell death, and worsened chronic motor function when compared with unsedated control subjects.

ETOMIDIATE

Etomidate is an ultra-short-acting nonbarbirturate hypnotic agent without analgesic effects. Intravenous administration of 0.3 mg/kg induces sleep for approximately 5 minutes. Cardiovascular and respirator adverse events are minimal.[26] Etomidate administration is associated with a transient 20% to 30% decrease in cerebral blood flow. Etomidate is rapidly metabolized in the liver to inactive metabolites. Approximately 75% of the administered dose is excreted in the urine during the first day after injection.[27] Involuntary muscle movements are a frequent occurrence. Etomidate may inhibit adrenal steroidgenesis, causing a decrease in cortisol plasma concentrations.[26] This has led to controversy regarding its use in the care of critically ill patients.[28]

DEXMEDETOMIDINE

Dexmedetomidine is a highly selective α_2-agonist with hypnotic and anxiolytic properties attributed to the α_{2A}-adrenoreceptors in the locus ceruleus. Analgesic properties are a result of stimulation of α_2-adrenoreceptors in the brain, spinal cord, and peripheral sites.[29] Sympatholysis disinhibits the arousal-suppressing neurons in the ventrolateral preoptic area ultimately leading to sedation.[30] Dexmedetomidine is used in the adult ICU setting because it allows postoperative patients to remain sedated, but arouse easily with gentle stimulation.[31] There is increasing off-label use in pediatrics, with published experiences[32–35] and pharmacokinetic data to help guide dosing.[36–38] In clinical studies the significant treatment-emergent adverse event reported in dexmedetomidine patients compared with placebo patients were hypotension and bradycardia.[39] Its 2-hour half-life allows for effective dose titration, and its absence of active metabolites prevents accumulation with extended use.

NEUROMUSCULAR BLOCKERS

Neuromuscular blockers or paralytics are often used in the PICU setting to minimize movement, and to facilitate procedures and mechanical ventilation. An important component of this adjunct to sedation is the ability to assess the patients' comfort while paralyzed. Surrogates for comfort, such as heart rate and blood pressure, must be assessed frequently. Paralytic interruptions should also be considered when administered as continuous infusion in the PICU setting. This helps to minimize muscle weakness, allow the determination of the lowest possible dose needed to achieve the desired effect, and facilitate spontaneous breathing.

During neurotransmission, the neurotransmitter acetylcholine is synthesized, stored in vesicles at the neuromuscular junction, released into the synapse, and bound to nicotinic receptors in the muscle end plate. The postsynaptic nicotinic receptor at the neuromuscular junction is the major site of action of depolarizing and nondepolarizing neuromuscular blockers.[40] Succinycholine, a depolarizing muscle relaxant, is used because of its favorable pharmacokinetic profile, with quick onset and short duration.[40] Administration is followed by muscle fasciculations and subsequent neuromuscular blockade approximately 60 seconds after intravenous dosing. The blockade remains for approximately 5 to 10 minutes.[41] Succinylcholine is eliminated by plasma cholinesterase, has a very short duration of action, and can be used independent of a patient's renal and hepatic status. Prolongation of blockade occurs in patients with conditions associated with plasma cholinesterase deficiency and with high doses.[40] Succinylcholine can cause severe, although uncommon, adverse drug reactions, such as malignant hyperthermia, increased intraocular pressure, masseter muscle rigidity, rhabdomyolysis, bradycardia, and hyperkalemia.[40,41]

Pancuronium is a nondepolarizing neuromuscular blocking agent. Onset of action occurs 4 to 6 minutes after administration and remains for 120 to 180 minutes.[26] Pancuronium is largely excreted unchanged in the urine, but a small percentage is metabolized to 3-desacetylpancuronium, which may accumulate after prolonged infusion. Although only 10% is eliminated by the liver, pancuronium also accumulates in fulminant hepatic failure.[41,42] Its administration causes tachycardia, largely because of the blocking of cardiac muscarinic cholinergic receptors.[41]

Vecuronium, a steroid-based compound derived from pancuronium, is a nondepolarizing neuromuscular blocker.[42] The onset of action occurs 2 to 4 minutes after administration and remains for 30 to 40 minutes.[26] Even though it is primarily metabolized, cumulative effects of vecuronium are evident in renal transplant recipients and patients with severe renal failure. This effect is attributable to its metabolite, 3-desacetyl vecuronium, which has 80% of the activity of the parent drug and reportedly accumulates to a greater degree in patients with renal failure. Vecuronium may also accumulate in patients with hepatic failure because of decreased biliary up-take.[41]

Atracurium is a nondepolarizing neuromuscular blocker of intermediate action.[42] Onset of action occurs 2 to 4 minutes after administration and remains for 30 to 40 minutes. Atracurium (and cisatracurium) are eliminated by Hofmann elimination, which is a spontaneous nonenzymatic degradation at physiologic pH and temperature. Atracurium is a good choice for patients with multiorgan dysfunction.[40]

Mivacurium is a nondepolarizing neuromuscular blocker.[42] Onset of action occurs 2 to 4 minutes after administration, similar to succinylcholine, and remains for 12 to 18 minutes.[26] Mivacurium is eliminated by plasma cholinesterase, has short duration of action, and can be used independent of a patient's renal and hepatic status.[40] Higher doses are associated with histamine release.[26]

Rocuronium is another nondepolarizing neuromuscular blocking agent, administered in doses of 0.6 to 1.2 mg/kg, with an onset of action in approximately 2 minutes. It is primarily metabolized by the liver, with an elimination half-life of approximately 1 hour in children.[43]

SPECIAL CONSIDERATIONS

In 2013, a review of preclinical and clinical evidence suggesting the possibility of neurotoxicity from neonatal exposure to general anesthetics was published.[44] The review identified 55 rodent studies, seven primate studies, and nine clinical studies, with the preclinical data consistently demonstrating robust apoptosis in the nervous system after anesthetic exposure, with limited studies having performed cognitive follow-up. A 2015 perspective discussed potential sedative-related neurotoxicity in preclinical studies,[45] calling to attention the evidence that anesthetic and sedative medications are associated with neurotoxic effects in the developing brains of laboratory animals, and was supported by a small number of observational studies in children who underwent anesthesia. This perspective emphasized the need and urgency for large-scale clinical studies to address whether this phenomenon existed in humans. As such, many clinical studies have attempted to address this issue.

In 2016 the GAS study was published[46] and examined whether general anesthesia in infancy had any effect on neurodevelopmental outcome. This was performed through an international assessor-masked randomized controlled equivalence trial of infants younger than 60 weeks postmenstrual age, born at greater than 26 weeks' gestation, and who had inguinal herniorrhaphy, from 28 hospitals in Australia, Italy, the United States, the United Kingdom, Canada, the Netherlands, and New Zealand. Infants were randomly assigned (1:1) to receive either awake-regional anesthesia or sevoflurane-based general anesthesia. The primary outcome of the trial was the Wechsler Preschool and Primary Scale of Intelligence Third Edition Full Scale Intelligence Quotient score at age 5 years. The secondary outcome was the composite cognitive score of the Bayley Scales of Infant and Toddler Development III, assessed at 2 years, and published in the 2016 paper. For the secondary outcome, the authors found no evidence that just less than 1 hour of sevoflurane anesthesia in infancy increased the risk of adverse neurodevelopmental outcome at 2 years of age compared with awake-regional anesthesia.

The PANDA study[47] was also published in 2016. This study also explored whether a single anesthesia exposure in otherwise healthy young children was associated with impaired neurocognitive development and abnormal behavior in later childhood and included sibling pairs within 36 months in age. The primary outcome was global cognitive function (IQ). Secondary outcomes included domain-specific neurocognitive functions and behavior. A detailed neuropsychological battery assessed IQ and domain-specific neurocognitive functions. Among the 105 sibling pairs, the exposed siblings (mean age, 17.3 months at surgery/anesthesia; 9.5% female) and the unexposed siblings (44% female) had IQ testing at mean ages of 10.6 and 10.9 years, respectively. All exposed children received inhaled anesthetic agents, and anesthesia duration ranged from 20 to 240 minutes, with a median duration of 80 minutes. Mean IQ scores between exposed siblings and unexposed siblings were not statistically significantly different. No statistically significant differences in mean scores were found between sibling pairs in memory/learning, motor/processing speed, visuospatial function, attention, executive function, language, or behavior. The authors concluded that among healthy children with a single anesthesia exposure before age 36 months, compared with healthy siblings with no anesthesia exposure, there were no statistically significant differences in IQ scores in later childhood.

In yet another recent 2016 study,[48] 138 preterm neonates (24–32 weeks of gestation) underwent MRI and diffusion tensor imaging and at term equivalent age. Cognitive, language, and motor abilities were assessed using the Bayley Scales of Infant Development–III. Multivariate modeling revealed that total midazolam dose predicted decreased hippocampal volumes ($P<.001$), whereas invasive procedures did not ($P>.5$). Lower cognitive scores were associated with hippocampal growth, midazolam dose, and surgery. It was concluded that midazolam exposure was associated with macrostructural and microstructural alterations in hippocampal development and poorer outcomes consistent with hippocampal dysmaturation. The authors concluded that the use of midazolam in preterm neonates, particularly those not undergoing surgery, is cautioned.

More recently, in December 2016, the Food and Drug Administration issued a "Drug Safety Communication" (www.fda.gov/Drugs/DrugSafety/ucm532356.htm) warning that general anesthesia and sedation drugs used in children younger than 3 years of age "may affect the development of children's brains." This warning includes 11 - common general anesthetics and sedative agents that bind to GABA or N-methyl-D-aspartate receptors, including all anesthetic gases in addition to propofol, ketamine, barbiturates, and benzodiazepines. Opiates and dexmedetomidine are not included in the list; however, they are not adequate by themselves to meet the sedation needs of most critically ill children.[49] The impact of this warning on drug prescribing and patient care in the PICU setting is yet to be seen, but emphasizes the need for research in this area, targeting alterative sedative agents and neuroprotective strategies.

The Society of Critical Care Medicine released updated practice guidelines about the management of pain, agitation, and delirium (PAD) in 2013 for adult patients.[50] These guidelines used the GRADE methodology (Grading of Recommendations, Assessment, Development, and Evaluation) in their development. Based on randomized controlled trials, the 2013 PAD guidelines emphasized the importance of minimizing sedation use, and recommended strategies that include targeted sedation and daily sedative interruption. The guidelines recommend treating pain first and then sedatives as needed. Based on a meta-analysis performed during the development of the PAD guidelines that compared ICU outcomes in patients who received benzodiazepines versus nonbenzodiazepines (propofol or dexmedetomidine), there was a weak recommendation for preferential use of nonbenzodiazepines for the sedation of critically ill patients. Single-agent sedative strategies are not readily used in the setting of prolonged sedation in critically ill children to minimize doses and the risk of tolerance. As such, a sedation regimen that does not include a benzodiazepine or propofol presents a challenge in the PICU, warranting the development of alternative sedatives.

Sedative drugs used in the ICU can have deleterious effects on sleep, and lead to loss of circadian rhythm. The disruption in sleep architecture that occurs during continuous sedation in the PICU is a contributing factor to the development of delirium. Recent research focuses on the disruption of circadian rhythms in critical illness as a result of the severity of their underlying diseases, the treatments required for these illnesses, and the environment in the ICU.[51] Midazolam and lorazepam do not promote physiologic sleep. Although diazepam causes sleep architecture changes similar to other benzodiazepines, ICU studies of its influence on sleep when used for sedation are lacking.[52] Rapid eye movement suppression is the most consistent effect of opiates, such as morphine methadone, on sleep architecture.[53]

Propofol causes regional, dose-dependent electroencephalogram effects, with a greater than 50% reduction in cerebral glucose metabolism during deep sedation.[54] Propofol has been found to result in a decrease in rapid eye movement sleep, but no differences in sleep efficiency, sleep fragmentation, or non–rapid eye movement sleep distribution.[55] In addition, a 2-hour propofol infusion for 5 nights has been demonstrated to aid in normalization of sleep in patients with chronic primary insomnia.[56]

Dexmedetomidine is associated with less delirium risk than midazolam or propofol.[57] In a 24-hour polysomnography study of ventilated ICU patients, dexmedetomidine was associated with relative preservation of gross sleep-wake cycle.[58] Patients sedated with dexmedetomidine are more easily aroused than patients on most other sedatives.[59] Further research is need in an approach to sedation in the PICU that could include rotation of sedative agents throughout the day and night cycle, with sleep-promoting agents administered at night.

The effects of sedatives on other organ systems are often not considered. As an example, sedatives are known to impact immune function. Because of the high prevalence of sedative and analgesic use in critically ill patients, the effects of sedatives on the immune response should be fully understood. The immune system is a complicated balance of effectors from the innate and adaptive systems. Such drugs as propofol, opiates, and benzodiazepines are known to be implicated in depression of the innate immune system and to some extent the adaptive immune system.[60] Likewise, critical illness itself has been found to be an important determinant on the pharmacokinetics of drugs, such as midazolam.[12,61]

Given the concerns and potential for adverse effects, much effort has been placed on the need to administer minimal yet optimal sedation to the critically ill child. The recent RESTORE study (Randomized Evaluation of Sedation Titration for Respiratory Failure) addressed this. RESTORE is a cluster randomized trial conducted in 31 US PICUs. The trial enrolled 2449 children (mean age, 4.7 years; range, 2 weeks to 17 years) who were mechanically ventilated for acute respiratory failure to evaluate whether children managed with a nurse-implemented, goal-directed sedation protocol experience fewer days of mechanical ventilation than patients receiving usual care.[62] "Intervention" PICUs (17 sites; n = 1225 patients) used a protocol that included targeted sedation, arousal assessments, extubation readiness testing, sedation adjustment every 8 hours, and sedation weaning. "Control" PICUs (14 sites; n = 1224 patients) managed sedation per usual care. Duration of mechanical ventilation was not different between the two groups. Sedation-related adverse events including inadequate pain and sedation management, clinically significant iatrogenic withdrawal, and unplanned endotracheal tube/invasive line removal were also not significantly different between the two groups. Intervention patients experienced fewer stage 2 or worse immobility-related pressure ulcers (<1% vs 2%; $P = .001$). In an exploratory analyses, intervention patients had fewer days of opioid administration, were exposed to fewer sedative classes, and were more often awake and calm while intubated than control patients.

SUMMARY

There remains a large armamentarium of agents that can be used for the sedation of the critically ill child. Many factors contribute to the pharmacokinetics and dynamics of sedation, whereas sedation itself is associated with some harm (**Fig. 1**). Recent studies concerning sedation-associated neurotoxicity, loss of circadian rhythm, and delirium have raised concerns for regarding the choices of agents and duration of exposure for these children. These concerns have resulted in studies targeting sedation scores and sedation interruptions to improve the administration of sedative agents to these vulnerable pediatric populations. A large knowledge gap remains regarding the relationship of sedation on immune function and the impact of critical illness on pharmacokinetics and pharmacodynamics. Likewise, current knowledge regarding the genetic influences on drug disposition and effect is poor, precluding a personalized approach to the sedation of the critically ill child. Further research on the impact of pharmacogenetics and critical illness on sedation, in addition to the risks of neurotoxicity, immunomodulation, sleep disruption, and delirium that are associated with sedation, is needed to allow for a tailored and safer approach to sedation in the PICU.

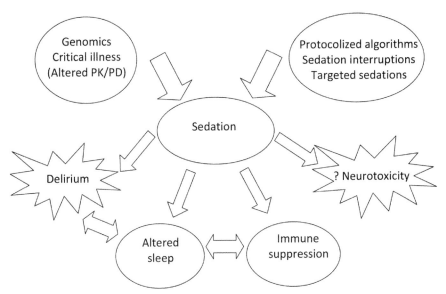

Fig. 1. Sedation-related adverse effects may include altered sleep, delirium, immunosuppression, and potential neurotoxicity. Inherited genetics and acquired critical illness can impact the pharmacokinetics and pharmacodynamics of sedation in the PICU setting. Likewise, informed strategies to sedation that include targeting sedation scores, sedation interruptions, and protocolized approaches to sedation management may allow for minimal yet optimal sedation strategies. PD, pharmacodynamics; PK, pharmacokinetics.

REFERENCES

1. Playfor S, Jenkins I, Boyles C, et al. Consensus guidelines on sedation and analgesia in critically ill children. Intensive Care Med 2006;32(8):1125–36.

2. Lucas SS, Nasr VG, Ng AJ, et al. Pediatric Cardiac Intensive Care Society 2014 consensus statement: pharmacotherapies in cardiac critical care: sedation, analgesia and muscle relaxant. Pediatr Crit Care Med 2016;17(3 Suppl 1):S3–15.

3. Mendelson WB. Neuropharmacology of sleep induction by benzodiazepines. Crit Rev Neurobiol 1992;6(4):221–32.

4. de Wildt SN, de Hoog M, Vinks AA, et al. Population pharmacokinetics and metabolism of midazolam in pediatric intensive care patients. Crit Care Med 2003; 31(7):1952–8.

5. Reed MD, Rodarte A, Blumer JL, et al. The single-dose pharmacokinetics of midazolam and its primary metabolite in pediatric patients after oral and intravenous administration. J Clin Pharmacol 2001;41(12):1359–69.

6. Young CC, Prielipp RC. Benzodiazepines in the intensive care unit. Crit Care Clin 2001;17(4):843–62.

7. Lacroix D, Sonnier M, Moncion A, et al. Expression of CYP3A in the human liver—evidence that the shift between CYP3A7 and CYP3A4 occurs immediately after birth. Eur J Biochem 1997;247(2):625–34.

8. Stevens JC. New perspectives on the impact of cytochrome P450 3A expression for pediatric pharmacology. Drug Discov Today 2006;11(9–10):440–5.

9. de Wildt SN, Kearns GL, Hop WC, et al. Pharmacokinetics and metabolism of oral midazolam in preterm infants. Br J Clin Pharmacol 2002;53(4):390–2.

10. Shelly MP, Mendel L, Park GR. Failure of critically ill patients to metabolise midazolam. Anaesthesia 1987;42(6):619–26.
11. Gehlbach BK, Kress JP. Sedation in the intensive care unit. Curr Opin Crit Care 2002;8(4):290–8.
12. Vet NJ, Brussee JM, de Hoog M, et al. Inflammation and organ failure severely affect midazolam clearance in critically ill children. Am J Respir Crit Care Med 2016;194(1):58–66.
13. Hubbard AM, Markowitz RI, Kimmel B, et al. Sedation for pediatric patients undergoing CT and MRI. J Comput Assist Tomogr 1992;16(1):3–6.
14. Greenberg SB, Adams RC, Aspinall CL. Initial experience with intravenous pentobarbital sedation for children undergoing MRI at a tertiary care pediatric hospital: the learning curve. Pediatr Radiol 2000;30(10):689–91.
15. Hall LG, Oyen LJ, Murray MJ. Analgesic agents. Pharmacology and application in critical care. Crit Care Clin 2001;17(4):899–923, viii.
16. Hagmeyer KO, Mauro LS, Mauro VF. Meperidine-related seizures associated with patient-controlled analgesia pumps. Ann Pharmacother 1993;27(1):29–32.
17. Volles DF, McGory R. Pharmacokinetic considerations. Crit Care Clin 1999;15(1): 55–75.
18. Zeiler FA, Teitelbaum J, West M, et al. The ketamine effect on ICP in traumatic brain injury. Neurocrit Care 2014;21(1):163–73.
19. Yip GM, Chen ZW, Edge CJ, et al. A propofol binding site on mammalian GABAA receptors identified by photolabeling. Nat Chem Biol 2013;9(11):715–20.
20. Guindon J, LoVerme J, Piomelli D, et al. The antinociceptive effects of local injections of propofol in rats are mediated in part by cannabinoid CB1 and CB2 receptors. Anesth Analg 2007;104(6):1563–9, table of contents.
21. Kam PC, Cardone D. Propofol infusion syndrome. Anaesthesia 2007;62(7): 690–701.
22. Cray SH, Robinson BH, Cox PN. Lactic acidemia and bradyarrhythmia in a child sedated with propofol. Crit Care Med 1998;26(12):2087–92.
23. Cremer OL, Moons KG, Bouman EA, et al. Long-term propofol infusion and cardiac failure in adult head-injured patients. Lancet 2001;357(9250):117–8.
24. Sebastiani A, Granold M, Ditter A, et al. Posttraumatic propofol neurotoxicity is mediated via the pro-brain-derived neurotrophic factor-p75 neurotrophin receptor pathway in adult mice. Crit Care Med 2016;44(2):e70–82.
25. Thal SC, Timaru-Kast R, Wilde F, et al. Propofol impairs neurogenesis and neurologic recovery and increases mortality rate in adult rats after traumatic brain injury. Crit Care Med 2014;42(1):129–41.
26. Hardman JG, editor. Goodman and Gilman's the pharmacologic basis of therapeutics. 9th edition. New York: McGraw-Hill Health Professions Division; 1996.
27. Katzung BG, editor. Basic and clinical pharmacology. 8th edition. New York: McGraw Hill; 2001.
28. Annane D. ICU physicians should abandon the use of etomidate! Intensive Care Med 2005;31(3):325–6.
29. Bhana N, Goa KL, McClellan KJ. Dexmedetomidine. Drugs 2000;59(2):263–8 [discussion: 269–70].
30. Nelson LE, Lu J, Guo T, et al. The alpha2-adrenoceptor agonist dexmedetomidine converges on an endogenous sleep-promoting pathway to exert its sedative effects. Anesthesiology 2003;98(2):428–36.
31. Venn RM, Grounds RM. Comparison between dexmedetomidine and propofol for sedation in the intensive care unit: patient and clinician perceptions. Br J Anaesth 2001;87(5):684–90.

32. Chrysostomou C, Schulman SR, Herrera Castellanos M, et al. A phase II/III, multi-center, safety, efficacy, and pharmacokinetic study of dexmedetomidine in preterm and term neonates. J Pediatr 2014;164(2):276–82.e1-3.

33. Chrysostomou C. Dexmedetomidine: should it be standard after pediatric cardiac surgery?*. Pediatr Crit Care Med 2012;13(6):696–7.

34. Chrysostomou C, Sanchez De Toledo J, Avolio T, et al. Dexmedetomidine use in a pediatric cardiac intensive care unit: can we use it in infants after cardiac surgery? Pediatr Crit Care Med 2009;10(6):654–60.

35. Weerink MA, Struys MM, Hannivoort LN, et al. Clinical pharmacokinetics and pharmacodynamics of dexmedetomidine. Clin Pharmacokinet 2017;56(8): 893–913.

36. Su F, Gastonguay MR, Nicolson SC, et al. Dexmedetomidine pharmacology in neonates and infants after open heart surgery. Anesth Analg 2016;122(5):1556–66.

37. Su F, Nicolson SC, Zuppa AF. A dose-response study of dexmedetomidine administered as the primary sedative in infants following open heart surgery. Pediatr Crit Care Med 2013;14(5):499–507.

38. Su F, Nicolson SC, Gastonguay MR, et al. Population pharmacokinetics of dexmedetomidine in infants after open heart surgery. Anesth Analg 2010;110(5): 1383–92.

39. Precedex Product Label. Abbott Laboratories: North Chicago (IL); 2003.

40. McManus MC. Neuromuscular blockers in surgery and intensive care, part 1. Am J Health Syst Pharm 2001;58(23):2287–99.

41. Chernow B, editor. The pharmacologic approach to the critically ill patient. 3rd edition. Baltimore (MD): Williams and Wilkins; 1994.

42. Power BM, Forbes AM, van Heerden PV, et al. Pharmacokinetics of drugs used in critically ill adults. Clin Pharmacokinet 1998;34(1):25–56.

43. Rocuronium bromide [package insert].

44. Sanders RD, Hassell J, Davidson AJ, et al. Impact of anaesthetics and surgery on neurodevelopment: an update. Br J Anaesth 2013;110(Suppl 1):i53–72.

45. Rappaport BA, Suresh S, Hertz S, et al. Anesthetic neurotoxicity: clinical implications of animal models. N Engl J Med 2015;372(9):796–7.

46. Davidson AJ, Disma N, de Graaff JC, et al. Neurodevelopmental outcome at 2 years of age after general anaesthesia and awake-regional anaesthesia in infancy (GAS): an international multicentre, randomised controlled trial. Lancet 2016;387(10015):239–50.

47. Sun LS, Li G, Miller TL, et al. Association between a single general anesthesia exposure before age 36 months and neurocognitive outcomes in later childhood. JAMA 2016;315(21):2312–20.

48. Duerden EG, Guo T, Dodbiba L, et al. Midazolam dose correlates with abnormal hippocampal growth and neurodevelopmental outcome in preterm infants. Ann Neurol 2016;79(4):548–59.

49. Andropoulos DB, Greene MF. Anesthesia and developing brains: implications of the FDA warning. N Engl J Med 2017;376(10):905–7.

50. Barr J, Fraser GL, Puntillo K, et al. Clinical practice guidelines for the management of pain, agitation, and delirium in adult patients in the intensive care unit. Crit Care Med 2013;41(1):263–306.

51. Chan MC, Spieth PM, Quinn K, et al. Circadian rhythms: from basic mechanisms to the intensive care unit. Crit Care Med 2012;40(1):246–53.

52. Oldham M, Pisani MA. Sedation in critically ill patients. Crit Care Clin 2015;31(3): 563–87.

53. Moore P, Dimsdale JE. Opioids, sleep, and cancer-related fatigue. Med Hypotheses 2002;58(1):77–82.

54. Herregods L, Rolly G, Mortier E, et al. EEG and SEMG monitoring during induction and maintenance of anesthesia with propofol. Int J Clin Monit Comput 1989; 6(2):67–73.

55. Kondili E, Alexopoulou C, Xirouchaki N, et al. Effects of propofol on sleep quality in mechanically ventilated critically ill patients: a physiological study. Intensive Care Med 2012;38(10):1640–6.

56. Xu Z, Jiang X, Li W, et al. Propofol-induced sleep: efficacy and safety in patients with refractory chronic primary insomnia. Cell Biochem Biophys 2011;60(3): 161–6.

57. Pasin L, Landoni G, Nardelli P, et al. Dexmedetomidine reduces the risk of delirium, agitation and confusion in critically ill patients: a meta-analysis of randomized controlled trials. J Cardiothorac Vasc Anesth 2014;28(6):1459–66.

58. Oto J, Yamamoto K, Koike S, et al. Sleep quality of mechanically ventilated patients sedated with dexmedetomidine. Intensive Care Med 2012;38(12):1982–9.

59. Hall JE, Uhrich TD, Barney JA, et al. Sedative, amnestic, and analgesic properties of small-dose dexmedetomidine infusions. Anesth Analg 2000;90(3):699–705.

60. Sanders RD, Hussell T, Maze M. Sedation & immunomodulation. Anesthesiol Clin 2011;29(4):687–706.

61. Ince I, de Wildt SN, Peeters MY, et al. Critical illness is a major determinant of midazolam clearance in children aged 1 month to 17 years. Ther Drug Monit 2012;34(4):381–9.

62. Curley MA, Wypij D, Watson RS, et al. Protocolized sedation vs usual care in pediatric patients mechanically ventilated for acute respiratory failure: a randomized clinical trial. JAMA 2015;313(4):379–89.

Delirium in Pediatric Critical Care

Anita K. Patel, MD[a], Michael J. Bell, MD[b,c,d], Chani Traube, MD[e,*]

KEYWORDS

- Delirium • Pediatric critical care • Pediatrics • Pain • Agitation • Sedation

KEY POINTS

- Delirium is a frequent and serious complication of pediatric critical illness.
- Pediatric delirium is associated with increased morbidity, including longer duration of mechanical ventilation, increased hospital length of stay, and higher resource utilization.
- Benzodiazepines likely increase the risk for development of pediatric delirium.
- Delirium in children is both treatable and preventable.

DELIRIUM IN PEDIATRIC CRITICAL ILLNESS

Introduction

As critical care medicine has matured over the decades, from a specialty fighting mortality from a myriad of diseases to one promoting recovery with as few disabilities as possible, mitigating complications of critical illness has become one of the intensivist's most important goals.[1] The sudden onset of unexplained deterioration of consciousness can be particularly worrisome. In critical illnesses such a deterioration of sensorium may represent delirium, which is characterized by an acute onset and fluctuating course with disturbances in awareness and cognition.[2] In adults, delirium occurs frequently and represents global cerebral dysfunction due to the direct physiologic effects of an underlying medical illness or its treatment.[2,3] Although delirium is generally a temporary state, it is strongly associated with poor outcomes, including increased mortality, and long-term cognitive impairment in survivors.[4,5] Because of the extensive research highlighting the morbidity associated with delirium, the Society of Critical Care Medicine (SCCM) released guidelines in 2013 that recommended routine

Disclosure Statement: All authors declare they have no relevant financial interests to disclose.
[a] Pediatrics, Children's National Medical Center, 111 Michigan Avenue Northwest Suite M4800, Washington, DC 20010, USA; [b] Critical Care Medicine, University of Pittsburgh, 3434 Fifth Avenue, Pittsburgh, PA 15260, USA; [c] Neurological Surgery, University of Pittsburgh, 3434 Fifth Avenue, Pittsburgh, PA 15260, USA; [d] Pediatrics, University of Pittsburgh, 3434 Fifth Avenue, Pittsburgh, PA 15260, USA; [e] Pediatrics, Weill Cornell Medical College, 525 East 68th Street, M-508, New York, NY 10065, USA
* Corresponding author.
E-mail address: chr9008@med.cornell.edu

monitoring for delirium in critically ill adults as standard of care.[3] A recent body of pediatric literature suggests that this recommendation should apply to children as well.[6,7]

Pathophysiology

The cause of delirium is complex, with many possible pathophysiologic pathways. Most researchers think that delirium results from a combination of predisposing and precipitating factors. Predisposing factors are patient related (for example, age, genetic susceptibility, or underlying disease). Precipitating factors include treatment effects (particularly sedative medications) and the intensive care unit (ICU) environment.[3,8,9] Here the authors highlight 3 processes that are thought to play important roles in the evolution of pediatric delirium.

The *neuroinflammatory* hypothesis suggests that systemic inflammation (commonly seen during critical illnesses, such as respiratory failure, sepsis, and others) leads to either compromise in the integrity of the blood-brain barrier or de novo production of inflammatory products within the brain.[10] Inflammation leads to endothelial activation, enhanced cytokine activity, and infiltration of leukocytes and cytokines into the central nervous system (CNS), producing local ischemia and neuronal apoptosis.[11] Several studies have demonstrated elevated levels of proinflammatory cytokines in delirious patients (such as C-reactive protein, tumor necrosis factor-alpha, and interleukin-6) compared with nondelirious patients, even after controlling for age and cognitive impairment.[12–14]

The *neurotransmitter* hypothesis was generated from clinical observations that delirium often followed the use of medications that change neurotransmitter function.[10] Studies show that impaired cholinergic function, coupled with an excess of dopaminergic transmission, leads to the development of delirium.[15–17] Notably, anticholinergic medications are tightly associated with development of delirium in the geriatric population, as the elderly have an age-related reduction in acetylcholine synthesis.[18,19] (Intriguingly, a similar phenomenon may exist in children less than 2 years of age, whereby functional MRIs have demonstrated sparse connectivity between control structures related to executive function. This sparse connectivity results in dependence on the cholinergic system to modulate attention and orientation. Like the elderly, these young children may be at particular risk of delirium with exposure to anticholinergic medication.)[20,21] In addition to dopamine and acetylcholine, dysregulation of melatonin, glutamate, norepinephrine, serotonin, histamine, and gamma-aminobutyric acid has also been suggested to contribute to delirium development.[10]

The *oxidative stress* hypothesis suggests that reduced oxygen delivery in critical illness, coupled with increased cerebral metabolism, leads to the production of reactive oxygen species that cause global CNS dysfunction.[10] Hypoxia has clearly been associated with delirium development.[22–24] For instance, a study of patients undergoing cardiac surgery found that intraoperative desaturation was an independent risk factor for postoperative delirium.[23] Demonstrating that overlapping sources of pathophysiology contribute to delirium, hypoxia also results in an excess of dopamine due to the failure of the oxygen-dependent conversion of dopamine to norepinephrine. The enzyme responsible for dopamine degradation, catechol-o-methyl transferase, is inhibited by toxic metabolites produced during oxidative stress.[22] An excess of dopamine has been evidenced in multiple studies to underlie the pathogenesis of hyperactive delirium.[10]

Regardless of the exact pathophysiology that triggers an episode of delirium, the end result is the same: altered neurotransmission that leads to a failure of integration and processing of sensory information and motor response. This final common pathway leads to the behaviors that we recognize as delirium.[25]

Clinical Presentation

There are 3 major subtypes of delirium recognized by the *Diagnostic and Statistical Manual of Mental Disorders*, Fifth Edition: hyperactive, hypoactive, and mixed-type delirium, with each having specific characteristics. Hyperactive delirium is characterized by agitation, restlessness, hypervigilance, and combative behavior. In contrast, hypoactive delirium is notable for lethargy, inattention, and decreased responsiveness. Mixed-type delirium exhibits aspects of both hyperactive and hypoactive delirium.[2,3] Importantly, hypoactive delirium can be easily misdiagnosed as oversedation or clinical depression without appropriate screening and diagnostic tools for assessment.[26–28] Unfortunately, hypoactive delirium has been associated with poorest prognosis and greatest frequency, emphasizing the need for diligent screening for delirium in patients with critical illnesses.[29,30] In a longitudinal study of pediatric delirium and its subtypes, involving 1547 children and more than 7500 patient days, hypoactive and mixed-type delirium were most common (46% and 45%, respectively), whereas the hyperactive subtype was only found in 8% of patients.[7] This profile of delirium is consistent with observations of adults with critical illnesses.

Delirium in children is often marked by changes in psychomotor activity, ranging from delayed responsiveness to constant, agitated movements. Emotional lability is also common, evidenced by inconsolableness or, alternatively, inappropriate calmness. Some pediatric patients (particularly adolescents) experience auditory and visual hallucinations. Disordered sleep is nearly always present in delirious children.[8,9,31,32]

Preliminary evidence suggests that delirium often occurs early in the ICU course of children with critical illnesses, with a median time to development of delirium of 1 to 3 days in pediatric studies.[7,33–35] Furthermore, the few studies that have been conducted to assess the duration of delirium suggest it is a relatively brief condition, with a median of 2 days.[7,33,34] A substantial portion (approximately one-third) of patients with early onset delirium will demonstrate recurrent episodes during their ICU stay.[7,33]

Regardless of its duration or timing, delirium has measurable effects on a variety of outcomes. In a recent study of postoperative delirium in children, 2 patterns of delirium were described. For approximately half of the children, delirium was diagnosed early in the course of their illness (within 24 hours), was of short duration (less than 24 hours), and was characterized by relatively low scores on the Cornell Assessment of Pediatric Delirium (CAPD). Within this series, these children were categorized as having mild delirium. In contrast, another cohort of children experienced delirium throughout the study period (5 days) and were categorized as having severe delirium. Compared with children who were never delirious, those with mild delirium had increased time on mechanical ventilation and longer hospital length of stay (LOS), whereas those with severe delirium had even longer hospitalizations, took longer to emerge from sedation, had longer time to extubation, and had higher resource utilization.[34]

Epidemiology

Delirium in adults is a well-known problem, with many hospitals implementing delirium scoring plans, because more than 30% of all critically ill adults develop delirium during their ICU stay.[3,36] Delirium research in pediatrics lagged behind because of the lack of validated screening tools and a decreased awareness of this condition among clinicians.

Recent reports have found that pediatric delirium is quite frequent, with prevalence rates between 12% and 65% in pediatric medical, surgical, and cardiac ICUs.[6] In one of the earliest series in the field, a prevalence of 12.3% was reported; but this cohort included only children older than 5 years and only 6% of the children were mechanically ventilated (MV).[37] In another cohort of children (0–21 years of age, 25% on MV), a delirium prevalence rate of 22% was observed. In this study, delirium was associated with age less than 5 years and preexisting developmental delay.[38] In a study of children with heart disease cared for in a cardiac ICU, a delirium prevalence of 49% was observed, largely comparable with adults with heart disease.[33] In the surgical population, a prevalence rate of 27% was described, with an overall delirium incidence of 65% in children within 5 days after surgery. (In this study, many subjects were infants after cardiac bypass procedures).[34] Another cohort study that included children within a limited age range (6 months to 5 years) found an overall prevalence of 47%; the highest rate (56%) was found in children younger than 2 years of age.[35] A large-scale, longitudinal study of delirium in all patients admitted to a single pediatric ICU (PICU) over a 1-year period of time, including more than 1500 patients, demonstrated a delirium rate of 17%.[7] It should be noted that this unit was an early adopter of delirium screening and had systematically changed its approach to sedation and management to minimize delirium risk. So it is likely that this 17% incidence is lower than rates in other institutions that have not been leaders in delirium screening.[7] In the largest multi-institutional pediatric delirium study to date, 994 children were assessed for delirium in 25 different PICUs. Delirium prevalence overall was 25%.[39]

Risk Factors

It is useful to separate risk factors for pediatric delirium into 2 categories: modifiable and nonmodifiable (**Table 1**). Independent risk factors for delirium development in critically ill adults include high severity-of-illness score on admission, elderly age, hypertension, dementia, alcoholism, and cigarette use. Hospital-related risk factors for delirium development in adults include depth of sedation, receipt of benzodiazepines, and use of restraints.[3]

Demographic risk factors for development of delirium in children include age less than 5 years and preexisting diagnosis of neurodevelopmental delay. It is not surprising that both the immature and abnormal brains, respectively, are more prone to development of delirium; this is similar to the finding of increased delirium in the elderly, and in those with underlying dementia.[7,25,33,35,39]

Children with higher severity-of-illness scores on admission are more likely to develop delirium. Delirium, in turn, then contributes to multiple organ dysfunction syndrome, as delirium itself is an indication of end-organ (brain) dysfunction.[7,33,34,40]

Duration of ICU stay likely contributes to delirium development, but this relationship is difficult to understand as a prolonged LOS likely exposes children to increased

Table 1	
Risk factors for development of delirium	
Predisposing Risk Factors	**Precipitating Risk Factors**
Age <2 y	Anticholinergic medications
Developmental delay	Benzodiazepines
High severity of illness	Cardiac bypass surgery
Low albumin	Immobilization
Mechanical ventilation	Prolonged ICU length of stay
Preexisting medical condition	Restraints

Risk factors for delirium can be separated into predisposing and precipitating risk factors. It is important to recognize that several risk factors are modifiable.

factors associated with delirium – and delirium also causes increased LOS.[7,25,33,34] To attempt to understand this relationship, an international study showed an increase in delirium rates after 5 days in the ICU (20% in children with LOS $\leq$5 days vs 38% in children with LOS >5 days, P<.001).[39]

Risk factors particular to children with congenital heart disease have been identified as well. Specifically, cardiac bypass surgery is thought to be a unique exposure, marked by a significant inflammatory response to the cardiotomy and bypass circuit, or possibly subclinical evidence of emboli during bypass.[41,42] Incidence of pediatric delirium after cardiotomy was strongly and independently associated with longer bypass times and greater complexity of the surgical repair. Children with cyanotic lesions were at increased risk for delirium, supporting several theories of delirium development, including those associated with hypoxia and oxidant stress. Poor nutritional status (using a preoperative albumin level <3 mg/dL as a surrogate marker for adequacy of nutrition) also strongly predicted delirium.[33]

Importantly, recent research has identified potentially modifiable risk factors for delirium development. A prospective observational study (n = 1540 children) used a multivariable model to demonstrate a 5-fold risk of delirium in children who were ever prescribed benzodiazepines (after controlling for severity of illness, developmental delay, mechanical ventilation, and other important confounders).[7] However, an assessment of the relationship between benzodiazepine use and delirium can be confounded by the fact that a child with hyperactive delirium could be prescribed benzodiazepines as a treatment of agitation. Therefore, it is important to assess the clinical context in much more detail. This was done in a longitudinal study that followed every child in a PICU throughout hospitalization. Each child was prospectively assigned a daily cognitive status of (1) delirium, (2) coma/deep sedation, or (3) delirium free/coma free. In this circumstance, and only considering children who developed next-day delirium (ie, a child who developed delirium after scoring delirium free/ coma free the previous day), benzodiazepines remained independently associated with delirium (odds ratio [OR] 3.14, confidence interval 2.08–4.74, P<.001) after controlling for multiple covariates. In addition, an analysis of benzodiazepine doses administered to 539 critically ill children showed a dose-response effect, with delirium rates of 79% in those who received greater than 0.82 mg/kg/d of midazolam equivalents as compared with a 27% delirium rate in children given less than 0.82 mg/kg/d (P<.001).[7]

A multi-institutional point prevalence study demonstrated that odds of delirium quadrupled in patients who were physically restrained. Although this analysis was controlled for mechanical ventilation and use of sedating medications, temporality was not assessed (and it is possible that children were restrained after developing delirium).[39] However, it is consistent with a large body of adult literature that shows a clear relationship between use of physical restraints and subsequent development of delirium.[3,36,43,44]

Outcomes

Delirium that develops in adults with critical illnesses has been associated with poor outcomes, including a 3-fold increased risk of mortality, increased ICU and hospital LOS, longer time on mechanical ventilation, long-term cognitive impairment, and post–intensive care syndrome.[3–5,45,46] Additionally, delirium has been linked to increased rates of auto-extubation and inadvertent removal of catheters.[3]

Preliminary studies strongly suggest a similar pattern in children with critical illnesses. Pediatric delirium has been linked to short-term morbidity, including increased duration of mechanical ventilation in children with delirium (median 4 vs 1 day, P<.001).[7]

Several studies have shown that delirium is associated with increased length of hospital stay. In fact, in a cardiac ICU cohort, delirium was independently associated with an increase in LOS of 60%.[33] In a general PICU, adjusted relative LOS was 2.3 in children with delirium, after controlling for mechanical ventilation and severity of illness on admission.[7] In yet another study, delirium predicted increased hospital LOS, increased duration of mechanical ventilation, and higher resource utilization; the extent of increases was directly related to duration of delirium.[34]

From a financial perspective, a diagnosis of delirium in children has been associated with increased health care costs. In a single-center study, daily PICU costs were 23% higher for an ICU day with delirium as compared with an ICU day without delirium. Incidence of delirium was associated with an overall 85% increase in hospital costs (relative costs 1.85 [1.51–2.26], $P<.001$), even after controlling for severity of illness, PICU LOS, and other important confounders. This increase translates into more than $500 million each year in US hospital costs alone.[47]

A prospective pediatric study has shown a strong and independent association between pediatric delirium and mortality, with an adjusted OR of 4.4 for in-hospital death in children who were diagnosed with delirium. In this cohort delirium was a stronger predictor of mortality than the Pediatric Index of Mortality 3 score (OR of 3.2 in patients in the highest severity-of-illness category). Delirium may be an important identifier of children who are most vulnerable to poor outcomes.[7] To date, there are no long-term studies published that describe the association between delirium and cognitive outcomes in children after discharge or the effect of delirium on the long-term psychological and emotional health of PICU survivors and their families.

Diagnosis

Until the advent of bedside screening tools, pediatric intensivists relied on consultation with pediatric psychiatrists to make the diagnosis of delirium. Not surprisingly, psychiatrists were usually only consulted in extreme cases, when delirium resulted in disruptive and aggressive behaviors that interfered with the medical team's management plans or the symptoms were so extreme as to require an expansion of the differential diagnosis to other possible neurologic conditions.[30,48,49] A psychiatric assessment, although reliable, is not available for point-of-care use in every child in the PICU.[50] As in adults, there was a need to establish delirium screens for nonpsychiatrists to use routinely at the patients' bedside.

It would not be possible to simply adopt delirium tools designed for adults, as diagnosing delirium in children is complicated by developmental variability. The behavior expected from a hospitalized 2-year-old child, as compared with a 16-year-old adolescent, are vastly different; appropriate developmental expectations are necessary.[51] As pediatric clinicians became aware of the significant burden of delirium in adult ICUs, it was clear that it was necessary to develop child-specific bedside screening tools.[8,9,52]

Two different versions of pediatric delirium screens were developed: the Pediatric Confusion Assessment Method for the ICU (pCAM-ICU or psCAM-ICU for preschool-age children) and the CAPD. Both have been proven to be valid and reliable for detection of delirium in critically ill children. Each requires that the child be arousable to verbal stimulation in order to be assessed. Both the pCAM-ICU and CAPD should take only minutes to complete.[6,35,37,38,53]

The pCAM-ICU/psCAM-ICU are interactive, cognitively oriented screens (**Fig. 1**). The pCAM-ICU is designed for patients older than 5 years, and the psCAM-ICU is designed for children aged 6 months to 5 years. These tools are point-in-time screens, designed to detect delirium that is present at the time of testing. The interactive nature of the tool should yield objective results (delirium present or absent).[35,37]

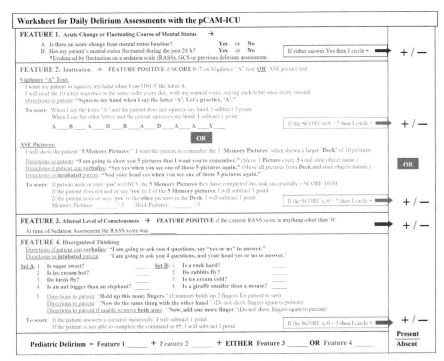

Fig. 1. pCAM-ICU. The pCAM-ICU is an interactive cognitively oriented tool validated in children from 5 to 18 years of age. (Available at: http://www.icudelirium.org/docs/ped_Instruction-Tool_pCAM-ICU_9-2016.pdf. Accessed July 10, 2017.)

The CAPD is an observational screen that provides a longitudinal picture of a pediatric patient over the course of a nursing shift (usually 8–12 hours) (**Table 2**). It is suitable for use in children 0 to 21 years of age and was validated in both developmentally delayed and developmentally typical children. A score of 9 or higher is consistent with a delirium diagnosis; the CAPD score can be trended within an individual patient over time, allowing for assessment of trajectory and response to interventions.[38]

With availability of rapid, valid, and reliable bedside tools for use in children of all ages, delirium screening has become feasible for use as standard of care in PICUs. In fact, 3 years after the publication of the SCCM's guidelines for adults, the European Society for Pediatric and Neonatal Intensive Care released consensus guidelines in 2016 calling for "use of CAPD as an instrument to assess pediatric delirium (grade of recommendation = A)" once each shift in critically ill children[6]. Routine monitoring will allow providers to detect and treat delirium earlier and potentially improve outcomes.[3,6]

Differential diagnosis

In children with underlying developmental delay, there is a need to establish alteration from cognitive baseline before diagnosing delirium. In addition to a positive delirium screen, the clinician needs to confirm that there is an acute process (ie, not merely static encephalopathy) with a fluctuating level of awareness over the course of the day.[50,51]

The classification of sedation-related delirium is controversial.[54] This type is a specific form of delirium that rapidly resolves once sedation is lifted and was noted in a protocol

Table 2
Cornell Assessment for Pediatric Delirium

Please answer these questions based on your interactions with the patient over the course of your shift:

	Never 4	Rarely 3	Sometimes 2	Often 1	Always 0	Score
1. Does the child make eye contact with the caregiver?						
2. Are the child's actions purposeful?						
3. Is the child aware of his or her surroundings?						
4. Does the child communicate needs and wants?						
	Never 0	Rarely 1	Sometimes 2	Often 3	Always 4	
5. Is the child restless?						
6. Is the child inconsolable?						
7. Is the child underactive: very little movement while awake?						
8. Does it take the child a long time to respond to interactions?						
TOTAL						

The CAPD is an observational longitudinal tool validated in children from birth to 21 years of age. (Available at: http://www.icudelirium.org/docs/capd.pdf. Accessed July 10, 2017.)

whereby adults were kept sedated for most of the day, with scheduled sedation breaks to allow for a period of wakefulness. In the subset of patients with delirium limited to rapidly reversible sedation-related delirium, outcomes were similar to patients who did not experience delirium,[55] suggesting that this was merely residual sedation and not delirium. This finding has not been replicated in a recent pediatric study using the CAPD, wherein delirium could be clearly distinguished from sedation by analysis of individual test items, and even mild delirium of short duration was associated with poor outcomes.[34] In fact, in a multicenter pediatric study, daily sedation interruption was associated with an overall increase in exposure to narcotics and benzodiazepines, increased time on mechanical ventilation, and increased length of hospital stay.[56] This finding highlights the importance of judicious sedation management in children.[57]

Iatrogenic withdrawal syndrome (IWS) can result in both the physiologic signs of abstinence and the behavioral symptoms of agitation, confusion, and motor activity that are consistent with hyperactive delirium. It is critically important to recognize and treat the physiologic signs of withdrawal (ie, dilated pupils, diarrhea) with judicious narcotic replacement.[58]

Treatment

When a child is diagnosed with delirium, the key to effective treatment is identifying the underlying cause. Clinically, delirium can be thought of as a product of the underlying illness, iatrogenic effects of treatment, and the ICU environment[9,25,31] (**Fig. 2**). With a stepwise approach, one should investigate for an underlying medical problem that

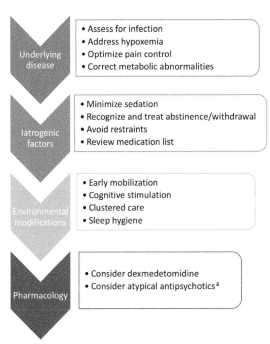

Fig. 2. Delirium treatment algorithm. With a systematic approach to targeting underlying triggers of delirium, most children will improve. If agitated behaviors persist, clinicians can consider pharmacologic treatment. [a] Note: This treatment is an off-label use of these drugs, as the Food and Drug Administration has not approved either dexmedetomidine or the atypical antipsychotics for treatment of pediatric delirium.

may have triggered the delirium episode. Delirium can be an early warning sign of an evolving infection or the result of hypoxia or acute metabolic derangements. A careful neurologic examination to exclude a primary CNS disease should be considered.[31,59,60]

After assessing for underlying illness, addressing iatrogenic causes of delirium is necessary. Optimizing pain control is essential, especially in preverbal children. Sedatives should be minimized, with consideration given to replacement of benzodiazepines with dexmedetomidine if possible, as several studies suggest that dexmedetomidine prevents and/or treats delirium.[61–65] (It is important to note that this is an off-label use, as the Food and Drug Administration has not approved dexmedetomidine for the treatment of pediatric delirium.) A careful review of the patients' medication list is warranted with consideration of discontinuing medications that might be associated with delirium, if possible (particularly sedatives, anticholinergics, and steroids).[3,9,25] Identification of IWS is necessary, with judicious narcotic replacement until the physiologic signs of withdrawal abate.[58] But after treating IWS, the agitated behavior of hyperactive delirium may persist and often requires environmental modifications (and sometimes pharmacologic alternatives) rather than a further increase in narcotics, which may just prolong the delirium.[66]

Careful attention to patients' environment is part of the process of treating delirium.[67] Repeated reorientation of patients, use of eye glasses or hearing aids when indicated, and minimization of excessive noise can be helpful. Keeping a child's favorite stuffed animal or blanket from home can normalize the ICU bed. Clustering care can dramatically reduce the frequency of stimulation.[9,25,39] Creating an environment less disruptive to sleep is important – ensuring lights off at night and on during the day helps to promote normal circadian rhythms.[68] Early mobilization has been an effective intervention in adult ICUs, not only in reducing poor functional outcomes, but also in decreasing delirium rates.[69] Progressive increase in activity levels can be safely achieved, even in extremely young and MV children.[70]

Most pediatric delirium will improve with management of underlying medical illness, minimizing iatrogenic triggers, and optimizing the PICU environment. However, if the delirium persists and the child has agitated behaviors that are distressful or interfering with the medical care plan, pharmacologic therapies are available. Most experts recommend use of the atypical antipsychotics because of their procognitive effects and favorable side effect profile.[3,71,72] This therapy is an off-label use, as this drug class is not approved for treatment of pediatric delirium. Nonetheless, a randomized controlled trial of quetiapine (an atypical antipsychotic) as treatment of adult delirium indicated a benefit; pediatric case series have suggested efficacy in children.[49,73–76] A retrospective safety study in 50 delirious children treated with quetiapine showed no serious adverse events.[77] Important when starting any form of antipsychotic is to monitor for QT prolongation, dysrhythmias, and extrapyramidal side effects.[72,78]

Prevention

Delirium can be conceptualized as a hospital-acquired complication that results in both short- and long-term adverse effects in survivors of pediatric critical illness. As such, prevention of delirium is an important goal.[3,6]

Anecdotally, the culture within critical care units, both adult and pediatric, seems to be changing. In years past, most critically ill children were sedated during their time in the ICU. They were often physically restrained, kept on strict bed rest, and exposed to noise and lights 24 hours a day. Although parents were allowed at the bedside, they were discouraged from physically interacting with their child. Cognitive stimulation was kept to a minimum. This practice was likely the result of the desire to spare children from a traumatic hospitalization and/or to allow them to rest. When children became agitated, they were labeled as difficult to sedate and sedating medications (usually benzodiazepines) were increased further.[53,54]

However, recent research on post-ICU outcomes (including myopathy and cognitive impairment) shows that neither the mind nor the body benefits from prolonged periods of inactivity.[3,79–81] In particular, use of deep sedation (specifically benzodiazepines) in children leads to increased delirium and decreased sleep and may be associated with delusional memories and posttraumatic stress disorder.[82–85]

The SCCM has endorsed an alternative approach in adult ICUs, termed *analgosedation*, that is now being adopted in PICUs as well (**Fig. 3**). For most patients, sedation is not necessary as first-line therapy. Rather, with an analgesic-first approach, the goal is to optimize pain control and minimize sedation. With less sedation on board, patients are less likely to develop iatrogenic delirium. They are better able to communicate pain, which in turn leads to better pain control. They are also more available to participate in early mobilization. Family members and child life specialists provide age-appropriate cognitive stimulation during the day, and the medical care team attempts to optimize the PICU environment for nighttime sleep.[3,83,86,87]

With heightened awareness as to the frequency and seriousness of pediatric delirium, implementation of an analgo-sedation approach, incorporation of early mobilization, and involvement of family members in daily care, we may be able to prevent delirium in at-risk children.

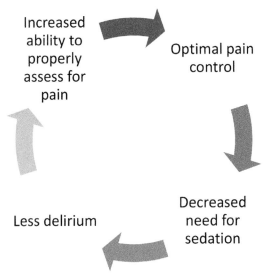

Fig. 3. Analgo-sedation. An analgesic-first approach avoids sedatives unless necessary. This approach decreases frequency of delirium.

SUMMARY

Delirium is a frequent complication of pediatric critical illness. Universal screening is feasible and necessary for early detection. This screening allows for targeted intervention and identification of children at risk for short-term morbidity and mortality. Further research is necessary to determine the long-term cognitive and psychological effects of pediatric delirium, and interventional studies are needed to establish best practices for treatment and prevention of delirium in critically ill children.

REFERENCES

1. Pollack MM, Holubkov R, Funai T, et al. Pediatric intensive care outcomes: development of new morbidities during pediatric critical care. Pediatr Crit Care Med 2014;15(9):821-7.
2. American Psychiatric Association: Diagnostic and Statistical Manual of Mental Disorders. Fifth Edition. Arlington, VA: American Psychiatric Association; 2013.
3. Barr J, Fraser GL, Puntillo K, et al. Clinical practice guidelines for the management of pain, agitation, and delirium in adult patients in the intensive care unit. Crit Care Med 2013;41(1):278-80.
4. Ely EW, Shintani A, Truman B, et al. Delirium as a predictor of mortality in mechanically ventilated patients in the intensive care unit. JAMA 2004;291(14):1753-62.
5. Girard TD, Jackson JC, Pandharipande PP, et al. Delirium as a predictor of long-term cognitive impairment in survivors of critical illness. Crit Care Med 2010; 38(7):1513-20.
6. Harris J, Ramelet A-S, van Dijk M, et al. Clinical recommendations for pain, sedation, withdrawal and delirium assessment in critically ill infants and children: an ESPNIC position statement for healthcare professionals. Intensive Care Med 2016;42(6):972-86.
7. Traube C, Silver G, Gerber L, et al. Delirium and mortality in critically ill children: epidemiology and outcomes of pediatric delirium. Crit Care Med 2017;45(5):891-8.

8. Silver G, Traube C, Kearney J, et al. Detecting pediatric delirium: development of a rapid observational assessment tool. Intensive Care Med 2012;38(6):1025–31.

9. Smith HAB, Brink E, Fuchs DC, et al. Pediatric delirium: monitoring and management in the pediatric intensive care unit. Pediatr Clin North Am 2013;60(3): 741–60.

10. Maldonado JR. Neuropathogenesis of delirium: review of current etiologic theories and common pathways. Am J Geriatr Psychiatry 2013;21(12):1190–222.

11. Cerejeira J, Firmino H, Vaz-Serra A, et al. The neuroinflammatory hypothesis of delirium. Acta Neuropathol 2010;119(6):737–54.

12. van Munster BC, Korevaar JC, Korse CM, et al. Serum S100B in elderly patients with and without delirium. Int J Geriatr Psychiatry 2010;25(3):234–9.

13. de Rooij SE, van Munster BC, Korevaar JC, et al. Cytokines and acute phase response in delirium. J Psychosom Res 2007;62(5):521–5.

14. McGrane S, Girard TD, Thompson JL, et al. Procalcitonin and C-reactive protein levels at admission as predictors of duration of acute brain dysfunction in critically ill patients. Crit Care 2011;15(2):R78.

15. Trzepacz PT. Is there a final common neural pathway in delirium? Focus on acetylcholine and dopamine. Semin Clin Neuropsychiatry 2000;5(2):132–48.

16. Hshieh TT, Fong TG, Marcantonio ER, et al. Cholinergic deficiency hypothesis in delirium: a synthesis of current evidence. J Gerontol A Biol Sci Med Sci 2008; 63(7):764–72.

17. Maldonado JR. Pathoetiological model of delirium: a comprehensive understanding of the neurobiology of delirium and an evidence-based approach to prevention and treatment. Crit Care Clin 2008;24(4):789–856, ix.

18. Flacker JM, Cummings V, Mach JR, et al. The association of serum anticholinergic activity with delirium in elderly medical patients. Am J Geriatr Psychiatry 1999;6(1):31–41.

19. Tune LE. Serum anticholinergic activity levels and delirium in the elderly. Semin Clin Neuropsychiatry 2000;5(2):149–53.

20. Posner MI, Rothbart MK, Sheese BE, et al. Control networks and neuromodulators of early development. Dev Psychol 2012;48(3):827–35.

21. Rothbart MK, Sheese BE, Rueda MR, et al. Developing mechanisms of self-regulation in early life. Emot Rev 2011;3(2):207–13.

22. Seaman JS, Schillerstrom J, Carroll D, et al. Impaired oxidative metabolism precipitates delirium: a study of 101 ICU patients. Psychosomatics 2006;47(1): 56–61.

23. Slater J, Guarino T, Stack J, et al. Cerebral oxygen desaturation predicts cognitive decline and longer hospital stay after cardiac surgery. Ann Thorac Surg 2009; 87(1):36–45.

24. Schoen J, Meyerrose J, Paarmann H, et al. Preoperative regional cerebral oxygen saturation is a predictor of postoperative delirium in on-pump cardiac surgery patients: a prospective observational trial. Crit Care 2011;15(5):R218.

25. Silver G, Traube C, Gerber LM, et al. Pediatric delirium and associated risk factors: a single-center prospective observational study. Pediatr Crit Care Med 2015; 16(4):303–9.

26. Peritogiannis V, Bolosi M, Lixouriotis C, et al. Recent insights on prevalence and correlations of hypoactive delirium. Behav Neurol 2015;2015:1–11.

27. Peterson JF, Pun BT, Dittus RS, et al. Delirium and its motoric subtypes: a study of 614 critically ill patients: delirium subtypes in the critically ill. J Am Geriatr Soc 2006;54(3):479–84.

28. Peitz GJ, Balas MC, Olsen KM, et al. Top 10 myths regarding sedation and delirium in the ICU. Crit Care Med 2013;41:S46–56.
29. Meagher DJ, O'Hanlon D, O'Mahony E, et al. Relationship between symptoms and motoric subtype of delirium. J Neuropsychiatry Clin Neurosci 2000;12(1): 51–6.
30. Ely EW, Siegel MD, Inouye SK. Delirium in the intensive care unit: an under-recognized syndrome of organ dysfunction. Semin Respir Crit Care Med 2002; 22(02):115–26.
31. Schieveld JNM, Leroy PLJM, Os J, et al. Pediatric delirium in critical illness: phe-nomenology, clinical correlates and treatment response in 40 cases in the pedi-atric intensive care unit. Intensive Care Med 2007;33(6):1033–40.
32. Turkel SB, Tavare CJ. Delirium in children and adolescents. J Neuropsychiatry Clin Neurosci 2003;15(4):431–5.
33. Patel AK, Biagas KV, Clarke EC, et al. Delirium in children after cardiac bypass surgery. Pediatr Crit Care Med 2017;18(2):165–71.
34. Meyburg J, Dill M-L, Traube C, et al. Patterns of postoperative delirium in chil-dren. Pediatr Crit Care Med 2017;18(2):128–33.
35. Smith HAB, Gangopadhyay M, Goben CM, et al. The preschool confusion assessment method for the ICU: valid and reliable delirium monitoring for criti-cally ill infants and children. Crit Care Med 2016;44(3):592–600.
36. Ouimet S, Kavanagh BP, Gottfried SB, et al. Incidence, risk factors and conse-quences of ICU delirium. Intensive Care Med 2006;33(1):66–73.
37. Smith HAB, Boyd J, Fuchs DC, et al. Diagnosing delirium in critically ill children: validity and reliability of the pediatric confusion assessment method for the inten-sive care unit. Crit Care Med 2011;39(1):150–7.
38. Traube C, Silver G, Kearney J, et al. Cornell assessment of pediatric delirium: a valid, rapid, observational tool for screening delirium in the PICU*. Crit Care Med 2014;42(3):656–63.
39. Traube C, Silver G, Reeder RW, et al. Delirium in critically ill children: an interna-tional point prevalence study. Crit Care Med 2017;45(4):584–90.
40. Schieveld JNM, Lousberg R, Berghmans E, et al. Pediatric illness severity mea-sures predict delirium in a pediatric intensive care unit. Crit Care Med 2008;36(6): 1933–6.
41. Brown CH. Delirium in the cardiac surgical ICU. Curr Opin Anaesthesiol 2014; 27(2):117–22.
42. Gosselt AN, Slooter AJ, Boere PR, et al. Risk factors for delirium after on-pump cardiac surgery: a systematic review. Crit Care 2015;19(1):346. Available at: http://ccforum.com/content/19/1/346. Accessed October 8, 2015.
43. Agarwal V, O'Neill PJ, Cotton BA, et al. Prevalence and risk factors for develop-ment of delirium in burn intensive care unit patients. J Burn Care Res 2010;31(5): 706–15.
44. Pandharipande P, Cotton BA, Shintani A, et al. Prevalence and risk factors for development of delirium in surgical and trauma intensive care unit patients. J Trauma 2008;65(1):34–41.
45. Ely EW, Gautam S, Margolin R, et al. The impact of delirium in the intensive care unit on hospital length of stay. Intensive Care Med 2001;27(12):1892–900.
46. Fann JR, Alfano CM, Roth-Roemer S, et al. Impact of delirium on cognition, distress, and health-related quality of life after hematopoietic stem-cell transplan-tation. J Clin Oncol 2007;25(10):1223–31.
47. Traube C, Mauer EA, Gerber LM, et al. Cost associated with pediatric delirium in the ICU. Crit Care Med 2016;44(12):e1175–9.

48. Schieveld JN, Staal M, Voogd L, et al. Refractory agitation as a marker for pediatric delirium in very young infants at a pediatric intensive care unit. Intensive Care Med 2010;36(11):1982–3.

49. Traube C, Augenstein J, Greenwald B, et al. Neuroblastoma and pediatric delirium: a case series: neuroblastoma and delirium. Pediatr Blood Cancer 2014;61(6):1121–3.

50. Silver G, Kearney J, Traube C, et al. Pediatric delirium: evaluating the gold standard. Palliat Support Care 2015;13(3):513–6.

51. Silver G, Kearney J, Traube C, et al. Delirium screening anchored in child development: the Cornell Assessment for Pediatric Delirium. Palliat Support Care 2015; 13(4):1005–11.

52. Schieveld JN, Janssen NJ. Delirium in the pediatric patient: on the growing awareness of its clinical interdisciplinary importance. JAMA Pediatr 2014; 168(7):595–6.

53. Daoud A, Duff JP, Joffe AR, Alberta Sepsis Network. Diagnostic accuracy of delirium diagnosis in pediatric intensive care: a systematic review. Crit Care 2014;18(5):489.

54. Fraser GL, Worby CP, Riker RR. Dissecting sedation-induced delirium. Crit Care Med 2013;41(4):1144–6.

55. Patel SB, Poston JT, Pohlman A, et al. Rapidly reversible, sedation-related delirium versus persistent delirium in the intensive care unit. Am J Respir Crit Care Med 2014;189(6):658–65.

56. Vet NJ, de Wildt SN, Verlaat CWM, et al. A randomized controlled trial of daily sedation interruption in critically ill children. Intensive Care Med 2016;42(2): 233–44.

57. Kollef MH. Less sedation in intensive care: the pendulum swings back. Am J Respir Crit Care Med 2000;162:505–11.

58. Best KM, Wypij D, Asaro LA, et al. Patient, process, and system predictors of iatrogenic withdrawal syndrome in critically ill children. Crit Care Med 2017;45(1): e7–15.

59. Karnik NS, Joshi SV, Paterno C, et al. Subtypes of pediatric delirium: a treatment algorithm. Psychosomatics 2007;48(3):253–7.

60. Skrobik Y. Delirium prevention and treatment. Anesthesiol Clin 2011;29(4):721–7.

61. Aydogan MS, Korkmaz MF, Ozgül U, et al. Pain, fentanyl consumption, and delirium in adolescents after scoliosis surgery: dexmedetomidine vs midazolam. Anderson B, editor. Pediatr Anesth 2013;23(5):446–52.

62. Carrasco G, Baeza N, Cabré L, et al. Dexmedetomidine for the treatment of hyperactive delirium refractory to haloperidol in nonintubated ICU patients: a nonrandomized controlled trial. Crit Care Med 2016;44(7):1295–306.

63. Jakob SM, Ruokonen E, Grounds RM, et al. Dexmedetomidine vs midazolam or propofol for sedation during prolonged mechanical ventilation: two randomized controlled trials. JAMA 2012;307(11):1151–60.

64. Pandharipande PP, Pun BT, Herr DL, et al. Effect of sedation with dexmedetomidine vs lorazepam on acute brain dysfunction in mechanically ventilated patients: the MENDS randomized controlled trial. JAMA 2007;298(22):2644–53.

65. Riker RR, Shehabi Y, Bokesch PM, et al. Dexmedetomidine vs midazolam for sedation of critically ill patients: a randomized trial. JAMA 2009;301(5):489–99.

66. Traube C, Greenwald B. Iatrogenic withdrawal syndrome, or undiagnosed delirium? Crit Care Med 2017;45(6):e622–3.

67. Hshieh TT, Yue J, Oh E, et al. Effectiveness of multicomponent nonpharmacological delirium interventions: a meta-analysis. JAMA Intern Med 2015;175(4):512.

68. Kudchadkar SR, Yaster M, Punjabi NM. Sedation, sleep promotion, and delirium screening practices in the care of mechanically ventilated children: a wake-up call for the pediatric critical care community. Crit Care Med 2014;42(7):1592–600.
69. The TEAM Study Investigators, Hodgson C, Bellomo R, Berney S, et al. Early mobilization and recovery in mechanically ventilated patients in the ICU: a bi-national, multi-centre, prospective cohort study. Crit Care 2015;19(1):81. Available at: http://ccforum.com/content/19/1/81. Accessed April 27, 2015.
70. Wieczorek B, Ascenzi J, Kim Y, et al. PICU Up!: impact of a quality improvement intervention to promote early mobilization in critically ill children. Pediatr Crit Care Med 2016;17(12):e559–66.
71. Boettger S, Breitbart W. Atypical antipsychotics in the management of delirium: a review of the empirical literature. Palliat Support Care 2005;3(3):227–37.
72. Turkel SB, Jacobson J, Munzig E, et al. Atypical antipsychotic medications to control symptoms of delirium in children and adolescents. J Child Adolesc Psychopharmacol 2012;22(2):126–30.
73. Devlin JW, Roberts RJ, Fong JJ, et al. Efficacy and safety of quetiapine in critically ill patients with delirium: a prospective, multicenter, randomized, double-blind, placebo-controlled pilot study. Crit Care Med 2010;38(2):419–27.
74. Tahir TA, Eeles E, Karapareddy V, et al. A randomized controlled trial of quetiapine versus placebo in the treatment of delirium. J Psychosom Res 2010;69(5):485–90.
75. Traube C, Witcher R, Mendez-Rico E, et al. Quetiapine as treatment for delirium in critically ill children: a case series. J Pediatr Intensive Care 2013;2(3):121–6.
76. Silver GH, Kearney JA, Kutko MC, et al. Infant delirium in pediatric critical care settings. Am J Psychiatry 2010;167(10):1172–7.
77. Joyce C, Witcher R, Herrup E, et al. Evaluation of the safety of quetiapine in treating delirium in critically ill children: a retrospective review. J Child Adolesc Psychopharmacol 2015;25(9):666–70. Available at: http://online.liebertpub.com/doi/10.1089/cap.2015.0093. Accessed October 18, 2015.
78. Rasimas JJ, Liebelt EL. Adverse effects and toxicity of the atypical antipsychotics: what is important for the pediatric emergency medicine practitioner? Clin Pediatr Emerg Med 2012;13(4):300–10.
79. Anderson BJ, Mikkelsen ME. Duration of delirium and patient-centered outcomes: embracing the short- and long-term perspective. Crit Care Med 2014;42(6):1558–9.
80. Herridge MS. Long-term outcomes after critical illness. Curr Opin Crit Care 2002;8(4):331–6.
81. Needham DM, Davidson J, Cohen H, et al. Improving long-term outcomes after discharge from intensive care unit: report from a stakeholders' conference. Crit Care Med 2012;40(2):502–9.
82. Kudchadkar SR, Aljohani OA, Punjabi NM. Sleep of critically ill children in the pediatric intensive care unit: a systematic review. Sleep Med Rev 2014;18(2):103–10.
83. Barnes SS, Kudchadkar SR. Sedative choice and ventilator-associated patient outcomes: don't sleep on delirium. Ann Transl Med 2016;4(2):34. Available at: https://www.ncbi.nlm.nih.gov/pmc/articles/PMC4731606/. Accessed February 10, 2017.
84. Colville G, Kerry S, Pierce C. Children's factual and delusional memories of intensive care. Am J Respir Crit Care Med 2008;177(9):976–82.
85. Colville GA, Pierce CM. Children's self-reported quality of life after intensive care treatment. Pediatr Crit Care Med 2013;14(2):e85–92.
86. Barnes-Daly MA, Phillips G, Ely EW. Improving hospital survival and reducing brain dysfunction at seven California community hospitals: implementing PAD

guidelines via the ABCDEF bundle in 6,064 patients. Crit Care Med 2017;45(2): 171–8.

87. Ely EW. The ABCDEF bundle: science and philosophy of how ICU liberation serves patients and families. Crit Care Med 2017;45(2):321–30.

Adjunctive Steroid Therapy for Treatment of Pediatric Septic Shock

 CrossMark

Jerry J. Zimmerman, PhD, MD

KEYWORDS

- Septic shock • Adjunctive sepsis therapy • Glucocorticoids/corticosteroids
- Aldosterone • Oxandrolone • 17β-estradiol • Cortisol • Hydrocortisone

KEY POINTS

- Mineralocorticoids, glucocorticoids, and gonadocorticoids are subject to individual synthetic regulation within the adrenal cortex and remote sites of steroid synthesis.
- In addition to governing sodium and potassium homeostasis, aldosterone mediates multiple aspects of hemodynamics that may be disrupted by endogenous and exogenous dopamine.
- Oxandrolone, an anabolic steroid, has been used to improve nitrogen balance and lean body mass among children with thermal burn injury, and this effect may be beneficial among children with sepsis.
- Estrogen analogs facilitate mitochondrial function and aspects of aerobic metabolism that logically might abrogate widespread energy failure as an antecedent to multiple organ dysfunction syndrome associated with severe sepsis.
- Corticosteroids have favorable hemodynamic and anti-inflammatory properties that may be invaluable among septic patients with recalcitrant septic shock, but immunosuppression and promotion of lean body catabolism associated with gluconeogenesis and hyperglycemia may ultimately mitigate any clinical benefit. A high-quality, prospective, double-blinded, randomized controlled interventional trial examining the potential benefits and risks of hydrocortisone as adjunctive therapy for pediatric sepsis is warranted.

ADRENAL STEROIDOGENESIS

With major involvement of cytochrome P450 isoforms, 3 classes of steroids are produced from cholesterol in the adrenal cortex. Generally mineralocorticoids are synthesized in the zona glomerulosa, glucocorticoids in the zona fasciculata, and

Disclosure Statement: J.J. Zimmerman receives research grant support from National Institutes of Health, Patient Centered Outcomes Research Institute and Immunexpress, Seattle, WA; he receives royalties from Elsevier Publishing, as coeditor of, Pediatric Critical Care; and he receives travel reimbursement from the Society of Critical Care Medicine to attend board meetings.
Pediatric Critical Care Medicine, Seattle Children's Hospital, Harborview Medical Center, University of Washington School of Medicine, 4800 Sand Point Way Northeast, Room FA.2.300-B, Seattle, WA 98105, USA
E-mail address: jerry.zimmerman@seattlechildrens.org

gonadocorticoids in the zona reticularis.[1] Synthesis of mineralocorticoids depends primarily on the renin-angiotensin-aldosterone (RAA) axis; synthesis of glucocorticoids is governed by activity of the hypothalamic-pituitary-adrenal (HPA) axis; and synthesis of gonadocorticoids is regulated by hypothalamic-derived gonadotropin-releasing hormone and pituitary-derived follicle stimulating hormone and luteinizing hormone with critical involvement of steroidogenic acute regulatory protein.[2] Steroid hormones are not stored at their sites of biosynthesis; rather, release of steroid hormones is controlled almost entirely through regulation of their synthesis. Although critical care medicine practitioners frequently prescribe glucocorticoids for their favorable hemodynamic as well as immunosuppression properties to patients with septic shock, the purpose of this review is to suggest that mineralocorticoids as well as gonadocorticoids may also represent potentially useful adjuncts for treatment of sepsis.

MINERALOCORTICOIDS

A schematic summary of aldosterone synthesis and regulation is provided in **Fig. 1**.

As an aspect of the RAA axis activation, angiotensin II production is enhanced by endothelial angiotensin-converting enzyme, particularly within the pulmonary vasculature.[3] Angiotensin II (a peptide not steroid hormone) mediates multiple activities also essential to the (sepsis) stress response:

- Increases systemic vascular resistance and blood pressure
- Stimulates aldosterone release
- Increases plasminogen activator inhibitor-1, facilitating a prothrombotic state
- Enhances thirst and salt craving
- Increases antidiuretic hormone, adrenocorticotropic hormone, and norepinephrine release
- Facilitates sodium reabsorption at proximal convoluted tubule
- Stimulates renal afferent/efferent vasoconstriction
- Increases nuclear factor κB (NF-κB), resulting in increased proinflammatory cytokine release

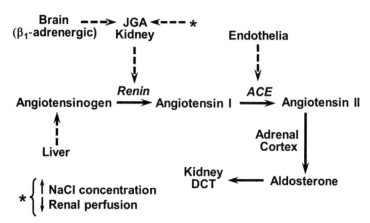

Fig. 1. RAA axis. ACE, angiotensin-converting enzyme; DCT, renal distal convoluted tubule; JGA, renal juxtaglomerular apparatus. In addition to monitoring local perfusion pressure and environmental Na$^+$ and Cl concentrations, the JGA receives β_1-adrenergic neural input from the brain.

The principal actions of aldosterone, the end product of the RAA axis, include the following[4]:

- Sodium reabsorption
- Potassium and hydrogen ion excretion
- Insulin resistance
- Hypertension
- Activation of nuclear transcription factor, NF-κB activation
- Arginine vasopressin release

More than 4 decades ago, hyperreninemic hypoaldosteronism was identified as a novel diagnostic entity among critically ill adults.[5] This syndrome was observed to occur primarily among patients with infection and hypotension who exhibited a normal serum potassium, increased plasma cortisol (averaging 40.1 ± 10.1 μg/dL), increased plasma renin, low concentrations of plasma aldosterone, and elevated concentrations of aldosterone's immediate precursor, 18-hydroxycorticosterone. Mortality with this constellation of findings was 78%. These patients were generally unresponsive to either adrenocorticotropic hormone or angiotensin II and were postulated to have a defect in the adrenal zona glomerulosa. Similar discordance between plasma renin and aldosterone concentrations has also been demonstrated in children with meningococcal sepsis[6]: among 29 nonseptic critically ill children, mean Pediatric Risk of Mortality (PRISM) score was 9.4 and mean aldosterone concentration, 1489 ± 2.44 pg/mL. Among 231 children with meningococcal sepsis with a mean PRISM score of 32.3, however, mean aldosterone concentration was only 428 pg/mL $\pm$ 88 pg/mL. In another study focused on children with meningococcemia, aldosterone concentrations tended to be higher among nonsurvivors compared with survivors, but plasma renin activity did not significantly differ.[7]

In ex vivo cell culture experiments, tumor necrosis factor (TNF)-a and interleukin-2 (IL-2) have been shown to inhibit synthesis of angiotensin II–induced aldosterone synthesis in a dose-response fashion.[8] Aldosterone production is known to be under tonic dopaminergic inhibition that can be overridden by infusion of angiotensin II. An infusion of dopamine can abrogate aldosterone production whereas metoclopramide, a dopamine antagonist, can reverse dopaminergic inhibition.[9] These findings suggest one reason why dopamine may not be the preferred vasoactive-inotropic agent among critically ill children.[10]

Aldosterone's role in hemodynamics and inflammation, as well as fluid and electrolyte balance, may be clinically relevant in the pediatric ICU, in view of the initial clinical trial that demonstrated a benefit of hydrocortisone in hastening resolution of septic shock as well as decreasing mortality, at least among patients demonstrating a seemingly inadequate (<9 μg/dL) increase in serum cortisol after corticotropin stimulation.[11] This trial included both hydrocortisone and fludrocortisone, an aldosterone agonist, in the treatment group. Although hydrocortisone also possesses mineralocorticoid activity, it may be that aldosterone plays a more protean role in maintaining hemodynamics than is currently acknowledged. In addition, perhaps aldosterone mediates a systemic proinflammatory response to balance to the broad systemic anti-inflammatory activity characteristic of sepsis and potentiated by endogenous and exogenous cortisol, perhaps modulating away from immune paralysis.[12]

GONADOCORTICOIDS

Two major classes of gonadocorticoids have been characterized for potential utilization in critical illness, namely the anabolic steroids exemplified by oxandrolone and the estrogens typified by 17β-estradiol.[13]

ANABOLIC STEROIDS

Critically ill patients, in particular those with severe sepsis, are at risk for proteolysis of lean body muscle as a result of a catabolic state induced by endogenous and exogenous corticosteroids as well as proinflammatory cytokines, IL-1, TNF-α, and IL-6, and the effect of immobilization.[14,15] These biochemical and clinical antecedents, common in the ICU, activate atrogene[16,17] as well as a variety of protease pathways[18] that ultimately release amino acids from skeletal muscle proteins.[19,20] These amino acids are used for 3 key aspects of the acute stress response[21]:

- Gluconeogenesis to generate carbohydrate energy substrate
- Protein synthesis focused on acute phase reactants
- Expansion of immune system components.

This catabolic state is perpetuated as long as the initiating proinflammatory stimuli remain in place. Electron microscopy of muscle biopsies from critically ill patients has demonstrated loss of the a-band due to loss of myosin thick filaments.[22] Computerized tomography[23–25] and ultrasonography[26] imaging have been used to document critical illness-associated lean body mass loss in real time.

Prolonged muscle catabolism has been extensively described among thermal burn patients, including children.[27] Muscle catabolism affects both skeletal and diaphragmatic muscle and may be associated with need for prolonged weaning from mechanical ventilation as well as long-term impaired functional status and health-related quality of life in the physical domain.[28–30] Patients with extensive loss of lean body mass may require prolonged rehabilitation.

During the first year after large thermal burns, both the fractional breakdown rate and the fractional synthesis rate for proteins have been documented.[27] This skeletal muscle protein turnover remains elevated for up to a year after burn injury and has been attributed to simultaneous increases in both protein anabolism and catabolism. Muscle breakdown generally exceeds synthesis during this time interval, however, resulting in a persistent negative net protein balance.[27,31]

Several potential therapeutic interventions have been suggested to counteract protein catabolism associated with prolonged critical illness, including

- Activation of phosphoinositide 3-kinase[32]
- Antiatrophy drugs specifically targeting muscle-specific ubiquitin ligases (MURF-1 and atrogin 1)[33]
- Insulin and insulin-like growth factor 1[34]
- Myostatin (growth factor differentiation factor 8)[35]
- Electrical muscle stimulation[36]
- Anabolic steroids[37]

Early clinical investigation demonstrated the benefits of both growth hormone and oxandrolone in promoting net positive nitrogen balance among thermal burn patients.[38] Similar anabolic effects of oxandrolone have been reported for children with severe burn injury with oxandrolone providing a stimulus for new protein synthesis with corresponding correction of negative protein balance.[39] Positive protein balance effects of oxandrolone translate clinically into improved weight gain after burn injury.[40] In addition, administering oxandrolone for up to 2 years after severe burn injury results in greater improvements in bone mineral content, bone mineral density, and height velocity.[41]

ESTROGENS

In multiple preclinical as well as human clinical studies, preferential survival of patients of the female gender has been reported. For example, in a clinically relevant mouse model of septic shock using cecal ligation and puncture, administration of an estrogen agonist markedly improved survival in a dose-response fashion.[42] Corresponding analysis of gene expression data derived in this study demonstrated reversal of proinflammatory gene expression in estrogen agonist–treated animals comparable to animals that underwent a sham operation.

Estrogen mediates regulation of a family of genes related to respiration, including[43]

- Aerobic glycolysis
- Respiratory efficiency
- ATP generation
- Calcium loading tolerance
- Antioxidant defenses
- Mitochondrial function in general

If the concept of mitochondrial dysfunction and widespread energy failure as a precursor for multiple organ dysfunction syndrome associated with sepsis is embraced,[44–47] estrogen agonist therapy seems attractive for additional investigation.

GLUCOCORTICOIDS, CORTICOSTEROIDS

Cortisol (hydrocortisone) represents the quintessential glucocorticoid that mediates alteration in gene expression for approximately 25% of the genome[48]. As summarized in **Fig. 2**, cortisol synthesis is under control of the HPA axis.[49] Multiple proinflammatory agents signal the hypothalamus to release corticotropin-releasing hormone, which stimulates the anterior pituitary to release adrenocorticotropin hormone (ACTH).[50] Corticotropin is released from the pituitary as proopiomelanocortin that is subsequently proteolytically cleaved to multiple small peptides. Corticotropin subsequently binds to class 2 melanocortin G protein–coupled receptors in the zona fasciculate cells of the adrenal cortex[51,52] (and other sites, including leukocytes[53,54]), stimulating synthesis and release of cortisol. Typical stimulants of the HPA axis include IL-1, IL-2, and IL-6. In addition to TNF-α, other inhibitors of cortisol synthesis

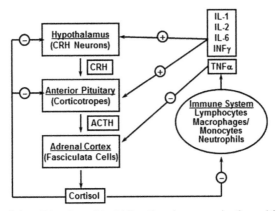

Fig. 2. Overview of the HPA axis and its bidirectional communication with the immune system. CRH, corticotropin-releasing hormone; INF, interferon.

include macrophage inhibition factor and corticostatin, a peptide defensin with anti-corticotropin activity.[55] Cortisol is transported to peripheral tissues by cortisol binding protein[56,57] as well as albumin.

Corticosteroids regulate gene expression through 2 major pathways.[49] After nonfacilitated transport across the plasma membrane and binding to the cytosol glucocorticoid receptor (composed of heat shock proteins),[58,59] the cortisol-receptor complex may: (1) traverse the nuclear membrane and directly bind to glucocorticoid responsive elements or (2) bind to NF-κB with subsequent binding of the complex to NF-κB responsive elements of the genome. Corticosteroids have the general effect of decreasing proinflammatory mediators and enhancing anti-inflammatory mediators.[50] For example, corticosteroids are known to inhibit chemotaxis; inhibit expression of adhesion molecules, such as ELAM-1 and ICAM-1; and inhibit inducible nitric oxide synthase, NADP oxidoreductase, and cyclooxygenase resulting in decreased production of nitric oxide, superoxide anion, and other reactive oxygen species and prostaglandins. In addition, corticosteroids increase the production of lipocortin-1 (annexin)[60] that similarly inhibits NADPH oxidoreductase and cyclooxygenase. Corticosteroids up-regulate the expression of IL-10 and IκB that both mediate anti-inflammatory activity. Finally, corticosteroids increase the production of macrophage inhibition factor that provides negative feedback for cortisol production.[61] As summarized in **Fig. 3**, based on in vitro animal and human studies, corticosteroids would be expected to favorably modulate all aspects related to unstable hemodynamics in septic shock.

Cortisol can be assessed as either total cortisol or free cortisol, with the free form representing typically only approximately 10% of the total but accounting for all of the biological activity.[62,63] Furthermore, cortisol can be assessed as a random concentration or a delta concentration change comparing baseline and stimulated states after administration of corticotropin.[64] True adrenal insufficiency is typically associated with random total cortisol concentrations less than 5 μg/dL.[65] Patients exhibiting an increase in circulating total cortisol from baseline less than 9 μg/dL after corticotropin administration have been viewed as having inadequate adrenal reserve and hence potential for relative adrenal insufficiency.[66–68] Neither random cortisol concentration nor the corticotropin stimulation test, however, has consistently identified a group of patients who might benefit from hydrocortisone replacement therapy.[69] In a general population of critically ill children, neither free cortisol nor total cortisol predicted signs or symptoms of adrenal insufficiency, such as hypotension, hypoglycemia, or hyponatremia.[70] In this study, 33% of children exhibited total cortisol less than 10, 57% exhibited free cortisol less than 2%, and 30% exhibited free cortisol less than 0.8 μg/dL, but none demonstrated clinical evidence of critical illness-related cortisol insufficiency.

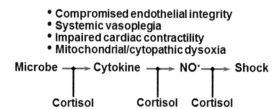

Fig. 3. Hemodynamic instability in sepsis and the biological plausible beneficial effects of adjunctive corticosteroids at multiple points along the natural history of septic shock. NO, nitric oxide (and other nitrogen and oxygen active species).

The 2014 Clinical Practice Parameters for Hemodynamic Support of Pediatric and Neonatal Septic Shock suggest adjunctive corticosteroid treatment of catecholamine-resistant shock if a patient is at risk for absolute adrenal insufficiency.[10] What constitutes catecholamine resistant shock and absolute adrenal insufficiency remains unclear. Patients receiving acute or chronic corticosteroid dosing, patients with disorders of the HPA axis, children with congenital adrenal hyperplasia[71,72] and multiple endocrinopathies, and patients who have had recent treatment with ketoconazole and etomidate are at risk for adrenal insufficiency. As discussed previously, however, laboratory testing of cortisol either with a random sample or corticotropin stimulation testing does not accurately predict which patients will respond favorably to hydrocortisone replacement.

In the twenty-first century, the practice of critical care medicine benefits from widespread vaccination for bacterial pathogens[73–75] as well as mandatory newborn screening for congenital adrenal hyperplasia.[76,77] Accordingly, the prevailing paranoia regarding risk for Addisonian crisis in pediatric sepsis is unfounded. Sepsis treatment guidelines previously recommended maintaining equipoise regarding the question of adjunctive steroid therapy for pediatric sepsis pending prospective randomized clinical trials.[78] This recommendation is appropriate given the contradicting results of the 2 large, high-quality adult trials examining adjunctive corticosteroid therapy for septic shock.[11,69] Currently, 2 large follow-up adult randomized controlled trials examining adjunctive corticosteroids for septic shock are in progress in Europe[79] and Australia/New Zealand.[80] In an important editorial related to prescription of corticosteroids for septic shock, clinicians were reminded that those who treat their patients with corticosteroids because they have observed a rapid reduction in the need for vasoactive inotropic support should be aware that more rapid weaning from this chemical hemodynamic support is an unreliable surrogate for clinically meaningful outcomes, because this intervention does not also improve survival.[81]

In addition to the 2 large adult clinical trials examining adjunctive corticosteroids for septic shock, multiple observational studies have also concluded that corticosteroids provide no benefit and are potentially harmful when used for this indication.[82–85] No high quality prospective randomized controlled clinical trials have examined the potential utility of adjunctive corticosteroids for pediatric septic shock. However, 7 good-quality, observational, cohort investigations have concluded no benefit or potential harm (increased mortality) related to adjunctive corticosteroids administered for pediatric septic shock:

- PHIS (Pediatric Health Information System) database investigation[86]
- Researching Severe Sepsis and Organ Dysfunction in Children: A Global Perspective (RESOLVE) database investigation[87]
- PERSEVERE (PEdiatRic SEpsis biomarkEr Risk modEl) database investigation[88]
- Pediatric septic shock personalized medicine[89]
- SPROUT (Sepsis Prevalence, Outcomes and Therapies Study) point prevalence investigation[90]
- STRIPES (Steroid Use in Pediatric Fluid and Vasoactive Infusion Dependent Shock) investigation[91]
- PALICC (Pediatric Acute Lung Injury Consensus Conference) database investigation[92]

As an example, one of these studies involved a follow-up investigation of the RESOLVE (NCT00049764) trial database.[87] In this retrospective analysis, 193 children who received adjunctive corticosteroids for septic shock were compared with 284 children who did not receive adjunctive corticosteroids. At baseline, the 2 groups were similar in terms of age, gender, illness severity per PRISM III scores, and number of organ dysfunctions as well as baseline Pediatric Overall Performance Category score. Several outcomes, including mortality, days of vasoactive-inotropic infusion, duration of mechanical ventilation, time to composite organ dysfunction resolution, Pediatric Overall Performance Category score, and duration of pediatric ICU and hospital lengths of stay were similar in children who did or did not receive corticosteroid intervention as adjunctive therapy in this largest pediatric sepsis interventional clinical trial conducted to date.

Although most clinicians readily cite the beneficial hemodynamic and anti-inflammatory properties of corticosteroids, the adverse effects of this drug class are typically underappreciated. Relevant corticosteroid side effects include widespread immunosuppression, hypertension, hyperglycemia, reduced somatic growth, impaired wound healing, neuromuscular weakness, hospital acquired infection, and possible altered neurodevelopment. When administering even a single dose of corticosteroids, it is important to realize that although the intervention may (or may not) improve clinical hemodynamics, the corticosteroid also alters expression of approximately 25% of the human genome.[48] Of particular relevance to treatment of pediatric septic shock with adjunctive corticosteroids is the observation that this intervention results in repression of multiple elements of adaptive immunity, including T-cell receptor signaling, T-helper cell signaling, overall regulation of the immune response, and signaling in T-lymphocytes and macrophages and cytotoxic T-lymphocytes as well as glucocorticoid receptor signaling.[88,93] With mounting evidence for an alternative paradigm for sepsis pathogenesis in which both proinflammatory and anti-inflammatory responses may be simultaneously operative, it makes little sense to administer potent anti-inflammatory agents to treat sepsis patients who are in a state of immune suppression and may well benefit from immune reconstitution.[94] Risks for ICU-acquired infections associated with hydrocortisone dosing have been clearly documented for both children and adults.[95,96]

Although a pediatric intensivist's gut reaction is to prescribe corticosteroids when a patient with (septic) shock is deteriorating, this instinctive approach may not be appropriate. The disconnect between improved hemodynamics after administration of the corticosteroids but lack of a benefit in terms of clinically meaningful outcome measures represents one of the most important research questions in pediatric critical care medicine, and, based on current evidence, it is difficult to argue either for or against the use of this drug class in children with septic shock.[97] Clinicians should be aware that the actions of corticosteroids are not just like those of vasoactive-inotropic drugs that are also commonly used to treat unstable hemodynamics in septic shock; the notion that "it can't hurt" is a misconception. There are passionate individuals on both sides of this important clinical controversy, but current guidelines are not supported by evidence in terms of whether corticosteroid therapy is beneficial for patients with severe sepsis.[98] Because corticosteroids may produce either benefit or harm, there is a scientific, ethical, and health economic imperative to conduct a randomized trial of adjunctive corticosteroids for pediatric septic shock.[80]

Design of such a trial is challenged by frequent (albeit unwarranted) lack of equipoise regarding the research question.[99] Pediatric intensivists may currently be practicing therapeutic illusion, wherein physicians believe that their actions or tools are more effective than they actually are. Therapeutic illusion facilitates continued use of inappropriate tests and treatments.[100,101] The results of such actions may be unnecessary and costly or dangerous care. Before concluding that a treatment is effective, physicians should consider other explanations, including natural history of the disease. If there exists some evidence for benefit, it is also important to look for evidence of risk.[100]

Pediatric intensivists need to acknowledge that evidence is not the plural of anecdotes and the need to practice with intellectual honesty. A randomized controlled trial of adjunctive corticosteroids for pediatric septic shock has been waiting offstage for decades. Science requires testing of ideas, including the potential risks and benefits of all types of steroid treatment of sepsis. This testing will determine if predictions are supported by the experiment. This testing of theories and generating evidence are what distinguish science, including medicine, from other creative fields and ultimately provide a platform for best practice.[102]

REFERENCES

1. Stocco DM, Clark BJ. Regulation of the acute production of steroids in steroidogenic cells. Endocr Rev 1996;17:221–44.

2. Stocco DM. StAR protein and the regulation of steroid hormone biosynthesis. Annu Rev Physiol 2001;63:193–213.

3. Caldwell PR, Seegal BC, Hsu KC, et al. Angiotensin-converting enzyme: vascular endothelial localization. Science 1976;191:1050–1.

4. Kubzansky LD, Adler GK. Aldosterone: a forgotten mediator of the relationship between psychological stress and heart disease. Neurosci Biobehav Rev 2010; 34:80–6.

5. Zipser RD, Little TE, Wilson W, et al. Dual effects of antidiuretic hormone on urinary prostaglandin E2 excretion in man. J Clin Endocrinol Metab 1981;53:522–6.

6. Lichtarowicz-Krynska EJ, Cole TJ, Camacho-Hubner C, et al. Circulating aldosterone levels are unexpectedly low in children with acute meningococcal disease. J Clin Endocrinol Metab 2004;89:1410–4.

7. den Brinker M, Joosten KF, Liem O, et al. Adrenal insufficiency in meningococcal sepsis: bioavailable cortisol levels and impact of interleukin-6 levels and intubation with etomidate on adrenal function and mortality. J Clin Endocrinol Metab 2005;90:5110–7.

8. Natarajan R, Ploszaj S, Horton R, et al. Tumor necrosis factor and interleukin-1 are potent inhibitors of angiotensin-II-induced aldosterone synthesis. Endocrinology 1989;125:3084–9.

9. Carey RM, Thorner MO, Ortt EM. Dopaminergic inhibition of metoclopramide-induced aldosterone secretion in man. Dissociation of responses to dopamine and bromocriptine. J Clin Invest 1980;66:10–8.

10. Carcillo JA, et al. 2014 ACCM clinical practice parameters for hemodynamic support of pediatric and neonatal septic shock. Pediatr Crit Care Med, in press.

11. Annane D, Sebille V, Charpentier C, et al. Effect of treatment with low doses of hydrocortisone and fludrocortisone on mortality in patients with septic shock. JAMA 2002;288:862–71.

12. Hotchkiss RS, Coopersmith CM, McDunn JE, et al. The sepsis seesaw: tilting toward immunosuppression. Nat Med 2009;15:496–7.

13. Mechanick JI, Nierman DM. Gonadal steroids in critical illness. Crit Care Clin 2006;22:87–103, vii.

14. Tiao G, Hobler S, Wang JJ, et al. Sepsis is associated with increased mRNAs of the ubiquitin-proteasome proteolytic pathway in human skeletal muscle. J Clin Invest 1997;99:163–8.

15. Lecker SH, Jagoe RT, Gilbert A, et al. Multiple types of skeletal muscle atrophy involve a common program of changes in gene expression. FASEB J 2004;18: 39–51.

16. Menconi M, Fareed M, O'Neal P, et al. Role of glucocorticoids in the molecular regulation of muscle wasting. Crit Care Med 2007;35:S602–8.

17. Truong AD, Fan E, Brower RG, et al. Bench-to-bedside review: mobilizing patients in the intensive care unit–from pathophysiology to clinical trials. Crit Care 2009;13:216.

18. Mitch WE. Robert H Herman Memorial Award in Clinical Nutrition Lecture, 1997. Mechanisms causing loss of lean body mass in kidney disease. Am J Clin Nutr 1998;67:359–66.

19. Gelfand RA, Matthews DE, Bier DM, et al. Role of counterregulatory hormones in the catabolic response to stress. J Clin Invest 1984;74:2238–48.

20. Levine S, Biswas C, Dierov J, et al. Increased proteolysis, myosin depletion, and atrophic AKT-FOXO signaling in human diaphragm disuse. Am J Respir Crit Care Med 2011;183:483–90.

21. Mitch WE, Goldberg AL. Mechanisms of muscle wasting. The role of the ubiquitin-proteasome pathway. N Engl J Med 1996;335:1897–905.

22. Banwell BL, Mildner RJ, Hassall AC, et al. Muscle weakness in critically ill children. Neurology 2003;61:1779–82.

23. Gruther W, Benesch T, Zorn C, et al. Muscle wasting in intensive care patients: ultrasound observation of the M. quadriceps femoris muscle layer. J Rehabil Med 2008;40:185–9.

24. Poulsen JB, Moller K, Jensen CV, et al. Effect of transcutaneous electrical muscle stimulation on muscle volume in patients with septic shock. Crit Care Med 2011;39:456–61.

25. Casaer MP, Langouche L, Coudyzer W, et al. Impact of early parenteral nutrition on muscle and adipose tissue compartments during critical illness. Crit Care Med 2013;41:2298–309.

26. Seymour JM, Ward K, Sidhu PS, et al. Ultrasound measurement of rectus femoris cross-sectional area and the relationship with quadriceps strength in COPD. Thorax 2009;64:418–23.

27. Chao T, Herndon DN, Porter C, et al. Skeletal muscle protein breakdown remains elevated in pediatric burn survivors up to one-year post-injury. Shock 2015;44:397–401.

28. De Jonghe B, Bastuji-Garin S, Durand MC, et al, Groupe de Reflexion et d'Etude des Neuromyopathies en R. Respiratory weakness is associated with limb weakness and delayed weaning in critical illness. Crit Care Med 2007;35: 2007–15.

29. Garnacho-Montero J, Amaya-Villar R, Garcia-Garmendia JL, et al. Effect of critical illness polyneuropathy on the withdrawal from mechanical ventilation and the length of stay in septic patients. Crit Care Med 2005;33:349–54.

30. Puthucheary Z, Harridge S, Hart N. Skeletal muscle dysfunction in critical care: wasting, weakness, and rehabilitation strategies. Crit Care Med 2010;38: S676–82.

31. Kazi AA, Pruznak AM, Frost RA, et al. Sepsis-induced alterations in protein-protein interactions within mTOR complex 1 and the modulating effect of leucine on muscle protein synthesis. Shock 2011;35:117–25.

32. Murgia M, Serrano AL, Calabria E, et al. Ras is involved in nerve-activity-dependent regulation of muscle genes. Nat Cell Biol 2000;2:142–7.

33. Tawa NE Jr, Odessey R, Goldberg AL. Inhibitors of the proteasome reduce the accelerated proteolysis in atrophying rat skeletal muscles. J Clin Invest 1997; 100:197–203.

34. Hermans G, Wilmer A, Meersseman W, et al. Impact of intensive insulin therapy on neuromuscular complications and ventilator dependency in the medical intensive care unit. Am J Respir Crit Care Med 2007;175:480–9.

35. Otto A, Patel K. Signalling and the control of skeletal muscle size. Exp Cell Res 2010;316:3059–66.

36. Gerovasili V, Stefanidis K, Vitzilaios K, et al. Electrical muscle stimulation preserves the muscle mass of critically ill patients: a randomized study. Crit Care 2009;13:R161.

37. Bhasin S, Storer TW, Berman N, et al. The effects of supraphysiologic doses of testosterone on muscle size and strength in normal men. N Engl J Med 1996; 335:1–7.

38. Demling RH. Comparison of the anabolic effects and complications of human growth hormone and the testosterone analog, oxandrolone, after severe burn injury. Burns 1999;25:215–21.

39. Hart DW, Wolf SE, Ramzy PI, et al. Anabolic effects of oxandrolone after severe burn. Ann Surg 2001;233:556–64.

40. Demling RH, DeSanti L. Oxandrolone induced lean mass gain during recovery from severe burns is maintained after discontinuation of the anabolic steroid. Burns 2003;29:793–7.

41. Reeves PT, Herndon DN, Tanksley JD, et al. Five-year outcomes after long-term oxandrolone administration in severely burned children: a randomized clinical trial. Shock 2016;45:367–74.

42. Christaki E, Opal SM, Keith JC Jr, et al. Estrogen receptor beta agonism increases survival in experimentally induced sepsis and ameliorates the genomic sepsis signature: a pharmacogenomic study. J Infect Dis 2010;201:1250–7.

43. Sanchez MI, Shearwood AM, Chia T, et al. Estrogen-mediated regulation of mitochondrial gene expression. Mol Endocrinol 2015;29:14–27.

44. Brealey D, Brand M, Hargreaves I, et al. Association between mitochondrial dysfunction and severity and outcome of septic shock. Lancet 2002;360: 219–23.

45. Singer M. Mitochondrial function in sepsis: acute phase versus multiple organ failure. Crit Care Med 2007;35:S441–8.

46. Weiss SL, Cvijanovich NZ, Allen GL, et al. Differential expression of the nuclear-encoded mitochondrial transcriptome in pediatric septic shock. Crit Care 2014; 18:623.

47. Weiss SL, Selak MA, Tuluc F, et al. Mitochondrial dysfunction in peripheral blood mononuclear cells in pediatric septic shock. Pediatr Crit Care Med 2015;16: e4–12.

48. Galon J, Franchimont D, Hiroi N, et al. Gene profiling reveals unknown enhancing and suppressive actions of glucocorticoids on immune cells. Faseb J 2002;16:61–71.

49. Rhen T, Cidlowski JA. Antiinflammatory action of glucocorticoids–new mechanisms for old drugs. N Engl J Med 2005;353:1711–23.

50. Annane D, Cavaillon JM. Corticosteroids in sepsis: from bench to bedside? Shock 2003;20:197–207.

51. Slawik M, Reisch N, Zwermann O, et al. Characterization of an adrenocorticotropin (ACTH) receptor promoter polymorphism leading to decreased adrenal responsiveness to ACTH. J Clin Endocrinol Metab 2004;89:3131–7.

52. Yang Y. Structure, function and regulation of the melanocortin receptors. Eur J Pharmacol 2011;660:125–30.

53. Fluck CE, Martens JW, Conte FA, et al. Clinical, genetic, and functional characterization of adrenocorticotropin receptor mutations using a novel receptor assay. J Clin Endocrinol Metab 2002;87:4318–23.

54. Catania A. The melanocortin system in leukocyte biology. J Leukoc Biol 2007;81:383–92.

55. Zhu Q, Bateman A, Singh A, et al. Isolation and biological activity of corticostatic peptides (anti-ACTH). Endocr Res 1989;15:129–49.

56. Chan WL, Carrell RW, Zhou A, et al. How changes in affinity of corticosteroid-binding globulin modulate free cortisol concentration. J Clin Endocrinol Metab 2013;98:3315–22.

57. Hammond GL, Smith CL, Underhill DA. Molecular studies of corticosteroid binding globulin structure, biosynthesis and function. J Steroid Biochem Mol Biol 1991;40:755–62.

58. Guerrero J, Gatica HA, Rodriguez M, et al. Septic serum induces glucocorticoid resistance and modifies the expression of glucocorticoid isoforms receptors: a prospective cohort study and in vitro experimental assay. Crit Care 2013;17:R107.

59. Briassoulis G, Damjanovic S, Xekouki P, et al. The glucocorticoid receptor and its expression in the anterior pituitary and the adrenal cortex: a source of variation in hypothalamic-pituitary-adrenal axis function; implications for pituitary and adrenal tumors. Endocr Pract 2011;17:941–8.

60. Flower RJ. Eleventh Gaddum memorial lecture. Lipocortin and the mechanism of action of the glucocorticoids. Br J Pharmacol 1988;94:987–1015.

61. Baugh JA, Bucala R. Macrophage migration inhibitory factor. Crit Care Med 2002;30:S27–35.

62. Arafah BM. Hypothalamic pituitary adrenal function during critical illness: limitations of current assessment methods. J Clin Endocrinol Metab 2006;91:3725–45.

63. Hamrahian AH, Oseni TS, Arafah BM. Measurements of serum free cortisol in critically ill patients. N Engl J Med 2004;350:1629–38.

64. Ospina NS, Al Nofal A, Bancos I, et al. ACTH stimulation tests for the diagnosis of adrenal insufficiency: systematic review and meta-analysis. J Clin Endocrinol Metab 2016;101:427–34.

65. Charmandari E, Nicolaides NC, Chrousos GP. Adrenal insufficiency. Lancet 2014;383:2152–67.

66. Chrousos GP, O'Dowd L, Uryniak T, et al. Basal and cosyntropin-stimulated plasma cortisol concentrations, as measured by high-performance liquid chromatography, in children aged 5 months to younger than 6 years. J Clin Endocrinol Metab 2007;92:2125–9.

67. Hatherill M, Tibby SM, Hilliard T, et al. Adrenal insufficiency in septic shock. Arch Dis Child 1999;80:51–5.

68. Hebbar KB, Stockwell JA, Leong T, et al. Incidence of adrenal insufficiency and impact of corticosteroid supplementation in critically ill children with systemic inflammatory syndrome and vasopressor-dependent shock. Crit Care Med 2011;39:1145–50.

69. Sprung CL, Annane D, Keh D, et al. Hydrocortisone therapy for patients with septic shock. N Engl J Med 2008;358:111–24.

70. Zimmerman JJ, Donaldson A, Barker RM, et al. Real-time free cortisol quantification among critically ill children. Pediatr Crit Care Med 2011;12:525–31.

71. Hsieh S, White PC. Presentation of primary adrenal insufficiency in childhood. J Clin Endocrinol Metab 2011;96:E925–8.
72. Turcu AF, Rege J, Chomic R, et al. Profiles of 21-Carbon Steroids in 21-hydroxylase deficiency. J Clin Endocrinol Metab 2015;100:2283–90.
73. Pollard AJ, Perrett KP, Beverley PC. Maintaining protection against invasive bacteria with protein-polysaccharide conjugate vaccines. Nat Rev Immunol 2009;9: 213–20.
74. Peltola H, Kilpi T, Anttila M. Rapid disappearance of Haemophilus influenzae type b meningitis after routine childhood immunisation with conjugate vaccines. Lancet 1992;340:592–4.
75. McIntyre PB, O'Brien KL, Greenwood B, et al. Effect of vaccines on bacterial meningitis worldwide. Lancet 2012;380:1703–11.
76. van der Kamp HJ, Wit JM. Neonatal screening for congenital adrenal hyperplasia. Eur J Endocrinol 2004;151(Suppl 3):U71–5.
77. White PC. Neonatal screening for congenital adrenal hyperplasia. Nat Rev Endocrinol 2009;5:490–8.
78. Brierley J, Carcillo JA, Choong K, et al. Clinical practice parameters for hemodynamic support of pediatric and neonatal septic shock: 2007 update from the American College of Critical Care Medicine. Crit Care Med 2009;37:666–88.
79. Annane D, Buisson CB, Cariou A, et al, APROCCHSS Investigators for the TRIGGERSEP Network. Design and conduct of the activated protein C and corticosteroids for human septic shock (APROCCHSS) trial. Ann Intensive Care 2016;6:43.
80. Venkatesh B, Myburgh J, Finfer S, et al, ANZICS CTG investigators. The ADRENAL study protocol: adjunctive corticosteroid treatment in critically ill patients with septic shock. Crit Care Resusc 2013;15:83–8.
81. Finfer S. Corticosteroids in septic shock. N Engl J Med 2008;358:188–90.
82. Ferrer R, Artigas A, Suarez D, et al. Effectiveness of treatments for severe sepsis: a prospective, multicenter, observational study. Am J Respir Crit Care Med 2009;180:861–6.
83. Beale R, Janes JM, Brunkhorst FM, et al. Global utilization of low-dose corticosteroids in severe sepsis and septic shock: a report from the PROGRESS registry. Crit Care 2010;14:R102.
84. Kalil AC, Sun J. Low-dose steroids for septic shock and severe sepsis: the use of Bayesian statistics to resolve clinical trial controversies. Intensive Care Med 2011;37:420–9.
85. Funk D, Doucette S, Pisipati A, et al, Cooperative Antimicrobial Therapy of Septic Shock Database Research Group. Low-dose corticosteroid treatment in septic shock: a propensity-matching study. Crit Care Med 2014;42:2333–41.
86. Markovitz BP, Goodman DM, Watson RS, et al. A retrospective cohort study of prognostic factors associated with outcome in pediatric severe sepsis: what is the role of steroids? Pediatr Crit Care Med 2005;6:270–4.
87. Zimmerman JJ, Williams MD. Adjunctive corticosteroid therapy in pediatric severe sepsis: observations from the RESOLVE study. Pediatr Crit Care Med 2011; 12:2–8.
88. Atkinson SJ, Cvijanovich NZ, Thomas NJ, et al. Corticosteroids and pediatric septic shock outcomes: a risk stratified analysis. PLoS One 2014;9:e112702.
89. Wong HR, Cvijanovich NZ, Anas N, et al. Developing a clinically feasible personalized medicine approach to pediatric septic shock. Am J Respir Crit Care Med 2015;191:309–15.

90. Weiss SL, Fitzgerald JC, Pappachan J, et al, Sepsis Prevalence, Outcomes, and Therapies (SPROUT) Study Investigators and Pediatric Acute Lung Injury and SepsisInvestigators (PALISI) Network. Global epidemiology of pediatric severe sepsis: the sepsis prevalence, outcomes, and therapies study. Am J Respir Crit Care Med 2015;191:1147–57.

91. Menon K, McNally JD, Choong K, et al, Canadian Critical Care Trials Group STRIPES Investigators. A cohort study of pediatric shock: frequency of corticosteriod use and association with clinical outcomes. Shock 2015;44:402–9.

92. Yehya N, Vogiatzi MG, Thomas NJ, et al. Cortisol correlates with severity of illness and poorly reflects adrenal function in pediatric acute respiratory distress syndrome. J Pediatr 2016;177:212–8.e1.

93. Wong HR, Cvijanovich NZ, Allen GL, et al. Corticosteroids are associated with repression of adaptive immunity gene programs in pediatric septic shock. Am J Respir Crit Care Med 2014;189:940–6.

94. Hotchkiss RS, Opal S. Immunotherapy for sepsis–a new approach against an ancient foe. N Engl J Med 2010;363:87–9.

95. Costello JM, Graham DA, Morrow DF, et al. Risk factors for central line-associated bloodstream infection in a pediatric cardiac intensive care unit. Pediatr Crit Care Med 2009;10:453–9.

96. van Vught LA, Klein Klouwenberg PM, Spitoni C, et al, MARS Consortium. Incidence, risk factors, and attributable mortality of secondary infections in the intensive care unit after admission for sepsis. JAMA 2016;315:1469–79.

97. Kissoon N. Yes, SIRS–I think we have come full circle. Crit Care Med 2011;39: 1232–3.

98. Patel GP, Balk RA. Systemic steroids in severe sepsis and septic shock. Am J Respir Crit Care Med 2012;185:133–9.

99. Holubkov R, Dean JM, Berger J, et al. Is "rescue" therapy ethical in randomized controlled trials? Pediatr Crit Care Med 2009;10:431–8.

100. Casarett D. The science of choosing wisely–overcoming the therapeutic illusion. N Engl J Med 2016;374:1203–5.

101. Thomas KB. The consultation and the therapeutic illusion. Br Med J 1978;1: 1327–8.

102. Giancoli DC. Physics: principles and applications. Englewood Cliffs (NJ): Prentice Hall; 1995.

Morbidity

Changing the Outcome Paradigm for Pediatric Critical Care

Julia A. Heneghan, MD[a], Murray M. Pollack, MD[a,b],*

KEYWORDS

- Morbidity • Functional status • Quality • Outcomes • Outcomes research
- Critical care • Pediatric critical care • Pediatric intensive care

KEY POINTS

- Morbidity is an important outcome that can be measured even for large studies. There are many measures of morbidity that can be selected based on the context of the study.
- In pediatric critical care, functional status is an "intermediate" outcome on the pathway to death that is significantly associated with physiologic instability (measured by the Pediatric Risk of Mortality [PRISM] score).
- Morbidity risk in pediatric critical care can be measured using physiologic profiles (PRISM) and other case-mix factors and used for quality assessment in a manner similar to death.
- New functional status morbidity rates are approximately double mortality rates.
- The Functional Status Scale (FSS) developed by the Collaborative Pediatric Critical Care Research Network is a granular method of measuring functional status and new functional status morbidity that is applicable to large-sample studies.

INTRODUCTION

The primary focus of critical care has evolved from saving lives by monitoring and maintaining physiologic status to placing greater emphasis on the prevention of secondary injuries and preservation of function. Current pediatric ICU (PICU) mortality rates approximate 2.5% to 5%, decreased from 8% to 18% during the early years of pediatric critical care,[1] and it has been suggested that a portion of the reduced mortality rates has been an exchange for higher morbidity rates.[2]

Pediatric critical care does not have a consensus concept of morbidity. Despite the low mortality rates and changing primary focus of pediatric critical care to include

[a] Critical Care Medicine, Children's National Health System, 111 Michigan Avenue Northwest, Washington, DC 20010, USA; [b] Department of Pediatrics, George Washington University School of Medicine and Health Sciences, Critical Care Medicine, Children's National Health system, 111 Michigan Avenue Northwest, Washington, DC 20010, USA
* Corresponding author.
E-mail address: mpollack@childrensnational.org

Pediatr Clin N Am 64 (2017) 1147–1165
http://dx.doi.org/10.1016/j.pcl.2017.06.011
0031-3955/17/© 2017 Elsevier Inc. All rights reserved.

morbidity prevention, the primary outcome for many critical care studies and assessments remains mortality. Studies that formerly could be accomplished with mortality as a legitimate and meaningful outcome are now difficult or impossible due to sample size considerations. If mortality is the primary outcome for research, quality, or other studies, the sample size required may be very large and the time required to obtain these samples may be so long as to make the results less meaningful when the study is completed.

This article's aims are

- To review the conceptual framework of morbidity most relevant to pediatric critical care
- Describe the uses of morbidity in research, quality, and other types of studies
- Describe measures of morbidity, especially those that measure functional status
- Review the foundational evidence that strongly supports the use of functional status morbidity as an equivalent or separate outcome to mortality
- Summarize the current pediatric critical care morbidity literature and the methods used to assess morbidity

WHAT IS MORBIDITY?

Morbidity is often difficult to define. Although mortality is simple (alive or dead), morbidity is usually conceptualized as an important deviation from baseline and/or a deviation from the expected result of care. In the context of critical care, morbidity is frequently thought of as the ramifications of both the disease process and the care provided in the ICU. It may encompass events during the inpatient stay, discharge status, or the long-term effects of the disease and the ensuing critical care interventions.

Morbidity during intensive care includes a diverse group of indicators, including the development of multisystem organ dysfunction, need for vasoactive medications, days on the ventilator, length of stay, hospital-acquired infections, and other medically focused outcomes. Morbidity, especially in the surgical literature, has increasingly been focused on inpatient complications or an unexpected hospital course associated with a procedure or its subsequent care, including length of stay, adverse events, and errors. An excellent example of using inpatient complications has been developed by using the congenital heart Society of Thoracic Surgeons Congenital Heart Surgery Database.[3] The selected complications of specific interest and relevance to congenital heart surgery patients include renal failure requiring dialysis, neurologic deficits at discharge, atrioventricular block requiring a permanent pacemaker, mechanical circulatory support, phrenic nerve injury or paralyzed diaphragm, and unplanned operation. The result of combining these complications with postoperative length of stay has been standardized for specific operations, resulting in a morbidity index specifically relevant to these patients' inpatient course, and suitable for use as a quality assessment method. Research by Kronman et al used more global measures of inpatient care such as cost.[4] Contemporary trends, such as patient-centered care and family-centered care and cost, may be may also be converted to morbidity indicators, such as family-related and patient-related changes in stress, mental health, financial status, and family functioning.[5]

Despite the traditional emphasis on inpatient metrics, there is growing recognition that the most important morbidities are decreases in functional status, which persist or develop after the hospital stay. These may be general, such as changes to activities of daily living, or organ-specific changes measured by functional tests, such as maximum oxygen consumption after cardiac surgery or pulmonary function tests after thoracic disease. Both types of morbidities are important. A recent review found that new functional impairment at the time of ICU discharge was reported from 10% to 36% of discharges depending on the methodology used.[6] Evidence detailed in this article indicates that changes to functional status in critically ill children are tightly linked to physiologic dysfunction (severity of illness).

THE RELATIONSHIP OF PHYSIOLOGIC DYSFUNCTION TO MORBIDITY

Morbidity often represents an intermediate outcome in a critically ill patient's progression toward death and is likely the result of the same physiologic dysfunctions that are associated with mortality (**Fig. 1**). Therefore, the conceptual foundation of intensive care, maintaining physiologic stability to prevent mortality, can be extended to morbidity, indicating that morbidity is a suitable and generalizable outcome measure for critical care quality assessments and research studies.

Although it has been well known for decades that physiologic dysfunction early in the PICU course is strongly associated with mortality risk, the association of physiologic dysfunction with morbidity has only recently been evaluated.[7] The Collaborative Pediatric Critical Care Research Network (CPCCRN) of the Eunice Kennedy Shriver National Institute of Child Health and Human Development assessed the relationship of physiologic profiles measured within the first 4 hours of admission to the ICU to both mortality and the development of significant, new functional status morbidity at hospital discharge. This study is the Trichotomous Outcome Prediction in Critical Care (TOPICC) study. The measure of physiologic profiles is the Pediatric Risk of Mortality (PRISM) score and the measure of morbidity is the Functional Status Scale (FSS [discussed later]).[8,9]

The CPCCRN study first identified a similar relationship between physiologic profiles and the development of new functional status morbidities as the relationship between physiologic profiles and mortality. As the physiologic instability increased, there was an increasing risk of both morbidity and mortality (**Fig. 2**A, B). Next, the TOPICC study determined the factors associated with the development of morbidity and mortality for critically ill children. **Table 1** compares the univariate odds ratios of developing either morbidity or mortality given the descriptive or physiologic factors. In

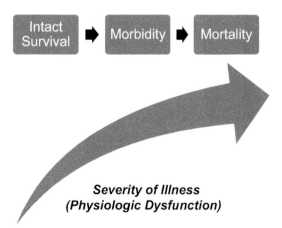

Fig. 1. The conceptual framework for critical care functional morbidity. The risks of both morbidity and mortality increase as severity of illness (physiologic profiles) increases. In this conceptual framework, morbidity is an intermediate outcome on the pathway to mortality.

A

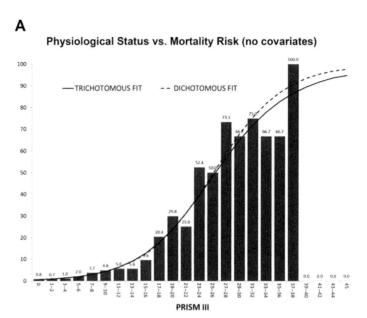

B

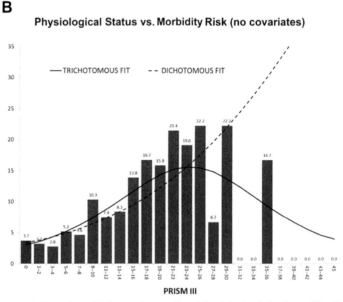

Fig. 2. The association of morbidity and mortality risk with physiologic profiles (PRISM). (*A*) Illustrates the relationship of PRISM with mortality risk and this relationship changes little when the prediction model is dichotomous (survival/death) or trichotomous (functional status morbidity/intact survival/death). (*B*) Illustrates the association of functional status morbidity with PRISM. In the dichotomous model (functional status morbidity/other), the relationship of morbidity risk to PRISM is similar to mortality risk. With the trichotomous model, however, morbidity risk increases until morbidity risk decreases as patients with high risks die. (*From* Pollack MM, Holubkov R, Funai T, et al. Simultaneous prediction of new morbidity, mortality, and survival without new morbidity from pediatric intensive care: a new paradigm for outcomes assessment. Crit Care Med 2015;43[8]:1699–1709.)

Table 1
Significant risk factors for developing new functional status morbidity and mortality

Variable	New Morbidity (%)	Death (%)	Odds Ratios: New Morbidity vs No New Morbidity (Odds Ratio [95% CI])	Odds Ratios: Death vs No New Morbidity (Odds Ratio [95% CI])
Age at PICU admission[a]				
0 d to <7 d	7.10	11.30	1.93 (1.12, 3.35)	5.12 (3.09, 8.50)
7 d to <14 d	12.00	9.60	3.40 (1.88, 6.15)	4.53 (2.31, 8.88)
Primary system of dysfunction[b]				
Respiratory	4.40	2.20	0.88 (0.55, 1.39)	0.24 (0.16, 0.37)
Cancer	5.70	2.50	1.16 (0.60, 2.23)	0.28 (0.12, 0.63)
Cardiovascular disease — congenital	4.50	4.20	0.92 (0.56, 1.51)	0.47 (0.31, 0.71)
Endocrine	0	0.40	<0.01 (<0.01, >999)	0.04 (0.01, 0.30)
Gastrointestinal disorder	5.70	3.40	1.18 (0.61, 2.31)	0.39 (0.19, 0.81)
Musculoskeletal condition	3.10	0.30	0.61 (0.29, 1.30)	0.03 (0.00, 0.24)
Neurologic	7.10	2.40	1.47 (0.93, 2.34)	0.27 (0.17, 0.43)
Miscellaneous	1.80	1.30	0.34 (0.15, 0.77)	0.14 (0.06, 0.33)
Intervention category[c]				
Neurosurgery	3.40	0.80	0.59 (0.36, 0.96)	0.20 (0.07, 0.54)
Orthopedic	2.60	0	0.45 (0.21, 0.97)	<0.01 (<0.01, >999)
Otolaryngology	1.70	0	0.29 (0.14, 0.63)	<0.01 (<0.01, >999)
Miscellaneous	1.60	1.20	0.27 (0.10, 0.74)	0.31 (0.10, 0.98)
Acute (nonprimary) or chronic diagnosis of cancer[d]				
Yes	5.90	7.40	1.37 (0.81, 2.30)	2.95 (1.83, 4.76)
Trauma[e]				
Trauma	11.90	3.50	3.14 (2.32, 4.24)	1.40 (0.84, 2.32)

(continued on next page)

Table 1
(continued)

Variable	New Morbidity (%)	Death (%)	Odds Ratios: New Morbidity vs No New Morbidity (Odds Ratio [95% CI])	Odds Ratios: Death vs No New Morbidity (Odds Ratio [95% CI])
Admission source[f]				
Inpatient unit from same hospital	6.60	5.60	2.15 (1.52, 3.02)	3.79 (2.49, 5.76)
Direct admission from referring hospital	7.20	4.90	2.33 (1.75, 3.09)	3.31 (2.27, 4.83)
PICU admission status[g]				
Elective (scheduled)	3.20	1.30	0.57 (0.44, 0.72)	0.33 (0.23, 0.48)
Cardiac arrest[h]				
Yes	15.40	38.50	6.91 (3.88, 12.3)	33.3 (21.3, 52.0)
4-Hour PRISM score[i]				
PRISM III (total)			1.11 (1.09, 1.13)	1.23 (1.21, 1.25)
PRISM III cardiovascular variables			1.12 (1.06, 1.20)	1.44 (1.37, 1.52)
PRISM III Metabolic Variables			1.16 (1.12, 1.21)	1.35 (1.30, 1.41)
PRISM III chemistry variables			1.14 (1.07, 1.21)	1.46 (1.38, 1.55)
PRISM III Hematological variables			1.16 (1.10, 1.23)	1.39 (1.32, 1.46)
PRISM III neurologic variables			1.17 (1.13, 1.21)	1.30 (1.27, 1.34)

Univariate odds ratios to develop morbidity (N = 351) and mortality (N = 214) based on 7560 PICU admissions. Only statistically significant factors are shown. Nonsignificant factors for both morbidity and mortality within each category are detailed in the footnotes.

[a] Reference is age ≥144 months. Nonsignificant age categories were 14 days to less than 21 days, 21 days to less than 1 month, 1 month to less than 12 months, 12 months to less than 60 months, and 60 months to less than 144 months.

[b] Reference is acquired cardiovascular disease. Nonsignificant systems of dysfunction were hematological and renal.

[c] Intervention category. Reference is no intervention. Nonsignificant intervention categories included cardiovascular surgery, interventional catheterization, and general surgery.

[d] Cancer. Reference is no acute or chronic cancer.

[e] Trauma. Reference is no trauma.

[f] Admission source. Reference is operating room or postanesthesia care unit. Nonsignificant categories are admissions from the emergency department of the same hospital.

[g] Admission status. Reference is emergency.

[h] Cardiac arrest. Reference is no cardiac arrest.

[i] PRISM. Data shown are for each change of 1 PRISM point.

From Pollack MM, Holubkov R, Funai T, et al. Simultaneous prediction of new morbidity, mortality, and survival without new morbidity from pediatric intensive general, the risk factors for dying are also the risk factors for development of morbidity and when a variable is significant for one outcome, it is often significant for the other. Because the morbidity rate is twice as high as the mortality rate, most of the variables have higher odds ratios for morbidity than mortality. Importantly, physiologic profiles measured by the 4-hour PRISM score were significant for the risk of developing both morbidity and mortality, and they are even a more powerful predictor of morbidity than mortality.

Next, the TOPICC study developed a model to predict the 3 critical care outcomes—intact survival, survival with a functional status morbidity, and death at hospital discharge—simultaneously using multivariate trichotomous logistic regression (see **Fig. 2**A, B). When the relationships of morbidity and mortality to physiologic profiles measured by the PRISM score are modeled separately, they were similar, with the risk of either mortality or morbidity increasing as physiologic instability increases. But, the relationship changes when both outcomes were considered simultaneously. As physiologic instability increased, both morbidity and mortality risk increased in parallel until mortality risk became dominant and the risk of morbidity decreased as those patients with a high mortality risk die. The association of morbidity risk to physiologic status, when mortality risk is factored in, is an inverted U shape. Morbidity risk first increased in parallel with mortality and then decreased.

This TOPICC study demonstrated that the same relationships underlying the association of mortality to physiologic status strongly influence the development of new, functional status morbidities at hospital discharge, as illustrated in **Fig. 1**. The implications are important: just as providers have the ability to influence mortality risk by appropriately identifying and treating physiologic dysfunction, they have the ability to influence morbidity through the same mechanisms.

Importantly, this study was also able to develop and validate a predictor of the aforementioned 3 outcomes from critical care simultaneously (**Table 2**). The relative risks for developing morbidity or mortality are reflected in the coefficients and odds ratios. Therefore, there is the potential to use both morbidity as well as mortality as meaningful ICU outcomes for quality assessments and researching new interventions because morbidity can be adjusted for using physiologic profiles and risk factors in the same way as mortality.

WHY DOES ASSESSING MORBIDITY MATTER FOR PEDIATRIC CRITICAL CARE?

Using morbidity with or without mortality as a critical care outcome presents opportunities. First, morbidity and morbidity plus mortality represent much larger signals for quality assessment and research. New functional status morbidity at hospital discharge, significant enough that parents and health care providers would understand that life has changed at least temporarily for that child and family, is twice as common as mortality. Studies using both outcomes will take less time and be more relevant to ensuring quality of care standards or relevant research outcomes.

The most important potential use for morbidity is as a new measure of quality of care. For almost 3 decades, ICUs have used measures of mortality adjusted for physiologic profiles and/or case-mix variables to assess the quality of care provided within an individual institution over time (internal benchmarking) or across a range of institutions using a known standard (external benchmarking). These methods compare the observed number of outcomes to the expected number of outcomes based on the physiologic and case-mix profiles of the patients (standardized ratios). Low mortality rates limit the utility of mortality as an outcome for quality studies because measuring quality using mortality may require long time periods to acquire a sufficient number

Table 2
Simultaneous prediction of morbidity and mortality

Predictors	Morbidity Coefficients (Standard Error)	Odds Ratios: New Morbidity vs No New Morbidity (95% CI)	Mortality Coefficients (Standard Error)	Odds Ratios: Death vs No New Morbidity (95% CI)
Intercept	−3.92 (0.17)	NA	−5.51 (0.27)	NA
Age at PICU admission				
0 d to <14 d	0.80 (0.23)	2.23 (1.43, 3.49)	1.64 (0.27)	5.14 (3.00, 8.79)
14 d to <1 mo	0.47 (0.44)	1.61 (0.68, 3.79)	1.26 (0.56)	3.53 (1.19, 10.50)
1 mo to <12 mo	0.39 (0.14)	1.48 (1.13, 1.93)	0.42 (0.21)	1.52 (1.02, 2.28)
>12 mo	Reference	Reference	Reference	Reference
Admission source				
Direct admission: referral hospital	0.76 (0.15)	2.15 (1.59, 2.90)	1.09 (0.24)	2.96 (1.87, 4.70)
Inpatient unit: same hospital	0.87 (0.18)	2.38 (1.67, 3.39)	1.70 (0.25)	5.46 (3.33, 8.95)
Emergency department: same hospital	0.11 (0.16)	1.12 (0.81, 1.53)	0.64 (0.25)	1.90 (1.16, 3.14)
Operating room or postanesthesia care unit for postoperative care	Reference	Reference	Reference	Reference
Cardiac arrest[a]	0.97 (0.33)	2.63 (1.38, 5.00)	1.52 (0.33)	4.56 (2.40, 8.66)
Acute (nonprimary) or chronic diagnosis of cancer[a]	0.25 (0.28)	1.28 (0.74, 2.21)	0.89 (0.30)	2.44 (1.36, 4.40)
Trauma[a]	1.18 (0.19)	3.26 (2.23, 4.77)	0.81 (0.35)	2.26 (1.13, 4.51)

Primary system of dysfunction				
Cardiovascular/respiratory	Reference	Reference	Reference	Reference
Cancer	0.73 (0.28)	2.07 (1.20, 3.59)	0.90 (0.43)	2.47 (1.06, 5.74)
Low risk (diabetic ketoacidosis, hematological, musculoskeletal, renal)	−0.93 (0.31)	0.39 (0.21,0.72)	−1.69 (0.61)	0.18 (0.06, 0.61)
Neurologic	0.38 (0.15)	1.46 (1.08, 1.98)	−0.07 (0.25)	0.93 (0.57, 1.54)
Other	−0.21 (0.23)	0.81 (0.52, 1.28)	0.11 (0.31)	1.11 (0.61, 2.03)
Baseline FSS score categorized as good[a,b]	−0.23 (0.13)	0.80 (0.61, 1.03)	−0.66 (0.19)	0.52 (0.36, 0.74)
PRISM III neurologic score[c,d]	0.11 (0.02)	1.12 (1.08, 1.16)	0.21 (0.02)	1.24 (1.19, 1.29)
PRISM III non-neurological score[d]	0.09 (0.01)	1.09 (1.07, 1.12)	0.18 (0.01)	1.19 (1.16, 1.23)

Abbreviation: NA, not applicable.

[a] Reference is absence of the factor.
[b] Baseline FSS score = 6 or 7.
[c] PRISM III neurologic components are pupillary reactions and mental status.
[d] For each 1 point change.

From Pollack MM, Holubkov R, Funai T, et al. Simultaneous prediction of new morbidity, mortality, and survival without new morbidity from pediatric intensive care: a new paradigm for outcomes assessment. Crit Care Med 2015;43(8):1699–1709.

deaths for a reliable quality assessment. Detecting sequential changes over time will be enhanced when the outcomes are both more relevant and more frequent.

A second important and contemporary use of morbidity is for pediatric critical care research trials. Pediatric critical care trials have been stymied by the need for large patient samples or a long enrollment period to capture an adequate number of events. Using mortality as a primary outcome in intervention trials requires very large samples to avoid "fragility," the concept that represents the number of deaths that, if changed to survivors, would have changed the statistical conclusion of the trial from significant to negative. A recent study noted that the statistical conclusions of more than half of the identified randomized clinical trials could be flipped either by using a more conservative statistical test or just changing the number of deaths to survivors by 2, even in multicentered trials in adult ICUs where mortality rates are approximately 3 to 4 times as high as pediatric units.[10] Critical care in general—especially pediatric critical care, due to the relatively low mortality rate—needs a more frequent outcome than mortality for robust and reliable studies.

Measures of morbidity are already prominent in pediatric critical care research studies. For example, the Therapeutic Hypothermia After Pediatric Cardiac Arrest (THAPCA) trial investigated whether the intervention of targeted temperature management to hypothermia after cardiac arrest would improve significant changes in adaptive functioning.[11] The primary outcome for THAPCA was survival with good functional status as assessed by the Vineland Adaptive Behavior Scale (VABS). The Approaches and Decisions in Acute Pediatric TBI Trial (ADAPT) is using the pediatric version of the Glasgow Outcome Scale–Extended (GOS-E).[12] The potential assessment methods for morbidity following head injury include detailed dissection of neurocognitive function but there is not agreement on the optimal method.[13] Other studies have assessed neurocognitive outcomes of tight glucose control in critically ill pediatric patients using a range of neuropsychological testing.[14] These studies demonstrate, however, the variability with which morbidity is defined and measured.

MEASURING MORBIDITY

Unlike mortality, which provides a clear dichotomous outcome, morbidity is a continuum of dysfunction. For many studies, documenting morbidity at a specific time point may be sufficient, but for other studies, assessments at a time when the morbidity has stabilized is most relevant. For example, prior work has shown that morbidity after trauma usually plateaus by 6 months postinjury.[15] For the general PICU population, however, recent evidence suggests that the incidence of significant morbidly and mortality determined at hospital discharge may double over the subsequent 3 years.[16]

A general method for measuring morbidity after critical care should include a broad range of function and be relevant to large populations in its practicality, specificity, and sensitivity. General measures of morbidity for pediatric critical care, especially if they are to be used for large population studies, such as quality studies requiring a general assessment of functional status should have as many of the following attributes as possible:

- Measure a clinically important outcome state
- Be relevant to long-term outcomes (can be used to project to medium-term and long-term outcomes)
- Can be completed relatively rapidly
- Can be completed without interaction with the family to allow studies to be done without informed consent and efficiently
- Is reliable across the sample even if some individual patients are misclassified

- Is age independent
- Is objective and sufficiently granular to limit subjective assessments
- Has strong inter-rater reliability

Historically, 3 broad categories of methods have been used to assess morbidity in critically ill children: global measurements; health-related quality of life (HRQOL) scales, including health utilities indices; and adaptive behavior scales, including neuropsychological and psychometric testing.[6] Depending on the method selected, a child's deficits in specific domain(s) (eg, motor ability and communication skills) that are relevant to the context of the study are objectively assessed.

Global Measures of Morbidity

Global outcome scales include the Glasgow Outcome Scale (GOS)[17] and its pediatric versions, the Pediatric Cerebral Performance Category (PCPC) and the Pediatric Overall Performance Category (POPC).[18] These scales assign a single score to classify overall functional level without examining specific domains beyond the PCPC's focus on cognitive performance. The GOS and POPC/PCPC are straightforward to administer but do not have uniformly objective and granular classifications for the assessment, leading to the potential for poor inter-rater reliability and poor precision. The second-generation GOSs are the GOS-E[19] and its pediatric version, the GOS-E Pediatrics (GOS-E Peds).[12] The GOS-E scores use a short structured interview with the patient or family to determine functional status.

The POPC and PCPC are intended to estimate short-term functioning based on a projection by health care providers at hospital discharge. They are widely used after critical illness because of their ease of assessment, face validity due to their similarity to the GOS, and statistically significant (but weak) relationship to long-term neuropsychological tests[20] and have been used in large pediatric critical care studies.[21] The scores include 1 for good, 2 for mild disability, 3 for moderate disability, 4 for severe disability, 5 for vegetative state or coma, and 6 for death. Completion of the POPC/PCPC generally takes only a few minutes and does not require parent/guardian or patient participation for completion. Unfortunately, the PCPC/POPC method lacks both precision and reproducibility. Inter-rater agreement of this system was only 76% to 80% when there was inclusion of a neighboring class.[21] That is, the agreements were only satisfactory if patients were classified as good to moderate disability, mild to severe disability, or moderate to very severe disability. Lack of precision was evident when the POPC/PCPC was compared with the more objective and granular FSS [discussed later].[22]

The GOS-E Peds is primarily used as an outcome for brain injury studies, although it has the potential for outcome assessment for other conditions. It has domains adapted to children (consciousness, independence in the home, independence outside the home, school/work, social and leisure activities, family and friendships, and return to normal life) and separates 2 age groups (younger and older patients) in an attempt to account for developmental stages. The GOS-E Peds was validated in 159 children (average age 81 ± 57 months) at a single site.[12] Overall, the GOS-E Peds was well-correlated with the GOS (correlation >0.8) and reasonably correlated with the composite VABS (correlation > 0.6), VABS domains (all correlations >0.45), Bayley (correlation >0.6), and other intelligence scores (correlations >0.55) but less well-correlated with parent ratings scales. The best results were obtained in older children with the worst head injuries. This suggests that it be further validated prior to use in any non-TBI group and in younger children with less severe TBI. The GOS-E Peds has not been assessed for inter-rater reliability (although the adult version has very good inter-rater reliability and has even been done with a mail questionnaire). Importantly, the validation assessments were done 3 months after the injury as a structured interview with professionals who were not blinded to other results. The GOS-E Peds was used as a secondary outcome in the Cool Kids trial, which was terminated after only 77 patients,[23] and is a primary outcome in the ADAPT.[24]

Health-Related Quality of Life

HRQOL measures attempt to gain an understanding of a child's overall functional status by using the concepts of quality of life. The most popular methods are the PedsQL and the Child Health Questionnaire.[25–28] Most HRQOL methods assess various combinations of different domains (eg, social, emotional, school functioning, and physical). The responses of children as young as 5 years of age may be used to complete the questionnaires. It is important to recognize that assessments are fundamentally subjective and patient, parent, and health care provider assessments often diverge.[29] HRQOL methods have multiple versions that may include interviews, in-person questionnaires/surveys, telephone surveys, long forms, short forms, and disease-specific or condition-specific versions. A recent review found that, overall, there is a significant decrease in HRQOL for PICU patients, although this has been measured by different methods and follow-up periods. This review also examined more than 20 different measures of HRQOL, concluding there are neither HRQOL tools specific to the post-PICU population nor a consensus as to the best method applicable to general post-ICU studies.[30]

Adaptive Behavior Scales

Adaptive behavior scales are commonly used and currently popular for research and for individual patient assessments. They focus on skill domains considered important to normal functioning and are adjusted for developmental age through evaluation of domains, such as social and cognitive skills. The most commonly used are the VABS and the Adaptive Behavior Assessment System (ABAS).[31,32] Both methods are available in different formats.

The ABAS is a questionnaire, and is commonly used by schools and in environments where questionnaires are more practical. The VABS is a psychometric instrument that is especially useful in the evaluation of children with intellectual disability, chronic disease, traumatic brain injury (TBI), mental health conditions, and many types of developmental delays as well as part of a battery of neuropsychological tests.

The VABS must be administered by a trained interviewer or psychologist. The VABS assesses personal independence and social responsibility using information relevant to day-to-day activities necessary to take care for oneself and to get along with others. There are multiple versions of the VABS that include short versions that can be administered by telephone. Unfortunately, despite its popularity, the VABS has not been assessed for validity in the peer-reviewed literature in several decades.[33,34] In general, the VABS is believed to function very well, especially in those with mild and moderate levels of functioning, but it may perform less well in those with severe and profound levels of dysfunction, and it can be logistically difficult to administer to large numbers of patients.

The Functional Status Scale

In an effort to develop a method using the principles of both activities of daily living and adaptive behavior that could be easily and accurately applied to larger patient populations, researchers with the CPCCRN developed the FSS. The FSS was developed by the CPCCRN based on consensus input from pediatricians, pediatric neurologists, pediatric developmental psychologists, pediatric nurses, pediatric intensivists, and pediatric respiratory therapists from 11 institutions. The FSS (**Table 3**) assesses functioning in the domains of mental status, sensory functioning, communication, motor functioning, feeding, and respiratory status.

Functional status for each domain is categorized from "normal" (1) to "very severe dysfunction" (6), with aggregate scores ranging from 6 (best) to 30 (worst). Construct validity was established by correlating the performance of the FSS with adaptive behavior as measured by the ABAS-II. Adaptive behavior was selected as a similar but not identical measure of function, recognizing that correlation between adaptive behavior scores purporting to measure the same functions is only moderate. Discriminant validity was established by receiver operating characteristic curve analysis. Other patient factors, including age, elective/emergency admission status, operative status, patient type, and study site, were investigated to determine if they were independently associated with FSS after adjusting for the ABAS-II using multivariable linear regression. FSS showed a consistent, moderate to strong association with ABAS-II across these other patient factors. The intraclass correlation of the total FSS was 0.95, indicating overall high reproducibility.

Because the FSS can be determined on admission based on parent recall or medical records, it enables a comparison of preillness with postillness functioning. The FSS was recently used in a CPCCRN study of greater than 10,000 PICU patients and was an excellent metric with sufficient precision and reliability for prediction based on physiologic profiles.[7] In this study, a new significant functional status change was defined as a change of 3 points or more for 2 major reasons. First, investigators thought that this magnitude of change would be very evident to both parents and providers. Second, 95% of the patients with a change of 3 points or more had a change of at least 2 points in a single FSS domain, indicating that the change had clearly occurred and was unlikely the result of a data collection error. This study established the practical advantages of the FSS for assessing hospitalized children by demonstrating that it can be assessed in less than 5 minutes from the medical record or conversations with health professions caring for the patient. Recently, the FSS was used to assess discharge status in a large pediatric trauma cohort.[35]

KNOWN MORBIDITY AFTER PEDIATRIC INTENSIVE CARE

Morbidity, including physical, psychosocial, and neurocognitive deficits, is common in intensive care conditions. A recent article found in a general, unselected population of PICU patients that new functional status morbidity assessed with the FSS was 33% higher than mortality at hospital discharge and both the morbidity and mortality rates doubled in the 3 years after initial hospital discharge.[16] Almost as many children demonstrated worsening of their functional status or died (38%) as survived without a change in functional status (44%). Less than 10% of children exhibited functional gains over time. Long-term function was associated with indicators of severity of illness including the need for invasive therapies, such as use of mechanical ventilation and use of vasoactive medications.

Although it is not possible to precisely compare morbidity and mortality rates over time because of the different research methods, data from several decades ago demonstrated a PICU mortality rate of 4.6% and a PICU morbidity rate of 3.1% (based on a 2-point or greater POPC change), whereas recent data from the TOPICC study (based on an FSS change of 3 or more points from baseline to hospital discharge) had a reversal of these percentages, with a hospital mortality rate of 2.4% and

Table 3
Functional status scale

	Normal (Score = 1)	Mild Dysfunction (Score = 2)	Moderate Dysfunction (Score = 3)	Severe Dysfunction (Score = 4)	Very Severe Dysfunction (Score = 5)
Mental status	Normal sleep/wake periods; appropriate responsiveness	Sleepy but arousable to noise/touch/movement and/or periods of social nonresponsiveness	Lethargic and/or irritable	Minimal arousal to stimuli (stupor)	Unresponsive, coma, and/or vegetative state
Sensory functioning	Intact hearing and vision and responsive to touch	Suspected hearing or vision loss	Not reactive to auditory stimuli or to visual stimuli	Not reactive to auditory stimuli and to visual stimuli	Abnormal responses to pain or touch
Communication	Appropriate noncrying vocalizations, interactive facial expressiveness, or gestures	Diminished vocalization, facial expression, and/ or social responsiveness	Absence of attention-getting behavior	No demonstration of discomfort	Absence of communication
Motor functioning	Coordinated body movements, normal muscle control, and awareness of action and reason	1 limb functionally impaired	≥2 limbs functionally impaired	Poor head control	Diffuse spasticity, paralysis, or decerebrate/decorticate posturing
Feeding	All food taken by mouth with age-appropriate help	Nothing by mouth or need for age-inappropriate help with feeding	Oral and tube feedings	Parenteral nutrition with oral or tube feedings	All parenteral nutrition
Respiratory status	Room air and no artificial support or aids	Oxygen treatment and/or suctioning	Tracheostomy	Continuous positive airway pressure treatment of all or part of the day and/or mechanical ventilatory support for part of the day	Mechanical ventilatory support for all of the day and night

Data from Pollack MM, Holubkov R, Glass P, et al. Functional status scale: new pediatric outcome measure. Pediatrics 2009;124(1):e18–28.

morbidity rate of 4.8%.[2,21] Thus, the "morbidity plus mortality rate" has decreased only from 7.7% to 7.2%, which has been mirrored in other studies.[2,21,36] These rates are not severity adjusted or risk adjusted, but the potential shift from mortality to morbidity is consistent with the clinical observations of many clinicians.

In the TOPICC study, morbidities affected essentially all types of patients and age groups in relatively equal measure. New morbidities occurred with relatively equal risk in those with all diagnostic groups and all degrees of baseline functional compromise. They also occurred in almost all operative groups, with the highest rates in cardiac surgery and general surgery and in only 3.1% of neurosurgical patients. Importantly, functional morbidity as well as mortality rates differed by more than 300% among the sites, indicating functional morbidity may be used as a robust and relevant measure of quality, effectiveness, and efficacy.

Prior research has used PCPC/POPC to determine risk factors for developing a new morbidity during critical illness. Using the VPS database, Bone and colleagues[37] identified children who survived their ICU admission but had worsening of PCPC/POPC scores. New functional or cognitive morbidities were noted in 10.3% and 3.4% of survivors, respectively. Multivariate analysis identified trauma, oncologic, and neurologic diagnoses as particularly high risk. As seen in other studies, patients who required significant invasive support (mechanical ventilation, renal replacement therapy, cardiopulmonary resuscitation, or extracorporeal membrane oxygenation) were also prone to development of new morbidities during admission, consistent with other studies using neuropsychological testing, VABS and HRQOL scales.[38–40]

In addition to the general knowledge about ICU-generated morbidities, some research has looked at development of new morbidities (or specific types of morbidities) in specific disease states.

Psychological Morbidity and Family Stress

In addition to the physical and cognitive outcomes associated with ICU care, researchers have also examined the psychiatric burden faced by children and families after critical illness. Given the physical and emotional stresses faced by patients and their families in critical care settings, it is unsurprising that there are psychological ramifications of these illnesses. A review by Davydow and colleagues[41] showed a patient incidence of posttraumatic stress disorder symptoms ranging from 10% to 28% and depression symptoms ranging from 7% to 13%. These rates are higher than have been seen in other patient populations, including the pediatric oncology population as well as children sustaining traumatic injury. Factors, such as ICU length of stay and severity of illness at the time of ICU admission, were associated with a higher prevalence of symptoms. This contrasts to studies in the adult population, where evidence is mixed as to whether these factors are associated with worse post-ICU psychiatric morbidity. This may be an instructive reminder as to the limitations of adapting research conducted in adults to the pediatric population.

Congenital Heart Surgery

Significant functional status morbidity at hospital discharge is approximately 50% greater than mortality for children after pediatric cardiac surgery. Discharge morbidity is associated with the same factors as mortality from congenital heart surgery, including the severity of the anatomic anomaly, the difficulty of the surgical palliation or repair, and the physiologic dysfunction in the immediately postoperative period. The TOPICC performs well predicting morbidity as well as mortality in congenital heart surgery patients as well the general ICU population.[42]

Trauma

The 2006 Institute of Medicine report, "Emergency Care for Children: Growing Pains," acknowledged the need for better outcomes including functional status at hospital discharge.[43] The National Trauma Data Bank, the leading US trauma registry and most commonly used database for injured children from more than 700 facilities, uses only mortality as a hospital discharge outcome for both ICU and non-ICU children even though mortality is substantially less than 3%.[44] In trauma research, most functional outcome studies have been used only in specific age groups, have been performed only among children with TBI, or have been assessed in a research setting, for example, the Pediatric Evaluation of Disability Inventory,[45] the Wee Functional Injury Measure For Children (WeeFIM),[46] and the GOS-E Peds. Few studies have evaluated functional measures of injury outcomes across a range of injury types and severity or have been validated across a wide age range.[47]

SUMMARY

Pediatric critical care has improved mortality rates over time but may have exchanged mortality for the development of new morbidities. Morbidity is linked to the same physiologic factors as mortality in critical illness. A variety of methods have been used to characterize morbidity in the pediatric critical care literature. Consensus on the most appropriate method to assess patient morbidities and integration of such a method into pediatric critical care research (including large database use) will offer the next step forward in caring for critically ill children. The FSS developed by the CPCCRN is a granular, age-independent, and validated method that has been valuable in large-sample critical care studies.

Morbidity assessments should be available from the medical record to ensure they are available for routine studies of quality and available for other large-scale studies. Similarly, databases must incorporate appropriate morbidity measures in their quality and research studies. Currently, large databases, such as those of the Society of Thoracic Surgeons, American College of Surgeons Trauma Registry, and the Pediatric Health Information System do not include a patient-level functional status morbidity assessment.

REFERENCES

1. Pollack MM, Ruttimann UE, Getson PR. Accurate prediction of the outcome of pediatric intensive care. A new quantitative method. N Engl J Med 1987;316(3): 134–9.
2. Pollack MM, Holubkov R, Funai T, et al. Pediatric intensive care outcomes: development of new morbidities during pediatric critical care. Pediatr Crit Care Med 2014;15(9):821–7.
3. Jacobs ML, O'Brien SM, Jacobs JP, et al. An empirically based tool for analyzing morbidity associated with operations for congenital heart disease. J Thorac Cardiovasc Surg 2013;145(4):1046–57.e1.
4. Kronman MP, Hall M, Slonim AD, et al. Charges and lengths of stay attributable to adverse patient-care events using pediatric-specific quality indicators: a multicenter study of freestanding children's hospitals. Pediatrics 2008;121(6): e1653–9.
5. Boyd JM, Burton R, Butler BL, et al. Development and validation of quality criteria for providing patient- and family-centered injury care. Ann Surg 2016. [Epub ahead of print].

6. Ong C, Lee JH, Leow MK, et al. Functional outcomes and physical impairments in pediatric critical care survivors: a scoping review. Pediatr Crit Care Med 2016; 17(5):e247–59.

7. Pollack MM, Holubkov R, Funai T, et al. Simultaneous prediction of new morbidity, mortality, and survival without new morbidity from pediatric intensive care: a new paradigm for outcomes assessment. Crit Care Med 2015;43(8):1699–709.

8. Pollack MM, Holubkov R, Funai T, et al. The pediatric risk of mortality score: update 2015. Pediatr Crit Care Med 2016;17(1):2–9.

9. Pollack MM, Holubkov R, Glass P, et al. Functional status scale: new pediatric outcome measure. Pediatrics 2009;124(1):e18–28.

10. Ridgeon EE, Young PJ, Bellomo R, et al. The fragility index in multicenter randomized controlled critical care trials. Crit Care Med 2016;44(7):1278–84.

11. Moler FW, Silverstein FS, Holubkov R, et al. Therapeutic hypothermia after out-of-hospital cardiac arrest in children. N Engl J Med 2015;372(20):1898–908.

12. Beers SR, Wisniewski SR, Garcia-Filion P, et al. Validity of a pediatric version of the Glasgow Outcome Scale-Extended. J Neurotrauma 2012;29(6):1126–39.

13. McCauley SR, Wilde EA, Anderson VA, et al. Recommendations for the use of common outcome measures in pediatric traumatic brain injury research. J Neurotrauma 2012;29(4):678–705.

14. Mesotten D, Gielen M, Sterken C, et al. Neurocognitive development of children 4 years after critical illness and treatment with tight glucose control: a randomized controlled trial. JAMA 2012;308(16):1641–50.

15. Polinder S, Meerding WJ, Toet H, et al. Prevalence and prognostic factors of disability after childhood injury. Pediatrics 2005;116(6):e810–7.

16. Pinto NP, Rhinesmith EW, Kim TY, et al. Long-term Function after pediatric critical illness: results from the survivor outcomes study. Pediatr Crit Care Med 2017; 18(3):e122–30.

17. Jennett B, Bond M. Assessment of outcome after severe brain damage. Lancet 1975;1:480–4.

18. Fiser DH. Assessing the outcome of pediatric intensive care. J Pediatr 1992;121: 69–74.

19. Jennett B, Snoek J, Bond MR, et al. Disability after severe head injury: observations on the use of the Glasgow outcome scale. J Neurol Neurosurg Psychiatry 1981;44(4):285–93.

20. Fiser DH, Long N, Roberson PK, et al. Relationship of pediatric overall performance category and pediatric cerebral performance category scores at pediatric intensive care unit discharge with outcome measures collected at hospital discharge and 1- and 6-month follow-up assessments. Crit Care Med 2000; 28(7):2616–20.

21. Fiser DH, Tilford JM, Roberson PK. Relationship of illness severity and length of stay to functional outcomes in the pediatric intensive care unit: a multi-institutional study. Crit Care Med 2000;28(4):1173–9.

22. Pollack MM, Holubkov R, Funai T, et al. Relationship between the functional status scale and the pediatric overall performance category and pediatric cerebral performance category scales. JAMA Pediatr 2014;168(7):671–6.

23. Adelson PD, Wisniewski SR, Beca J, et al. Comparison of hypothermia and normothermia after severe traumatic brain injury in children (Cool Kids): a phase 3, randomised controlled trial. Lancet Neurol 2013;12(6):546–53.

24. Larsen GY, Schober M, Fabio A, et al. Structure, process, and culture differences of pediatric trauma centers participating in an international comparative

effectiveness study of children with severe traumatic brain injury. Neurocrit Care 2016;24(3):353–60.

25. Varni JW, Seid M, Knight TS, et al. The PedsQL 4.0 generic core scales: sensitivity, responsiveness, and impact on clinical decision-making. J Behav Med 2002;25(2):175–93.

26. Varni JW, Limbers CA, Neighbors K, et al. The PedsQLTM infant scales: feasibility, internal consistency reliability, and validity in healthy and ill infants. Qual Life Res 2011;20(1):45–55.

27. Drotar D, Schwartz L, Palermo TM, et al. Factor structure of the child health questionnaire-parent form in pediatric populations. J Pediatr Psychol 2006; 31(2):127–38.

28. Raat H, Bonsel GJ, Essink-Bot ML, et al. Reliability and validity of comprehensive health status measures in children: the child health questionnaire in relation to the health utilities index. J Clin Epidemiol 2002;55(1):67–76.

29. Jardine J, Glinianaia SV, McConachie H, et al. Self-reported quality of life of young children with conditions from early infancy: a systematic review. Pediatrics 2014;134(4):e1129–48.

30. Aspesberro F, Mangione-Smith R, Zimmerman JJ. Health-related quality of life following pediatric critical illness. Intensive Care Med 2015;41(7):1235–46.

31. Sparrow S, Cicchetti D, Balla D. Vineland-II. Vineland adaptive behavior scales - survey forms manual. 2nd edition. Circle Pines, MN: AGS Publishing; 2005.

32. Harrison PL, Oakland T. ABAS II. Adaptive behavior assessment system. 2nd edition. San Antonio, TX: PsychCorp; 2003.

33. Raggio DJ, Massingale TW. Comparison of the vineland social maturity scale, the vineland adaptive behavior scales–survey form, and the bayley scales of infant development with infants evaluated for developmental delay. Percept Mot Skills 1993;77(3 Pt 1):931–7.

34. Raggio DJ, Massingale TW, Bass JD. Comparison of vineland adaptive behavior scales-survey form age equivalent and standard score with the bayley mental development index. Percept Mot Skills 1994;79(1 Pt 1):203–6.

35. Bennett TD, Dixon RR, Kartchner C, et al. Functional status scale in children with traumatic brain injury: a prospective cohort study. Pediatr Crit Care Med 2016; 17(12):1147–56.

36. Namachivayam P, Shann F, Shekerdemian L, et al. Three decades of pediatric intensive care: who was admitted, what happened in intensive care, and what happened afterward. Pediatr Crit Care Med 2010;11(5):549–55.

37. Bone MF, Feinglass JM, Goodman DM. Risk factors for acquiring functional and cognitive disabilities during admission to a PICU*. Pediatr Crit Care Med 2014; 15(7):640–8.

38. Ebrahim S, Singh S, Hutchison JS, et al. Adaptive behavior, functional outcomes, and quality of life outcomes of children requiring urgent ICU admission. Pediatr Crit Care Med 2013;14(1):10–8.

39. Als LC, Nadel S, Cooper M, et al. Neuropsychologic function three to six months following admission to the PICU with meningoencephalitis, sepsis, and other disorders: a prospective study of school-aged children. Crit Care Med 2013;41(4): 1094–103.

40. Als LC, Tennant A, Nadel S, et al. Persistence of neuropsychological deficits following pediatric critical illness. Crit Care Med 2015;43(8):e312–5.

41. Davydow DS, Richardson LP, Zatzick DF, et al. Psychiatric morbidity in pediatric critical illness survivors: a comprehensive review of the literature. Arch Pediatr Adolesc Med 2010;164(4):377–85.

42. Berger JT, Holubkov R, Reeder R, et al. Morbidity and mortality prediction in pe-diatric heart surgery: physiological profiles and surgical complexity. J Thorac Cardiovasc Surg 2017. [Epub ahead of print].
43. Committee on the future of emergency care. Future of emergency care: emer-gency care for children: growing pains. Washington, DC:The National Academies Press; 2006.
44. Amer Coll of Surgeon. ACS NTDB National trauma data standard: data dictio-nary. 2015. Available at: https://www.facs.org/quality-programs/trauma/ntdb/ntds. Accessed July 11, 2017.
45. Dumas HM, Haley SM, Carey TM, et al. The relationship between functional mobility and the intensity of physical therapy intervention in children with trau-matic brain injury. Pediatr Phys Ther 2004;16(3):157–64.
46. Shaklai S, Peretz R, Spasser R, et al. Long-term functional outcome after moderate-to-severe paediatric traumatic brain injury. Brain Inj 2014;28(7):915–21.
47. Gabbe BJ, Simpson PM, Sutherland AM, et al. Functional and health-related quality of life outcomes after pediatric trauma. J Trauma 2011;70(6):1532–8.

End-of-Life and Bereavement Care in Pediatric Intensive Care Units

Markita L. Suttle, MD[a],*, Tammara L. Jenkins, MSN, RN, PCNS-BC[b],
Robert F. Tamburro, MD, MSc[b]

KEYWORDS

- Pediatric death • End of life • Pediatric intensive care unit • Family support
- Parental grief

KEY POINTS

- Most childhood deaths in the United States occur in hospitals and most of these in intensive care settings. Thus, the ability to provide high-quality end-of-life (EOL) care is an essential component of successful pediatric critical care programs.
- The ability to anticipate, identify, and treat pain and suffering at EOL while concurrently attending to the psychosocial needs of dying children and their families may facilitate a peaceful death and help families adjust during bereavement.
- Parents often experience reduced mental and physical health following the loss of their child.
- EOL care in the pediatric intensive care unit is often associated with challenging ethical issues. Clinicians must maintain a sound and working understanding of these matters.

INTRODUCTION
Pediatric Death in the Pediatric Intensive Care Unit

Overall pediatric mortality is decreasing in the United States. In 1980, more than 64,000 infants and children less than 15 years of age died in the United States. In striking contrast, 2014 data show that number has almost decreased in half with only 32,295 reported deaths among this age group (**Fig. 1**).[1] Similarly, mortality rates among pediatric intensive care unit (PICU) admissions have also decreased over time (**Fig. 2**).[2–8] Three recent multicenter studies have reported PICU mortality rates less than 3%.[9–11]

No financial support was obtained for this review.
[a] Department of Critical Care Medicine, Nationwide Children's Hospital, 700 Children's Drive, Columbus, OH 43205, USA; [b] Pediatric Trauma and Critical Illness Branch, Eunice Kennedy Shriver National Institute of Child Health and Human Development
* Corresponding author.
E-mail address: markita.suttle@nationwidechildrens.org

Pediatr Clin N Am 64 (2017) 1167–1183
http://dx.doi.org/10.1016/j.pcl.2017.06.012
0031-3955/17/© 2017 Elsevier Inc. All rights reserved.

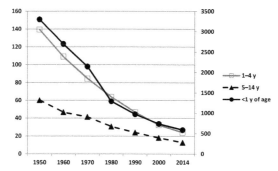

Fig. 1. Death rates among 3 pediatric cohorts for all causes in the United States. The image depicts the decreasing mortality rates among 3 pediatric cohorts from 1950 through 2014. The less-than-1-year-of-age cohort (*solid black circles, solid black line*) is plotted on the right-sided secondary axis. The 1- to 4-year-old cohort (*open squares, gray line*) and the 5- to 14-year-old cohorts are plotted on the left-sided, primary axis. Mortality rates are expressed in deaths per 100,000 resident population. (*Data from* National Center for Health Statistics. Health, United States, 2015: With Special Feature on Racial and Ethnic Health Disparities. Hyattsville, MD. 2016. Death rates for all causes, by sex, race, Hispanic origin, and age: United States, selected years 1950–2014.)

Approximately half of the deaths among US children 1 to 19 years of age occur in hospitals with an additional 14% occurring in emergency departments.[12,13] Of hospital deaths, most occur in intensive care settings.[14,15] Consequently, a sound understanding of the principles and practices of palliative and end-of-life (EOL) care should be maintained by all clinicians in the field.

Recent prospective, multicenter data suggest that approximately 70% of patients dying in a PICU do so in the context of withdrawal or withholding of life-sustaining therapies, with the remaining 30% being fairly equally divided between a diagnosis of brain death and failed cardiopulmonary resuscitation.[11,16] One study suggests that PICU deaths can be categorized into one of 2 groups based on the PICU length of stay at the time of the death.[11] Children who died within a week of PICU admission were characterized by the onset of a new illness or injury and were also more likely to die as a result of brain death or failed resuscitation. In contrast, those who died

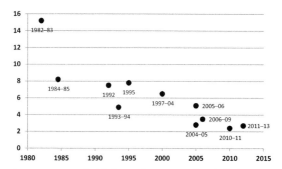

Fig. 2. Mortality rates among pediatric intensive care unit admissions over time. This image depicts the declining rates of mortality in the pediatric intensive care unit over the past 3 decades. The years next to each data point indicate the years that the data were collected. (*Data from* Refs.[2–7,9–11])

more than a week into their PICU course were characterized by preexisting conditions and technology dependence at baseline. Their deaths tended to follow the withdrawal of life-sustaining support.[11]

In terms of overall causes of death, congenital malformations and disorders related to prematurity accounted for most deaths in children less than 1 year of age in 2014, whereas unintentional injury was the leading cause of death in children 1 year of age and older.[1] Within the PICU, multiple organ failure has been reported to be the most common diagnosis at the time of death followed by neurologic and respiratory conditions.[11] Despite unintentional injuries being the leading overall cause of death in children older than 1 year, most deaths in the PICU are associated with a preexisting or chronic condition.[11] Given recent data that suggest more than half of the children admitted to a PICU have a chronic, complex medical condition,[17] this finding may merely reflect the population of patients currently being cared for in the PICU. Independent of the reasons, the findings that children with chronic conditions account for a large proportion of both the admissions to and the deaths within a PICU may have significant implications for the provision of palliative care within that setting. Both the Institute of Medicine[18] and the American Academy of Pediatrics[19] have long offered that palliative care should be initiated at the time of diagnosis of a life-limiting condition and be implemented concurrently with curative therapies. Consequently, palliative care services should not simply be provided at EOL for these children and their families but, rather, implemented from the time of diagnosis and throughout their often multiple admissions to the PICU. Data suggest that children with a life-limiting condition who are discharged from the PICU with palliative care services in place are more likely to die outside of the hospital than those without such provisions of care.[20]

DISCUSSION
End-of-Life Care

Although early implementation of palliative care has the potential to improve outcomes for many children with complex, chronic medical conditions, the provision of quality EOL care in the PICU is an essential pillar of any successful pediatric critical care program.[21] To provide such care, it is imperative to meet the physical needs of patients in terms of pain control and symptom management.[22] Survey data suggest that most PICU clinicians express confidence in their ability to treat acute symptoms of dying patients, including pain, agitation, dyspnea, secretions, and seizures; however, they seem less comfortable in their ability to treat more chronic issues, such as skin breakdown and constipation.[23] More than simply addressing physical suffering, effective EOL care must also address the children and their families' psychosocial and spiritual needs.[24] Clearly, critical illness in a child impacts the entire family and, independent of outcome, has the potential for long-standing dysfunction and detriment among family members.[25–27] The provision of such comprehensive and time-consuming care may be particularly challenging for PICU clinicians,[28,29] and current data purport wide variability in identifying and addressing these complex issues associated with EOL care in the PICU.[30,31] Clinicians must strive to develop a sound understanding of this field and its potential to impact the quality of life for patients, families, and clinicians alike.

The Needs of Children at the End of Life

The National Quality Forum, the Institute of Medicine, and the National Institutes of Health have all identified EOL care as a national priority, including medical care for children with advanced illness. At the EOL, children may have many needs across a vast array of domains; clinicians must be equipped with the skills necessary to address the needs of each individual in order to provide high-quality care. These needs are often divided into physical, psychosocial, spiritual, and environmental domains.[32] This discussion focuses on the physical and psychosocial needs of the dying child. However, if children do in fact hold certain religious or spiritual beliefs, particularly in the case of adolescents, understanding those beliefs is important, as is ensuring that children are allowed to die comfortably, in the family's chosen environment, surrounded by the people they love.

Physical needs

Although little is known about the personal priorities of children nearing death, adult patients have consistently endorsed pain and symptom management as a high priority with regard to their care.[33,34] Children at the EOL experience numerous physical symptoms and can suffer if their physical needs are not promptly recognized and addressed. Various pediatric palliative care experts have developed clinical practice guidelines and algorithms to manage EOL symptoms in children with cancer, which can be readily adapted for use in children with other advanced illnesses (**Tables 1 and 2**).[35]

Although rare, there are situations in which patients experience intractable physical and/or psychosocial suffering at EOL despite aggressive treatment regimens and escalating doses. These clinical scenarios are most likely to occur in the PICU and may require palliative sedation therapy with infusions, such as propofol, to achieve continuous deep sedation and relief of pain and distress.[35] In these difficult situations, other medications, such as ketamine and more recently dexmedetomidine, may play a vital role in the ease of suffering. Ketamine has been found to alleviate severe pain and decrease the use and escalation of opioids at EOL in both adults and children with cancer.[36,37] It has also been found to be effective for neuropathic pain in children at EOL.[38] Dexmedetomidine, an α_2-adrenoreceptor agonist, is a sedative frequently used in both adult ICUs and PICUs. It was recently evaluated as an adjuvant therapy to treat pain and agitation in children and adolescents with advanced illness at EOL, and a significant decrease in pain scores was observed after the initiation of a dexmedetomidine infusion.[39] Although further study is clearly needed, it seems that both ketamine and dexmedetomidine hold promise in treating refractory pain and distress at EOL for children.

In addition to pharmacologic methods of controlling pain at EOL, there are also nonpharmacologic measures. Complementary and alternative medicine (CAM) encompasses a wide range of modalities, such as acupuncture, massage, faith healing, and organic supplementation. Parents have reported that CAM benefitted their dying child and did not cause any additional suffering.[40] Although a detailed discussion of nonpharmacologic palliative care therapies is beyond the scope of this review, interest seems to be growing in the use of these modalities; thus, it is important for clinicians to be knowledgeable of their role.

Psychosocial needs

Children facing EOL often exhibit psychosocial distress linked to various illness-related factors.[41] A child's reaction to illness and their understanding of the concept of death is largely influenced by their cognitive and developmental level.[41] Clinical experience suggests that it is 3 losses that cause the most distress for children, including loss of control over their bodies and what is happening at any given moment, loss of personal identity, and finally loss of interpersonal relationships.[41] Identifying the extent to which each of these is affecting dying children can aid clinicians in meeting

Table 1
Pharmacologic management of pediatric pain at the end of life

Drug	Initial Dose	Route	Interval	Maximum Dosage[a]
Acetaminophen	10–16 mg/kg	PO/PR/IV	q 4 h	1 g per dose 4 g/d
Ibuprofen	5–10 mg/kg	PO	q 6 h	2.4 g per dose 3.4 g/d (adults)
Naproxen	5–7 mg/kg	PO	q 8–12 h	1 g per dose 4 g/d
Ketorolac	0.5 mg/kg	PO, IV	q 6 h	30 mg per dose (IV) 10 mg per dose (PO)
Tramadol	1–2 mg/kg	PO	q 6 h	100 mg per dose 400 mg/d
Morphine	0.2–0.5 mg/kg 0.1 mg/kg 0.3–0.6 mg/kg (LA)	PO, SL, PR IV, SQ PO	q 3–4 h q 2–4 h q 8–12 h	Titrate
Hydromorphone	0.03–0.08 mg/kg 0.015 mg/kg	PO, PR IV, SQ	q 3–4 h q 2–4 h	Titrate
Methadone	0.2 mg/kg 0.1 mg/kg	PO IV, SQ	q 8–12 h q 8–12 h	Titrate
Fentanyl	0.5–1.0 µg/kg/h 5–15 µg/kg (sed) 1–2 µg/kg	TD TM IV, SQ	q 48–72 h q 4–6 h q 1–2 h	Titrate
Oxycodone	0.05–0.15 mg/kg 0.1–0.3 mg/kg (LA)	PO PO	q 6 h q 12 h	Titrate

Abbreviations: IV, intravenous; LA, long acting; PO, by mouth; PR, per rectum; sed, sedative; SL, sublingual; SQ, subcutaneous; TD, transdermal; TM, transmucosal.

[a] Common maximum dosage; however, dose escalation may be necessary at EOL.

Adapted from Johnson LM, Snaman JM, Cupit MC, et al. End-of-life care for hospitalized children. Pediatr Clin North Am 2014;61:835–54.

the emotional needs of their patients. Some pediatric patients at EOL will experience significant emotional distress manifested by signs of anxiety and depression. These children may benefit from consultation with psychology and/or psychiatry teams.

Facilitating communication between parents and their children is a critical aspect of pediatric EOL care.[41] A Swedish study found that 100% of participating parents reported satisfaction with their decision to discuss death with their dying child, whereas a small percentage of those who chose not to have this discussion were dissatisfied with their decision.[42] The content and approach to these conversations will depend on the cognitive level of the child; however, it is recommended that these conversations occur in series and can be encouraged through various forums (eg, talking, writing, drawing).[41] Many palliative care experts believe that providing dying children the opportunity to openly discuss death, grief, and illness minimizes their confusion and fears.[41] Clinicians must be prepared to patiently and honestly answer the questions of dying children. In addition to the expertise of palliative medicine, ancillary teams, such as child life, can serve an extremely important role in helping explain concepts of death in developmentally appropriate ways to patients and their siblings.

For children with life-threatening illnesses, efforts to build memories and confirm that they will be remembered are important.[43] Legacy building encompasses actions to create items that are remembered, including artwork, photographs, and videos.[35]

Table 2
Pediatric symptom management (nonpain) at the end of life

Symptom	Medication	Common Pediatric Dosage (<60 kg)	Maximum Daily Dosage[a]
Agitation/delirium	Nonpharmacologic	Familiar objects, low lighting, soothing tones/music	
	Lorazepam	0.05 mg/kg per dose PO, SL (preferred for seizure), or PR every 4–6 h	2 mg per dose
	Chloral hydrate	25–50 mg/kg/d PO/PR divided every 6–8 h	1 g/d for infants, 2 g/d for children
	Haloperidol	0.01–0.02 mg/kg per dose PO, SL, or PR every 8–12 h	0.15 mg/kg/d
Dyspnea	Nonpharmacologic	Elevate head of bed, fluid restriction, suctioning, bedside fan, flowing air	
	Morphine	0.15 mg/kg PO/SL every 2 h as needed (titrate to effect)	
	Lorazepam[b]	0.05 mg/kg PO/SL every 4–6 h as needed (titrate to effect)	2 mg per dose
Nausea/vomiting	Nonpharmacologic	Avoid irritating foods or smells, relaxation, biofeedback, acupuncture, aromatherapy	
	Ondansetron	0.15 mg/kg per dose PO/IV every 8 h as needed	8 mg per dose
	Promethazine	>2 y: 0.25 mg/kg per dose PO/IV every 6–8 h as needed	1 mg/kg/d
	Scopolamine	8–15 kg: half patch TD every 3 d, >15 kg: 1 patch TD every 3 d	1 patch every 3 d
	Metoclopramide	0.01–0.02 mg/kg per dose per dose IV every 4 h	
	Lorazepam	0.05 mg/kg PO/SL every 4–6 h as needed (titrate to effect)	2 mg per dose
Secretions	Nonpharmacologic	Fluid restriction, gentle suctioning	
	Glycopyrrolate	0.04–0.1 mg/kg/d PO every 4–8 h	1–2 mg per dose or 8 mg per dose
		0.01–0.02 mg/kg/d IV every 4–6 h	

Abbreviations: IV, intravenous; PR, per rectum; SL, sublingual; SQ, subcutaneous.
[a] Common maximum dosage; however, dose escalation may be necessary at EOL.
[b] Lorazepam used for dyspnea associated with anxiety.
Adapted from Johnson LM, Snaman JM, Cupit MC, et al. End-of-life care for hospitalized children. Pediatr Clin North Am 2014;61:835–54.

Dying children in the PICU are often too sick to participate in legacy-building activities, but other forms of memory making do exist for parents and siblings. Regardless of the activity, legacy making may have positive effects for ill children and their families.[44]

The Needs of Parents at the End of a Child's Life

The needs of parents in the PICU at the end of a child's life warrant special attention. Evidence suggests that parents who perceive greater fulfillment of their needs during their child's PICU stay experience less symptoms of complicated grief during bereavement.[45] Communication remains an integral component of addressing bereaved parents' needs. Parents have reported a desire to receive honest communication that is given in a caring and sensitive tone.[46,47] Honest communication for parents includes frequent updates on their child's condition and prognosis, which facilitates decision-making.[47] Moreover, honest communication improves parental understanding and reduces conflict.[47] Evasive answers and incomplete information may undermine trust and interfere with the parents' ability to cope with the death of their child.[48] Parent-physician interactions with more patient-centered elements, such as increased proportions of empathetic statements, question asking, and emotional talk, positively influence parent satisfaction with care independent of the child's severity of illness.[49] Parents of dying children also desire simple language in lieu of medical jargon.[47] High-quality communication at the end of a child's life fosters trust between families and medical staff and helps to ensure that the dying child receives the best possible care.

Physical and emotional health

For parents facing the loss of their child, the relief of their child's pain and suffering is a critically important need; however, bereaved family members have historically reported poor management of distressful symptoms.[50–52] PICU clinicians should begin the process of symptom management and preparedness by first educating families on the anticipated physical symptoms associated with EOL and the potential therapies. Parents should be given a platform to express their concerns and to identify their unique preferences[35] and should be reassured that relieving their child's pain and suffering is a top priority of care.[53]

Although parents of dying children will largely be focused on the needs of their child, they themselves are at risk for physical and mental health issues. Numerous studies have highlighted the detrimental effects of child death on the physical health of bereaved parents[54–58] and even more have identified risks for emotional distress and mental illness.[59–67] Although often beyond the scope of the pediatric clinician, psychology or psychiatry services can be used to help parents cope more effectively and to assess for signs of psychopathology.

Psychosocial needs

Numerous psychosocial needs exist for parents at the end of a child's life, and clinicians should strive to provide care that is inclusive of a family's personal, cultural, religious, or spiritual beliefs.[35] Spirituality seems to play a significant role in adult grief reactions[68,69]; therefore, facilitating the expression of a family's religious or spiritual beliefs as a child approaches EOL may provide comfort and a sense of meaning.[35] Hospital chaplains may play an important role in helping clinicians identify a family's specific religious and spiritual needs.

One of the most prominent spiritual needs described by bereaved parents is that of maintaining a connection to their child at the EOL.[70] Clinicians may foster this connection by helping parents maintain the parent-child relationship at EOL. As parents struggle with the loss of their traditional roles of protector and provider,[53] maintenance of the parent-child relationship may be facilitated by encouraging active parent involvement in patient care, allowing parents to be present during invasive procedures or cardiopulmonary resuscitation,[71] providing the opportunity to stay with their child at the time of death, and by helping parents create memories that can bring comfort in the future.

Parents also need staff to be kind and compassionate,[45] and they want to know that the medical team genuinely cares about their child.[53] Although clinicians previously unknown to the family may be quickly incorporated into parents' support network, special effort should be made to include friends and family during the EOL process, as this facilitates continuity of support when the child dies and the parental support network abruptly shifts from the medical team to primarily family members and friends.[53]

Environmental

Parents experiencing their child's death have also identified environmental needs in the PICU, including the need for easy access to their child, privacy, facilities for self and sibling care, and the ability to accommodate family and friends at the time of death.[71] Memories of a welcoming environment can contribute to comfort during bereavement, whereas environmental frustrations may lead to negative interpersonal interactions and greater grief for parents.[71] Clinicians with a heightened awareness of a parent's environmental needs at EOL may enhance the quality of care provided, improve satisfaction with care, and create a supportive atmosphere for families preparing for their child's imminent death.

Parental Bereavement

Studies have demonstrated that bereaved parents suffer more intense grief after the death of a child as compared with the grief associated with the loss of a spouse or a parent.[72,73] This intense grief puts these parents at risk for long-term psychological issues, such as anxiety,[59] depression,[59–61] posttraumatic stress,[62–64] substance abuse,[65] suicide,[66] and increased risk for psychiatric hospitalization.[67] There is also evidence that bereaved parents may be at higher risk for physical morbidity, including certain types of cancer and response to cancer treatments,[54,55] multiple sclerosis,[74] diabetes,[56] and myocardial infarction.[75] Data not only suggest that this grief results in increased health service utilization and sick leave,[64] but also suggests higher rates of mortality for bereaved parents.[58]

Complicated grief

It is estimated that 7% of bereaved people will develop a severe and protracted grief response frequently referred to as complicated grief.[76,77] This response seems to be even more pronounced in parents who experience the death of a child; as many as 60% of parents whose children died in a PICU demonstrated high levels of complicated grief that persisted over time.[27] Individuals with complicated grief can experience a wide array of symptoms that interfere with daily function, including an intense longing or yearning for the person who died, avoidance of reminders of the deceased, intrusive thoughts, or a feeling of meaninglessness.[27,78] Individuals often feel stuck in a chronic state of mourning and are unable to move on with life.[27,78] Among parents who experience the death of a child in the PICU, several variables have been associated with an increased risk for complicated grief, including being the biological mother or female guardian, trauma as the cause of death, greater attachment-related anxiety and avoidance, and greater grief avoidance.[27]

Bereavement interventions

The evidence supporting bereavement prevention and intervention is ever growing; but the general consensus is that most cases of grief, though painful, are normative and self-limiting. Thus, only the highest-risk individuals and those with complicated grief are likely to show benefit from preventive or therapeutic intervention.[79,80] In one study, 60% of parents bereaved by child death in the PICU reported a desire to meet with their child's intensive care physician in the weeks following the death.[81] Parents wanted to revisit events and management at EOL, gain reassurance about decisions that were made, and provide feedback to the medical team.[81] A follow-up meeting between pediatric intensivists and bereaved parents after the death of a child could provide parents with greater clarity regarding EOL events as well as emotional support. These meetings may also enable clinicians to screen for parents and/or siblings exhibiting significant physical or emotional distress so that appropriate referrals can be made. Although further study is needed, these meetings may be a potential platform by which intensive care communication is made more complete, bereaved parental knowledge enhanced, and the risk for complicated grief decreased.

Ethical Issues in End-of-Life Care in the Pediatric Intensive Care Unit

As previously described, most childhood deaths in the PICU occur after withdrawal or withholding of life-sustaining therapies.[11,15,82] Decision-making in these situations is often complex and may be a source of conflict between families and clinicians. Frequently, the first and most common discussion under such circumstances is regarding withholding of cardiopulmonary resuscitation.

The do-not-resuscitate order

A do-not-resuscitate (DNR) (also referred to as a do-not-attempt-resuscitation) order in its purest form states that cardiopulmonary resuscitation will not be initiated if the child experiences cardiopulmonary arrest. In a study that assessed the meaning, implication, and timing of DNR orders for critically ill children, 67.0% of clinicians believed that a DNR order only limits care in the event of cardiopulmonary arrest, whereas one-third (33.0%) of respondents considered a DNR order to be the impetus to consider or implement limitation of other life-sustaining therapies not related to cardiopulmonary arrest; 6.2% of respondents believed that a DNR order means a transition to comfort care only.[83] Although most clinicians contend that DNR orders guide care only during a cardiopulmonary arrest, many believe that once a DNR order is written for a child, the level and type of care provided changes, frequently through an increased attention to comfort care measures but also through limitation or withdrawal of diagnostic tests and therapeutic interventions. As written by the President's Commission for the Study of Ethical Problems in Medicine and Biomedical and Behavioral Research, "Any DNR policy should ensure that the order not to resuscitate has no implications for any other treatment decisions. Patients with DNR orders on their charts may still be appropriate candidates for all other vigorous care."[84] The disconnect between clinician understanding and the actual intent of DNR orders can cause significant confusion for family members.

Differences between withdrawal and limiting of life-sustaining therapies

Ethical conflict and moral distress may occur when there is confusion regarding what is meant by the withdrawal of life-sustaining therapies versus the withholding, or limiting, of those therapies.[85] Both of these actions reflect a shift in patient care goals, typically occurring when there is a decision that the goal of curing the critical illness is no longer possible or that curing the illness is so improbable that the risk of pain and suffering and decreased quality of life far outweighs the benefits of life-sustaining therapies.

Optimally, such decisions are made by consensus after targeted discussions between family and clinicians so that all individuals involved are in agreement.[28,86,87]

Once there is a shift in care goals, decisions regarding whether to limit the initiation of any new life-sustaining therapies or to withdraw certain therapies can be made. The most common interventions to limit or withdraw include mechanical ventilation, vasoactive agents, blood products or antibiotics, and hydration or nutrition.[88] *Withholding* or limiting life-sustaining therapies means that no new life-sustaining intervention will be initiated based on the belief that the child is dying and the family and clinicians concur that the intervention will not enhance the probability of meaningful survival and may exacerbate or prolong suffering. *Withdrawal* of a life-sustaining therapy, on the other hand, refers to the active removal of a therapy that was previously initiated. Despite the physiologic differences in stopping a life-sustaining therapy versus never starting one, it is generally accepted that there is no ethical distinction between withdrawing and withholding life support.[89] It is important to educate clinicians and families that when death is the expected outcome for the child, clinicians are simply removing or not starting therapies that would artificially prolong life and that the underlying disease or condition is the cause of death.[89,90]

The doctrine of double effect

Management of pain and anxiety is key to providing compassionate EOL care[86]; however, clinicians are often concerned that by providing medications, such as opioids and anxiolytics, to mitigate these symptoms, they may hasten death.

The doctrine of double effect states that an action has 2 effects: one that is inherently good and one that is inherently bad but justifiable. In order to abide by the doctrine of double effect, the following conditions must be met. The nature of the act must be good or at least morally neutral, the clinician's intention must be to only provide the good effect, there must be distinction between means and effect such that the bad effect must not be a means to a good effect, and finally there must be proportionality between the good effect and the bad effect (i.e. the benefits of the good effect must outweigh the risk of the bad effect). Thus, the delivery of anxiolytics and opioid pain medications to a child at EOL, despite the risk of causing respiratory depression or hypotension, is clinically, morally, and ethically justifiable if the clinician's *intent* is strictly to relieve pain and suffering.[86]

Conflict over futile or potentially inappropriate therapies

One of the most ethically troubling events while caring for a critically ill child in the PICU occurs when conflict arises between the family and care providers during EOL decision-making. Typically, conflict occurs when a family requests the initiation of therapies that the clinician believes to be ineffective or inappropriate. Ethical controversy occurs as families believe they are acting in the best interest of their child and clinicians feel pressured to provide a therapy that they do not believe will help and may foster pain and discomfort.[86,91,92] Accordingly, clinicians are not obligated to provide truly futile therapies (defined as those therapies that are unable to meet physiologic goals) nor should they under the ethical principle of beneficence (*do no harm*). However, disagreements about the potential effectiveness of a given therapy often lead to distrust and ineffective communication between the family and clinician.

A recent consensus policy statement from the American Thoracic Society, the American Association for Critical Care Nurses, the American College of Chest Physicians, the European Society for Intensive Care Medicine, and the Society of Critical Care Medicine provides recommendations addressing the management of requests from patients and families for treatment that clinicians deem to be inappropriate and believe should not be administered.[93] These clinical recommendations include (1) creating institutional strategies, such as proactive communication and expert consultants, to minimize or prevent care disputes; (2) using the terms *potentially inappropriate* rather than *medically futile* or *futility* when discussing treatments that may have some chance of meeting a patient care goal, no matter how small, but that the clinicians believe are clinically not indicated and their nonuse ethically justified; (3) saving the term *futile* to use only in those specific occasions in which the family requests care that cannot achieve the intended goal in any way. Family meetings early in the PICU admission, in which clinicians listen to family perceptions and concerns and explain clinical situations in clear language, are instrumental in laying a foundation of trust and good communication.[87]

Brain death and organ donation

As more children are kept alive through life-saving technologies, the need for donated pediatric organs for transplantation has dramatically increased.[90,94] The Uniform Determination of Death Act (UDDA) of 1981 coded the concept of brain into law and helped establish the *dead donor rule*, which is neither a law nor a regulation, but rather a description of an ethical norm that says an organ donor must be dead before vital organs are removed.[95] However, the UDDA did not adequately discuss the unique aspects of declaring brain death in infants and children.[96] Subsequently, the guidelines for the determination of brain death in children were published in 1987 and updated in 2011.[97,98] Most transplanted organs in children have traditionally been procured from brain-dead donors.[90]

As the demand for healthy organs grows, alternative methods for procurement and transplantation have been developed. One controversial method is organ donation after cardiac death (DCD), previously referred to as "non-heart-beating organ donation."[90] DCD involves procurement of organs from donors who have cessation of circulation and who have been declared dead by circulatory standards, usually related to withdrawal of life-sustaining therapies.

Although DCD practices vary, the following conditions generally must be present before DCD donation. Informed written consent for DCD must be obtained from the parents or legal guardians, there must be irreversible and end-stage illness whereby a decision to withdraw life-sustaining therapies was made before the decision to donate, withdrawal of support must occur in the ICU or operating suite to assure adequate treatment of pain and anxiety, a specified observation period must be provided (generally 60–120 minutes), and finally if cardiac function and circulation stop within the observation period, patients may be declared dead and the organs procured after a waiting period of approximately 2 to 5 minutes.[90,99] However, if those conditions are not met during the observation period, EOL care is continued and patients are no longer considered a potential DCD donor.[90,99]

Although DCD has been endorsed by several professional organizations, controversy exists regarding the ethics of DCD.[99–102] Concerns include violation of the dead donor rule, including the concern that donors may endure pain and suffering if death is declared prematurely; irreversible damage to donated organs from ischemia if death is not pronounced within the necessary timeframe; and conflict of interest between the needs of the donor and the needs of the transplant recipient.[90,99] Additional research is warranted to address these ethical concerns.

REFERENCES

1. National Center for Health Statistics. Health, United States, 2015: with special feature on racial and ethnic health disparities. Hyattsville (MD): 2016. p. 111.

2. Conlon NP, Breatnach C, O'Hare BP, et al. Health-related quality of life after prolonged pediatric intensive care unit stay. Pediatr Crit Care Med 2009;10:41–4.
3. Visser IH, Hazelzet JA, Albers MJ, et al. Mortality prediction models for pediatric intensive care: comparison of overall and subgroup specific performance. Intensive Care Med 2013;39:942–50.
4. Gemke RJ, Bonsel GJ, van Vught AJ. Long-term survival and state of health after paediatric intensive care. Arch Dis Child 1995;73:196–201.
5. Pollack MM, Patel KM, Ruttimann UE. PRISM III: an updated pediatric risk of mortality score. Crit Care Med 1996;24:743–52.
6. Pollack MM, Ruttimann UE, Getson PR. Pediatric risk of mortality (PRISM) score. Crit Care Med 1988;16:1110–6.
7. Namachivayam P, Shann F, Shekerdemian L, et al. Three decades of pediatric intensive care: who was admitted, what happened in intensive care, and what happened afterward. Pediatr Crit Care Med 2010;11:549–55.
8. Aspesberro F, Mangione-Smith R, Zimmerman JJ. Health-related quality of life following pediatric critical illness. Intensive Care Med 2015;41:1235–46.
9. Typpo KV, Petersen NJ, Hallman DM, et al. Day 1 multiple organ dysfunction syndrome is associated with poor functional outcome and mortality in the pediatric intensive care unit. Pediatr Crit Care Med 2009;10:562–70.
10. Pollack MM, Holubkov R, Funai T, et al, Eunice Kennedy Shriver National Institute of Child Health and Human Development Collaborative Pediatric Critical Care Research Network. Simultaneous prediction of new morbidity, mortality, and survival without new morbidity from pediatric intensive care: a new paradigm for outcomes assessment. Crit Care Med 2015;43:1699–709.
11. Burns JP, Sellers DE, Meyer EC, et al. Epidemiology of death in the PICU at five U.S. teaching hospitals. Crit Care Med 2014;42:2101–8.
12. Feudtner C, Silveira MJ, Shabbout M, et al. Distance from home when death occurs: a population-based study of Washington State, 1989-2002. Pediatrics 2006;117:e932–9.
13. Chang E, MacLeod R, Drake R. Characteristics influencing location of death for children with life-limiting illness. Arch Dis Child 2013;98:419–24.
14. Angus DC, Barnato AE, Linde-Zwirble WT, et al, Robert Wood Johnson Foundation ICU End-of-Life Peer Group. Use of intensive care at the end of life in the United States: an epidemiologic study. Crit Care Med 2004;32:638–43.
15. Carter BS, Howenstein M, Gilmer MJ, et al. Circumstances surrounding the deaths of hospitalized children: opportunities for pediatric palliative care. Pediatrics 2004;114:e361–6.
16. Meert KL, Keele L, Morrison W, et al, Eunice Kennedy Shriver National Institute of Child Health and Human Development Collaborative Pediatric Critical Care Research Network. End-of-life practices among tertiary care PICUs in the United States: a multicenter study. Pediatr Crit Care Med 2015;16:e231–8.
17. Chan T, Rodean J, Richardson T, et al. Pediatric critical care resource use by children with medical complexity. J Pediatr 2016;177:197–203.e1.
18. Committee on Palliative and End-of-Life Care for Children and their Families. When children die: improving palliative and end-of-life care for children and their families. Washington, DC: National Academy Press; 2003.
19. American Academy of Pediatrics. Committee on Bioethics and Committee on Hospital Care. Palliative care for children. Pediatrics 2000;106:351–7.
20. Fraser LK, Miller M, Draper ES, et al, Paediatric Intensive Care Audit Network. Place of death and palliative care following discharge from paediatric intensive care units. Arch Dis Child 2011;96:1195–8.

21. Boss R, Nelson J, Weissman D, et al. Integrating palliative care into the PICU: a report from the Improving Palliative Care in the ICU Advisory Board. Pediatr Crit Care Med 2014;15:762–7.
22. Mosenthal AC, Weissman DE, Curtis JR, et al. Integrating palliative care in the surgical and trauma intensive care unit: a report from the Improving Palliative Care in the Intensive Care Unit (IPAL-ICU) Project Advisory Board and the Center to Advance Palliative Care. Crit Care Med 2012;40:1199–206.
23. Jones PM, Carter BS. Pediatric palliative care: feedback from the pediatric intensivist community. Am J Hosp Palliat Care 2010;27:450–5.
24. WHO definition of palliative care. Available at: http://www.who.int/cancer/palliative/definition/en/. Accessed February 27, 2017.
25. Balluffi A, Kassam-Adams N, Kazak A, et al. Traumatic stress in parents of children admitted to the pediatric intensive care unit. Pediatr Crit Care Med 2004;5:547–53.
26. Meert KL, Slomine BS, Christensen JR, et al, Therapeutic Hypothermia after Pediatric Cardiac Arrest Trial Investigators. Family burden after out-of-hospital cardiac arrest in children. Pediatr Crit Care Med 2016;17:498–507.
27. Meert KL, Donaldson AE, Newth CJ, et al, Eunice Kennedy Shriver National Institute of Child Health and Human Development Collaborative Pediatric Critical Care Research Network. Complicated grief and associated risk factors among parents following a child's death in the pediatric intensive care unit. Arch Pediatr Adolesc Med 2010;164:1045–51.
28. Lee KJ, Dupree CY. Staff experiences with end-of-life care in the pediatric intensive care unit. J Palliat Med 2008;11:986–90.
29. Stayer D, Lockhart JS. Living with dying in the pediatric intensive care unit: a nursing perspective. Am J Crit Care 2016;25:350–6.
30. Keele L, Meert KL, Berg RA, et al, Eunice Kennedy Shriver National Institute of Child Health and Human Development Collaborative Pediatric Critical Care Research Network. Limiting and withdrawing life support in the PICU: for whom are these options discussed? Pediatr Crit Care Med 2016;17:110–20.
31. Lago PM, Piva J, Garcia PC, et al, Brazilian Pediatric Center of Studies on Ethics. End-of-life practices in seven Brazilian pediatric intensive care units. Pediatr Crit Care Med 2008;9:26–31.
32. Donnelly JP, Huff SM, Lindsey ML, et al. The needs of children with life-limiting conditions: a healthcare-provider-based model. Am J Hosp Palliat Care 2005;22:259–67.
33. Steinhauser KE, Christakis NA, Clipp EC, et al. Factors considered important at the end of life by patients, family, physicians, and other care providers. JAMA 2000;284:2476–82.
34. Patrick DL, Engelberg RA, Curtis JR. Evaluating the quality of dying and death. J Pain Symptom Manage 2001;22:717–26.
35. Johnson L-M, Snaman JM, Cupit MC, et al. End-of-life care for hospitalized children. Pediatr Clin North Am 2014;61:835–54.
36. Conway M, White N, St. Jean C, et al. Use of continuous intravenous ketamine for end-stage cancer pain in children. J Pediatr Oncol Nurs 2009;26:100–6.
37. Campbell-Fleming JM, Williams A. The use of ketamine as adjuvant therapy to control severe pain. Clin J Oncol Nurs 2008;12:102–7.
38. Taylor M, Jakaci R, May C, et al. Ketamine PCA for treatment of end-of-life neuropathic pain in pediatrics. Am J Hosp Palliat Med 2015;32:841–8.
39. Burns J, Jackson K, Sheehy K, et al. The use of dexmedetomidine in pediatric palliative care: a preliminary study. J Palliat Med 2017;20(7):779–83.

40. Heath JA, Oh LJ, Clark NE. Complementary and alternative medicine use in children with cancer at the end of life. J Palliat Med 2012;15:1218–21.

41. McSherry M, Kehoe K, Carroll JM, et al. Psychosocial and spiritual needs of children living with a life-limiting illness. Pediatr Clin North Am 2007;54:609–29.

42. Kreicbergs U, Valdimarsdottir U, Onelov E, et al. Talking about death with children who have severe malignant disease. N Engl J Med 2004;351:1175–86.

43. Levetown M, Liben S, Audet M. Palliative care in the pediatric intensive care unit. In: Carter BS, Levetown M, editors. Palliative care for infants, children, and adolescents: a practical handbook. Baltimore (MD): John Hopkins University Press; 2004. p. 273–91.

44. Allen RS, Hilgeman MM, Ege MA, et al. Legacy activities as interventions approaching the end of life. J Palliat Med 2008;11:1029–38.

45. Meert KL, Templin TN, Michelson KN, et al. The bereaved parent needs assessment: a new instrument to assess the needs of parents whose children died in the pediatric intensive care unit. Crit Care Med 2012;40:3050–7.

46. Mack JW, Hilden JM, Watterson J, et al. Parent and physician perspective on quality of life at the end of life in children with cancer. J Clin Oncol 2005;23: 9155–61.

47. Meert KM, Eggly S, Pollack M, et al, National Institute of Child Health and Human Development Collaborative Pediatric Critical Care Research Network. Parents' perspectives on physician-parent communication near the time of a child's death in the pediatric intensive care unit. Pediatr Crit Care Med 2008;9:2–7.

48. Bright KL, Huff MB, Hollon K. A broken heart – the physician's role: bereaved parents' perceptions of interactions with physicians. Clin Pediatr 2009;48: 376–82.

49. October TW, Hinds PS, Wang J, et al. Parent satisfaction with communication is associated with physician's patient-centered communication patterns during family conferences. Pediatr Crit Care Med 2016;17:490–7.

50. Homer CJ, Marino B, Cleary PD, et al. Quality of care at a children's hospital: the parents' perspective. Arch Pediatr Adolesc Med 1999;153:1123–9.

51. Wolfe J, Grier HE, Klar N, et al. Symptoms and suffering at the end of life in children with cancer. N Engl J Med 2000;342:326–33.

52. Teno JM, Clarridge BR, Casey V, et al. Family perspectives on end-of-life care at the last place of care. JAMA 2004;291:88–93.

53. Meyer EC, Burns JP, Griffith JL, et al. Parental perspectives on end-of-life care in the pediatric intensive care unit. Crit Care Med 2002;30:226–31.

54. Li J, Johansen C, Hansen D, et al. Cancer incidence in parents who lost a child: a nationwide study in Denmark. Cancer 2002;95:2237–42.

55. Levav I, Kohn R, Iscovich J, et al. Cancer incidence and survival following bereavement. Am J Public Health 2000;90:1601–7.

56. Olsen J, Li J, Precht DH. Hospitalization because of diabetes and bereavement: a national cohort study of parents who lost a child. Diabet Med 2005;22: 1338–42.

57. Lannen PK, Wolfe J, Prigerson HG, et al. Unresolved grief in a national sample of bereaved parents: impaired mental and physical health 4 to 9 years later. J Clin Oncol 2008;26:5870–6.

58. Rostila M, Saarela J, Kawachi I. Mortality in parents following the death of a child: a nationwide follow-up study from Sweden. J Epidemiol Community Health 2012;66:927–33.

59. Kreicbergs U, Valdimarsdottir U, Onelov E, et al. Anxiety and depression in parents 4–9 years after the loss of a child owing to a malignancy: a population-based follow-up. Psychol Med 2004;34:1431–41.
60. McCarthy MC, Clark NE, Ting CL, et al. Prevalence and predictors of parental grief and depression after the death of a child from cancer. J Palliat Med 2010;13:1321–6.
61. Rogers CH, Floyd FJ, Seltzer MM, et al. Long-term effects of the death of a child on parents' adjustment in midlife. J Fam Psychol 2008;22:203–11.
62. Murphy SA, Braun T, Tillery L, et al. PTSD among bereaved parents following the violent deaths of their 12- to 28-year-old children: a longitudinal prospective analysis. J Trauma Stress 1999;12:273–91.
63. Murphy SA, Johnson LC, Chung IJ, et al. The prevalence of PTSD following the violent death of a child and predictors of change 5 years later. J Trauma Stress 2003;16:17–25.
64. Dyregrov A, Dyregrov K. Long-term impact of sudden infant death: a 12- to 15-year follow-up. Death Stud 1999;23:635–61.
65. Vance JC, Najman JM, Boyle FM, et al. Alcohol and drug usage in parents soon after stillbirth, neonatal death or SIDS. J Paediatr Child Health 1994;30:269–72.
66. Qin P, Mortensen PB. The impact of parental status on the risk of completed suicide. Arch Gen Psychiatry 2003;60:797–802.
67. Li J, Laursen TM, Precht DH, et al. Hospitalization for mental illness among parents after the death of a child. N Engl J Med 2005;352:1190–6.
68. Walsh K, King M, Jones L, et al. Spiritual beliefs may affect outcome of bereavement: prospective study. BMJ 2002;324:1551–5.
69. Hawthorne DM, Youngblut JM, Brooten D. Parent spirituality, grief, and mental health at 1 and 3 months after their infant's/child's death in the intensive care unit. J Pediatr Nurs 2016;31:73–80.
70. Meert KL, Thurston CS, Briller SH. The spiritual needs of parents at the time of their child's death in the pediatric intensive care until and during bereavement: a qualitative study. Pediatr Crit Care Med 2005;6:420–7.
71. Meert KL, Briller SH, Meyers S, et al. Exploring parents' environmental needs at the time of a child's death in the pediatric intensive care unit. Pediatr Crit Care Med 2008;9:623–8.
72. Sanders CM. A comparison of adult bereavement in the death of a spouse, child, and parent. Omega 1979;10:303–22.
73. Middleton W, Raphael B, Burnett P, et al. A longitudinal study comparing bereaved spouses, adult children, and parents. Aust N Z J Psychiatry 1998;32:235–41.
74. Li J, Johansen C, Brønnum-Hansen H, et al. The risk of multiple sclerosis in bereaved parents: a nationwide cohort study in Denmark. Neurology 2004;62:726–9.
75. Li J, Hansen D, Mortensen PB, et al. Myocardial infarction in parents who lost a child: a nationwide prospective cohort study in Denmark. Circulation 2002;106:1634–9.
76. Kersting A, Brähler E, Glaesmer H, et al. Prevalence of complicated grief in a representative population-based sample. J Affect Disord 2011;131:339–43.
77. He L, Tang S, Yu W, et al. The prevalence, comorbidity and risks of prolonged grief disorder among bereaved Chinese adults. Psychiatry Res 2014;219:347–52.
78. Kacel E, Gao X, Prigerson HG. Understanding bereavement: what every oncology practitioner should know. J Support Oncol 2011;9:172–80.

79. Jordan J, Neimeyer R. Does grief counseling work? Death Stud 2003;27:765–86.
80. Schut H, Stroebe MS, van den Bout J, et al. The efficacy of bereavement interventions: determining who benefits. In: Stroebe MS, Hansson RO, Stroebe W, et al, editors. Handbook of bereavement research. 1st edition. Washington, DC: American Psychological Association; 1993. p. 705–38.
81. Meert KL, Eggly S, Pollack M, et al, National Institute of Child Health and Human Development Collaborative Pediatric Critical Care Research Network. Parents' perspectives regarding a physician-parent conference after their child's death in the pediatric intensive care unit. J Pediatr 2007;151:50–5.
82. Zawistowski CA, DeVita MA. A descriptive study of children dying in the pediatric intensive care unit after withdrawal of life-sustaining treatment. Pediatr Crit Care Med 2004;5:216–23.
83. Sanderson A, Zurakowski D, Wolfe J. Clinician perspectives regarding the do-not-resuscitate order. JAMA Pediatr 2013;167:954–8.
84. President's Commission for the Study of Ethical Problems in Medicine and Biomedical and Behavioral Research. Deciding to forgo life-sustaining treatment. Washington, DC: US Government Printing Office; 1983.
85. Garros D, Austin W, Carnevale FA. Moral distress in pediatric intensive care. JAMA Pediatr 2015;169:885–6.
86. Truog RD, Cist AFM, Brackett SE, et al. Recommendations for end-of-life care in the intensive care unit: the Ethics Committee of the Society of Critical Care Medicine. Crit Care Med 2001;29:2332–48.
87. Michelson KN, Patel R, Haber-Barker N, et al. End-of-life care decisions in the pediatric intensive care unit: roles professionals play. Pediatr Crit Care Med 2013;14:e34–44.
88. Prendergast TJ, Puntillo KA. Withdrawal of life support: intensive caring at the end of life. JAMA 2002;288:2732–40.
89. Solomon MZ, Sellers DE, Heller KS, et al. New and lingering controversies in pediatric end-of-life care. Pediatrics 2005;116:872–83.
90. Sarnaik AA, Clark JA, Meert KL, et al. Views of pediatric intensive care physicians on the ethics of organ donation after cardiac death. Crit Care Med 2013;41:1733–44.
91. De Vos MA, Bos AP, Plötz FB, et al. Talking with parents about end-of-life decisions for their children. Pediatr 2015;135:e465–76.
92. Morparia K, Dickerman M, Hoehn KS. Futility: unilateral decision making is not the default for pediatric intensivists. Pediatr Crit Care Med 2012;13:e311–5.
93. Bosslet GT, Pope TM, Rubenfeld GD, et al, on behalf of The American Thoracic Society ad hoc Committee on Futile and Potentially Inappropriate Treatment. An Official ATS/AACN/ACCP/ESICM/SCCM policy statement: responding to requests for potentially inappropriate treatments in intensive care units. Am J Respir Crit Care Med 2015;191:1318–30.
94. Webster PA, Markham L. Pediatric organ donation: a national survey examining consent rates and characteristics of donor hospitals. Pediatr Crit Care Med 2009;10:500–4.
95. Sade R. Brain Death, Cardiac Death, and the Dead Donor Rule. J S C Med Assoc 2001;107(4):146–9.
96. Robertson JA. The dead donor rule. Hastings Cent Rep 1999;29:6–14.
97. Report of Special Task Force. Guidelines for the determination of brain death in children. American Academy of Pediatrics Task Force on Brain Death in Children. Pediatrics 1987;80:298–300.

98. Nakagawa TA, Ashwal S, Mathur M, et al, and the Society of Critical Care Medicine, Section on Critical Care and Section on Neurology of the American Academy of Pediatrics, and the Child Neurology Society. Clinical report—Guidelines for the determination of brain death in infants and children: an update of the 1987 task force recommendations. Pediatrics 2011;128:e720–40.
99. American Academy of Pediatrics Committee on Bioethics. Ethical controversies in organ donation after circulatory death. Pediatrics 2013;131:1021–6.
100. Potts JT. Non-heart-beating organ transplantation: medical and ethical issues in procurement. Washington, DC: National Academy Press; 1997.
101. American Academy of Pediatrics Committee on Hospital Care, Section on Surgery, and Section on Critical Care. Policy statement - pediatric organ donation and transplantation. Pediatrics 2010;125:822–8.
102. Ethics Committee, American College of Critical Care Medicine, Society of Critical Care Medicine. Recommendations for nonheartbeating organ donation. A position paper by the Ethics Committee, American College of Critical Care Medicine, Society of Critical Care Medicine. Crit Care Med 2001;29:1826–31.

UNITED STATES POSTAL SERVICE ® Statement of Ownership, Management, and Circulation (All Periodicals Publications Except Requester Publications)

1. Publication Title	2. Publication Number		3. Filing Date
PEDIATRIC CLINICS OF NORTH AMERICA	424 – 66		9/18/2017

4. Issue Frequency	5. Number of Issues Published Annually	6. Annual Subscription Price
FEB, APR, JUN, AUG, OCT, DEC	6	$208.00

7. Complete Mailing Address of Known Office of Publication (Not printer) (Street, city, county, state, and ZIP+4®)

ELSEVIER INC.
230 Park Avenue, Suite 800
New York, NY 10169

Contact Person
STEPHEN R. BUSHING
Telephone (Include area code)
215-239-3688

8. Complete Mailing Address of Headquarters or General Business Office of Publisher (Not printer)

ELSEVIER INC.
230 Park Avenue, Suite 800
New York, NY 10169

9. Full Names and Complete Mailing Addresses of Publisher, Editor, and Managing Editor (Do not leave blank)

Publisher (Name and complete mailing address)

ADRIANNE BRIGIDO, ELSEVIER INC.
1600 JOHN F KENNEDY BLVD. SUITE 1800
PHILADELPHIA, PA 19103-2899

Editor (Name and complete mailing address)

KERRY HOLLAND, ELSEVIER INC.
1600 JOHN F KENNEDY BLVD. SUITE 1800
PHILADELPHIA, PA 19103-2899

Managing Editor (Name and complete mailing address)

PATRICK MANLEY, ELSEVIER INC.
1600 JOHN F KENNEDY BLVD. SUITE 1800
PHILADELPHIA, PA 19103-2899

10. Owner (Do not leave blank. If the publication is owned by a corporation, give the name and address of the corporation immediately followed by the names and addresses of all stockholders owning or holding 1 percent or more of the total amount of stock. If not owned by a corporation, give the names and addresses of the individual owners. If owned by a partnership or other unincorporated firm, give its name and address as well as those of each individual owner. If the publication is published by a nonprofit organization, give its name and address.)

Full Name	Complete Mailing Address
WHOLLY OWNED SUBSIDIARY OF REED/ELSEVIER, US HOLDINGS	1600 JOHN F KENNEDY BLVD. SUITE 1800 PHILADELPHIA, PA 19103-2899

11. Known Bondholders, Mortgagees, and Other Security Holders Owning or Holding 1 Percent or More of Total Amount of Bonds, Mortgages, or Other Securities. If none, check box ▶ ☐ None

Full Name	Complete Mailing Address
N/A	

12. Tax Status (For completion by nonprofit organizations authorized to mail at nonprofit rates) (Check one)
The purpose, function, and nonprofit status of this organization and the exempt status for federal income tax purposes:
☒ Has Not Changed During Preceding 12 Months
☐ Has Changed During Preceding 12 Months (Publisher must submit explanation of change with this statement)

PS Form **3526**, July 2014 [Page 1 of 4 (see instructions page 4)] PSN: 7530-01-000-9931   PRIVACY NOTICE: See our privacy policy on www.usps.com.

---

13. Publication Title	14. Issue Date for Circulation Data Below
PEDIATRIC CLINICS OF NORTH AMERICA	JUNE 2017

15. Extent and Nature of Circulation		Average No. Copies Each Issue During Preceding 12 Months	No. Copies of Single Issue Published Nearest to Filing Date
a. Total Number of Copies (Net press run)		1175	823
b. Paid Circulation (By Mail and Outside the Mail)	(1) Mailed Outside-County Paid Subscriptions Stated on PS Form 3541 (Include paid distribution above nominal rate, advertiser's proof copies, and exchange copies)	519	455
	(2) Mailed In-County Paid Subscriptions Stated on PS Form 3541 (Include paid distribution above nominal rate, advertiser's proof copies, and exchange copies)	0	0
	(3) Paid Distribution Outside the Mails Including Sales Through Dealers and Carriers, Street Vendors, Counter Sales, and Other Paid Distribution Outside USPS®	365	307
	(4) Paid Distribution by Other Classes of Mail Through the USPS (e.g., First-Class Mail®)	0	0
c. Total Paid Distribution (Sum of 15b (1), (2), (3), and (4))	▶	884	762
d. Free or Nominal Rate Distribution (By Mail and Outside the Mail)	(1) Free or Nominal Rate Outside-County Copies included on PS Form 3541	69	61
	(2) Free or Nominal Rate In-County Copies Included on PS Form 3541	0	0
	(3) Free or Nominal Rate Copies Mailed at Other Classes Through the USPS (e.g., First-Class Mail)	0	0
	(4) Free or Nominal Rate Distribution Outside the Mail (Carriers or other means)	0	0
e. Total Free or Nominal Rate Distribution (Sum of 15d (1), (2), (3) and (4))	▶	69	61
f. Total Distribution (Sum of 15c and 15e)	▶	953	823
g. Copies not Distributed (See Instructions to Publishers #4 (page #3))	▶	222	0
h. Total (Sum of 15f and g)	▶	1175	823
i. Percent Paid (15c divided by 15f times 100)		92.76%	92.59%

* If you are claiming electronic copies, go to line 16 on page 3. If you are not claiming electronic copies, skip to line 17 on page 3.

16. Electronic Copy Circulation		Average No. Copies Each Issue During Preceding 12 Months	No. Copies of Single Issue Published Nearest to Filing Date
a. Paid Electronic Copies	▶	0	0
b. Total Paid Print Copies (Line 15c) + Paid Electronic Copies (Line 16a)	▶	884	762
c. Total Print Distribution (Line 15f) + Paid Electronic Copies (Line 16a)	▶	953	823
d. Percent Paid (Both Print & Electronic Copies) (16b divided by 16c × 100)	▶	92.76%	92.59%

☒ I certify that 50% of all my distributed copies (electronic and print) are paid above a nominal price.

17. Publication of Statement of Ownership
☒ If the publication is a general publication, publication of this statement is required. Will be printed ☐ Publication not required
in the OCTOBER 2017 issue of this publication.

18. Signature and Title of Editor, Publisher, Business Manager, or Owner

Stephen R. Bushing   Date 9/18/2017

STEPHEN R. BUSHING - INVENTORY DISTRIBUTION CONTROL MANAGER

I certify that all information furnished on this form is true and complete. I understand that anyone who furnishes false or misleading information on this form or who omits material or information requested on the form may be subject to criminal sanctions (including fines and imprisonment) and/or civil sanctions (including civil penalties).

PS Form **3526**, July 2014 (Page 3 of 4)   PRIVACY NOTICE: See our privacy policy on www.usps.com.

Moving?

Make sure your subscription moves with you!

To notify us of your new address, find your **Clinics Account Number** (located on your mailing label above your name), and contact customer service at:

Email: journalscustomerservice-usa@elsevier.com

800-654-2452 (subscribers in the U.S. & Canada)
314-447-8871 (subscribers outside of the U.S. & Canada)

Fax number: 314-447-8029

Elsevier Health Sciences Division
Subscription Customer Service
3251 Riverport Lane
Maryland Heights, MO 63043

*To ensure uninterrupted delivery of your subscription,
please notify us at least 4 weeks in advance of move.

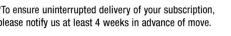